LIVER BIOPSY - INDICATIONS, PROCEDURES, RESULTS

Edited by **Nobumi Tagaya**

Liver Biopsy - Indications, Procedures, Results
http://dx.doi.org/10.5772/46113
Edited by Nobumi Tagaya

Contributors

Firpi, Alpna Limaye, Lisa Dixon, Ludmila Viksna, Ilze Strumfa, Janis Vilmanis, Andrejs Vanags, Zane Simtniece, Dzeina Sulte, Arnis Abolins, Janis Gardovskis, Ervins Vasko, Javier Crespo, Joaquín Cabezas, Marta Mayorga, Hiroyasu Morikawa, Jean-François Cadranel, Jean-Baptiste Nousbaum, Ivan Tokin, Anna Mania, Pawel Kemnitz, Magdalena Figlerowicz, Wojciech Sluzewski, Aldona Woźniak, Nobumi Tagaya, Nana Makino, Masatoshi Oya, Yoshitake Sugamata, Claudia Randazzo, Anna Licata, Piero Luigi Almasio, Teresa Casanovas, Costin Teodor Teodor Streba, Letitia Adela Maria Streba, Daniela Dumitrescu, Eugen Florin Georgescu, Monica Lupsor, Horia Stefanescu, Diana Feier, Radu Ion Badea

Published by InTech

Janeza Trdine 9, 51000 Rijeka, Croatia

Publishing Process Manager Viktorija Zgela
Technical Editor InTech DTP team
Cover InTech Design team

Additional hard copies can be obtained from orders@intechopen.com

Liver Biopsy - Indications, Procedures, Results, Edited by Nobumi Tagaya
p. cm.
ISBN 978-953-51-0853-5

For EU product safety concerns:
IN TECH d.o.o., Prolaz Marije Krucifikse Kozulić 3, 51000 Rijeka, Croatia,
info@intechopen.com or visit our website at intechopen.com.

Meet the editor

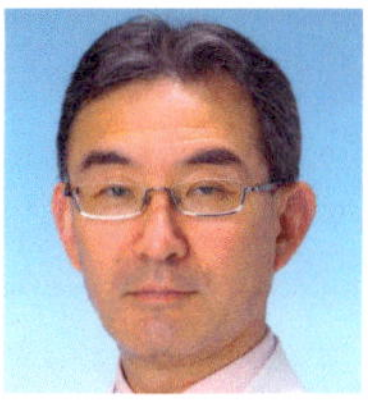

Dr. Tagaya is an Associate Professor of Surgery in Dokkyo Medical University Koshigaya Hospital. He is presently working as a leading laparoscopic and endoscopic surgeon, and has been accumulating an extremely vast experience with hepatobiliary and gastrointestinal operations, as well as adrenal and bariatric surgery. He also studied liver transplantation at Queensland Liver Transplant Service in Brisbane, Australia from April 1994 to March 1996. This technique is useful for performing laparoscopic liver resection and vascular reconstruction. He is a recipient of a Video Award by the European Association for Endoscopic Surgery in 2007 with regards to double-balloon endoscopy. He is now investigating the technique of fluorescence imaging using indocyanine green during laparoscopic procedures and image overlay surgery as a navigation surgery.

Contents

Preface

Liver biopsy is a procedure that involves obtaining a small piece of liver tissue, which is then analyzed in the laboratory. Liver biopsy may be used to evaluate a mass seen on ultrasound, CT or MRI images, diagnose unexplained liver diseases or abnormal liver function tests, determine the severity of the liver diseases including non-alcoholic liver disease, certain liver disease such as chronic hepatitis B or C, primary biliary cirrhosis, primary sclerosing cholangitis, autoimmune hepatitis, hemochromatosis or Wilson's disease, and monitor the liver after a liver transplantation. Liver biopsy is a safe procedure when performed by an experienced doctor. However, it is an invasive procedure, and the common problems include mild pain and a decrease in blood pressure. Although more serious complications such as bleeding, infection, and injury of nearby organs are rare but potentially lethal, the monitoring within 24 hours after the liver biopsy is important. This book describes the role, indication, contraindication, technique and evaluation of outcome of liver biopsy. I believe that it will be greatly useful to the readers. Furthermore, this book introduces transgastric liver biopsy using NOTES technique and non-invasive alternatives including elastography and computer analysis of liver fibrosis as new tools for the evaluation of liver diseases.

Nobumi Tagaya, M.D., Ph.D.
Department of Surgery,
Dokkyo Medical University Koshigaya Hospital,
Koshigaya, Saitama,
Japan

Section 1

An Overview and Future Aspects of Liver Biopsy

Chapter 1

Liver Biopsy - Indications, Procedures, Results

Claudia Randazzo, Anna Licata and
Piero Luigi Almasio

Additional information is available at the end of the chapter

http://dx.doi.org/10.5772/52616

1. Introduction

Liver biopsy (LB) is the most common procedure performed in clinical hepatology. Histological assessment of the liver, and thus, LB is traditionally the "reference standard" in the diagnosis and management of parenchymal liver diseases. Definitive diagnosis often depends on LB, and much of understanding of the characteristic features and natural history of liver diseases is based on information obtained by serial liver biopsies. During the last 60 years as the result of a better understanding of liver disorders, appearance of newer entities and advent of novel hepatic imaging techniques, the indications for LB have evolved. Whereas in the past LB was often performed as the initial investigation in the workup of liver disease of unknown aetiology, today the most common indication for LB includes staging of chronic hepatitis. A variety of methods exist for getting a liver tissue specimen. These take account of a percutaneous method, a transvenous (transjugular or transfemoral) approach, and intra-abdominal biopsy (laparoscopic or laparotomic). All LB techniques require specific training so as to ensure appropriate-sized specimen retrieval and the lowest rate of complications. However, because LB is an invasive procedure that carries a definite, albeit small, risk of complications, controversy persists with regard to its precise indications in various clinical situations, its clear contraindications, the optimal technique for its performance (and whether certain modifications improve its safety), and training requirements for clinicians. The aim of this chapter will be summarize the existing clinical practice of LB with an emphasis on the technique, indications, contraindications, quality of LB specimens and risk of complications.

2. Indications

Historically, LB was applied almost exclusively as a diagnostic tool [1]. Nevertheless, as the result of natural history data and the introduction of many new therapies for patients with liver disease, histological assessment of the liver has now got on an important role in clinical management. Therefore, LB currently has three major indications: for diagnosis, for assessment of prognosis and/or to assist in the management of patient with known liver disease.

Diagnosis
•Identification and staging of parenchymalandcholestatic liver diseases
-alcoholic liver disease
-non-alcoholic steatohepatitis
-autoimmune hepatitis
-primary biliary cirrhosis
-primary sclerosing cholangitis
-metabolic and mitochondrial storage liver diseases such as Wilson's disease, hemochromatosis, Gaucher's disease
•Evaluation of persistent abnormal liver biochemical tests after negative or inconclusive serologic workup
•Evaluation of the type and extent of drug-induced liver injury
•Evaluation of fever of unknown origin or immunocompromised patients with hepatomegaly or elevated liver enzymes levels
•Diagnosis of multisystem infiltrative disorders
- Identification and determination of the nature of focal/ diffuse intrahepatic abnormalities on imaging studies
Prognosis - Staging of known liver disease
•Evaluation of pre-transplant living-related donor
•Evaluation of post-transplant patient with abnormal liver tests (rejection vs. infectious aetiology)
Management – Developing treatment plans based on histologic analysis
•Pre-treatment evaluation and staging of chronic hepatitis
•Evaluation of effectiveness of therapies for liver diseases (*eg*, autoimmune hepatitis)

Table 1. Indications for liver biopsy

LB is performed to evaluate diffuse parenchymal or focal liver disease (see table 1). LB is mainly helpful in patients with diagnostic uncertainty(eg, in patients with atypical features). Available data show that liver histology will, in a proportion of patients, point to a specific diagnosis [2] and lead to a change in patient management [3,4]. LB has long been considered as an important diagnostic adjunct in the evaluation of otherwise unexplained abnormalities of liver biochemical tests. For example, LB may exclude serious liver disease or detect unsuspected non-alcoholic fatty liver disease (NAFLD) or intrahepatic sclerosing cholangitis after an otherwise negative biochemical, serologic and radiologic evaluation [3]. Needle LB for diagnosis remains important in cases of coexisting disorders such as steatosis and HCV [5] or an "overlap" syndrome of primary biliary cirrhosis (PBC) with autoimmune hepatitis (AIH) [6].

Other indications for LB include documentation of alcoholic liver disease and assessment of its severity; evaluation of otherwise unexplained fever, particularly in patients with Acquired Immune Deficiency Syndrome (AIDS); detection of underlying granulomatous liver disease. LB also provides important diagnostic information regarding drug-induced liver injury. Liver histology is appropriately considered in conjunction with clinical and laboratory data in case of hereditary disorders, eg hemochromatosis (quantitation of the level of iron), Wilson's disease (quantitation of the level of copper), and alpha-1 antitrypsin deficiency.

Liver histology may also be useful in detection of infiltrative processes such as amyloidosis [7]. Moreover, liver histology is often helpful in the setting of acute liver failure (ALF) [8].

An additional main use of LB is in assessing disease severity, particularly fibrosis, which, as a precursor to cirrhosis, may predict the emergence of complications of portal hypertension and also liver-related morbidity and mortality.

Owing to the wide use and superior resolution of cross-sectional imaging such as ultrasonography (US), computed tomography, and magnetic resonance imaging, focal lesions are being detected more often. Fortunately, the same technologic advances allow us to confidently establish a diagnosis without biopsy in most cases. Nevertheless, sometimes a biopsy of a suspected neoplasm will help change management. In this case, careful consideration of biopsy technique is important, as neoplasms have a higher bleeding risk and the potential to seed other sites along the biopsy tract or in the abdominal cavity [9]. At present, most biopsies currently performed for parenchymal disease are not to make a specific diagnosis but to assess liver damage, particularly in situations where (prognostic) information about fibrosis may guide consequent treatment. For example, histological analysis of the liver in patients with chronic HCV-induced liver disease gives information about the grading (inflammatory activity) and the staging (degree of fibrosis) that predict the course of disease; the treatment is often advocated for those with at least moderate to severe staging, but may be withheld when fibrosis is minimal or absent [10]. Liver histology is also generally used in disease monitoring of patients with AIH [11]. Monitoring the plasma cell score on LB may help predict relapse when a physician is considering reducing or discontinuing immunosuppressive therapy [12]. For further information on the role of histological analysis in the management of individual liver diseases, is possible to see guidelines for HCV [10], HBV [13], hemochromatosis [14], cholestatic liver diseases [15], AIH [11], and Wilson's disease [16].

Assessment of liver histology after orthotopic liver transplantation (OLT) is highly valuable to assess for allograft rejection and the presence and intensity of disease recurrence. Controversy persists regarding the precise indications for LB. Among these controversies are the following:

- The precise cut-off of serum aminotransferase levels that should prompt a LB: any persistent elevation, 1.5 times the upper normal limit, or 2 standard deviations above the mean [17,18]. Even the definition of the upper limit of normal is controversial [19-21].
- The need for LB in patients presumed to have NAFLD. Whereas imaging studies are sensitive for detecting steatosis, they are relatively not sensitive and nonspecific for detecting inflammation and fibrosis. Only on liver histology can distinguish fatty liver from steato-

hepatitis, which can lead to fibrosis and cirrhosis. LB is often considered if serum alanine aminotransferase (ALT) levels remain elevated after a modification of lifestyle and risk factors [22].

- The need for LB in all patients with PBC and primary sclerosing cholangitis (PSC). In most cases the diagnosis can be established on the basis of a cholestatic pattern of liver chemistries and either anti-mitochondrial antibodies in PBC [6] or endoscopic retrograde cholangiopancreatography (ERCP) in PSC [23]; scoring systems based on quickly established clinical variables could be used to assess prognosis and response to therapy.
- The need for protocol liver biopsies in all liver transplant recipients. A high rate of histologic abnormalities in the absence of liver biochemical test abnormalities has been described as late as 10 years after transplantation [24].

Overall, in patients without a definitive pre-biopsy diagnosis, LB has been shown to change the clinical diagnosis in 8% to 10% and to change the management in 12% of patients [25]. However, changes in management are often of minor importance [3].

3. Biopsy technique

Performance of LB requires an adequate sized and dedicated space suitable for focused physician effort as well as safe patient recovery. There are different approaches for obtaining liver tissue: percutaneous, transjugular, laparoscopic, and intraoperative, each having advantages and disadvantages. The biopsy technique is chosen on the basis of the indication, risks, and benefits in the individual patient. The most common approach for collecting a liver sample is percutaneous LB, either blinded or under US guidance. It is quick and safe procedures commonly performed by gastroenterologists or hepatologists in out-patient settings.

A variety of needles are available for percutaneous LB; they are broadly classified into suction needles (Menghini, Klatskin, Jamshidi), cutting needles (Vim-Silverman, Tru-cut), and spring-loaded cutting needles that have a triggering mechanism. The choice of a specific type of needle depends in part on local preference. Cutting needles usually produce a larger sample and are less likely to yield inadequate specimens than are suction needles, but they probably result in more complications [26], probably because the needle remains in the liver longer. Cutting needles can be useful in patients with cirrhosis. Suction needles are quicker (in the liver for a briefer time), easier to use, and less expensive, but tend to produce more fragmented samples. Disposable biopsy needles and biopsy guns are often used. A typical biopsy gun uses a modified 18-, 16-, or 14-gauge Tru-cut needle that is fired by a fast and powerful spring mechanism.

If the patient is not relaxed, a mild sedative should be administered just before the biopsy [27]. The current data on the use of prophylactic antibiotics is inconclusive. Prophylactic antibiotics have been recommended for patients at increased risk of endocarditis or with biliary sepsis [28]. However, recent results suggest that prophylactic administration of antibiotics following apercutaneous liver biopsy does not have a significant impact on the post-procedure results or incidence of infection [29]. During the procedure, patients placed in the supine position with the right hand resting behind the head [30]. For the blind approach (also referred to as the percussion-palpation approach), caudal percussion is helpful in selecting the site for the biopsy over the hemithorax between the anterior and mid-axillary lines, until an intercostal space is reached where dullness is maximal at the end of expiration. The intercostal space below this point (usually in the 7th-8th intercostal space) is used. A local anesthetic, typically lidocaine (without adrenaline), is administered with a 25-gauge needle first subcutaneously and into the intercostal muscle and finally down to the diaphragm and the capsule of the liver to reduce pain. The biopsy is performed while the patient holds a breath in full expiration [31]. With a suction needle, aspiration is applied, and the needle is rapidly introduced perpendicularly to the skin into the liver and withdrawn quickly (within 1 second). This is the critical step in performing the biopsy to minimize the risk of lacerating the liver and inducing bleeding. If insufficient tissue is obtained on the first pass [32], a second pass is performed at a different angle. After the biopsy, the patients is usually kept on the right lateral decubitus position for up to 2 hours to reduce the risk of bleeding and the pulse and blood pressure are monitored. Post-procedure monitoring has evolved over time. Most complications manifest within the first few hours [26], and under certain circumstances more and more patients are being discharged just 1 or 2 hours after imaging-guided biopsy. Rightly, the recommended observation time after biopsy is between 2 to 4 hours. To direct the needle away from other organs and large vascular structures, physicians often use US guidance. The US has been used either throughout the entire procedure (real-time) or immediately before (site marking) through a technique in which the patient subsequently has LB performed at the marked site. US guidance is the most controversial issue associated with LB [33-35]. Potential LB sites marked by percussion were changed in between 3 and 15% of patients after US was performed [36,37]. In an uncontrolled Italian study, routine identification of the puncture site by US led to a diagnostic tissue sample in 99% of patients [35]. In diffuse liver disease, US marking or guidance has been associated with lower rates of pain, hypotension, and bleeding [31]. In a survey of 2084 liver biopsies in France, US guidance is used in 56% of cases (in 34% to determine the puncture site and in 22% to guide the biopsy) and is thought to reduce the frequency of severe complications [38]. Cost-effectiveness analyses have suggested that routine US guidance in clinical practice increases the cost of LB but may be cost-effective, with an incremental cost of $2731 to avoid one major complication [39,40]. In addition, a large, randomized, prospective trial found that US use lowered the rate of post-biopsy hospitalization (most common reason for hospital admission was pain). Indeed there is a long track record of safety for performing percutaneous LB without imaging guidance. Thus, the role of US to guide percutaneous LB remains controversial. Use of ultrasound is not mandatory. A transjugular biopsy route offers a reasonable alternative to standard biopsy in high-risk patients (eg presence of massive ascites, severe coagulopathy, morbid obesity with a difficult to identify flank site or fulminant hepatic failure) [41]. With transjugular LB, the liver tissue is obtained from within the vascular system, which minimizes the risk of bleeding [42,43]. The procedure is performed by interventional radiologists or hepatologists under X-ray videofluoroscopy. Electrocardiographic monitoring is required to detect arrhythmias induced by passage of the catheter through the heart [41,44]. The patient is positioned supinely, with the head rotated opposite to that of the right internal jugular vein to be punctured, under local anesthesia using the Seldinger technique; then, a catheter is introduced into the hepatic vein under fluoroscopic control, and a needle biopsy of the liver performed through the catheter. Samples are retrieved from a Menghini or Tru-cut needle passed through the catheter into the liver. The transjugular approach permits concomitantly measurement of hepatic venous pressure gradient or opacification and imaging of the hepatic veins and inferior vena cava [45] helping in the diagnosis and management of select group of patients, particularly those with cirrhosis. In the past, a drawback of transjugular biopsy was the small and fragmented samples obtained. Better needles and more experience have led to improved quality of specimens. However, a transjugular LB is available only at a limited number of tertiary care facilities. Mortality is low (0.09%) [41], but perforation of the liver capsule can be fatal [46]. With laparoscopic approach, specific lesions can be identified and targeted precisely; thus it is especially useful in the diagnosis of peritoneal disease, the evaluation of ascites of unknown origin and abdominal mass, the staging of abdominal cancer. Laparoscopic LB is a safe procedure that can be performed under local anesthesia with conscious sedation, although it requires expertise that is not readily available. Absolute contraindications include severe cardiopulmonary failure, intestinal obstruction, bacterial peritonitis; relative contraindications are severe coagulopathy, morbid obesity, and a large ventral hernia [33]. For most parenchymal liver diseases, the extra time and cost required for laparoscopy are not justified by the increased yield. Liver biopsies (needle or wedge) can also be obtained during abdominal surgery whenever liver disease is suspected. In many instances, an abnormal appearance of the liver during surgery for an unrelated procedure (most often cholecystectomy) is the first indication of an underlying liver disease. It is generally performed either with typical needle devices or by wedge resection by those with special expertise. While intraoperatively obtained liver biopsies have the added advantage of obtaining adequate tissue sampling under direct vision from grossly visible/suspicious lesions, they are suboptimal for assessment of liver fibrosis and inflammation, due to preponderance of Glissen's capsule, wider portal tracts in the subcapsular area, and frequent but inconsequential surgically induced hepatitis. Other advantages are the ability to evaluate for potential extrahepatic spread of malignancy and to look for a cause of unexplained ascites (peritoneal biopsy). The major disadvantages are cost and the added risk of anesthesia. Therefore, needle biopsy should be the technique of choice at laparotomy.

4. Contraindications

Although LB is often essential in the management of patients with liver disease, physicians and patients may find it to be a difficult undertaking because of the associated risks.

The consensus guidelines of contraindications for percutaneous LB are listed in Table 2.

Absolute
•Uncooperative patient
•History of unexplained bleeding
•Tendency to bleed
-Prothrombin time "/> 3-4 sec over control
-Platelet counts < 50.000/mm3
-Prolonged bleeding time (≥10 min)
•Unavailability of blood transfusion support
•Recent use of aspirin or other nonsteroidal anti-inflammatory drugs (within last 7-10 days)
Relative
•Ascites
•Morbid obesity
•Infection in the right pleural cavity or below the right hemidiphragm
•Suspected hemangioma or other vascular tumor
•Hydatid disease (Echinococcal cysts)

Table 2. Contraindications to percutaneous LB

Percutaneous LB with or without image guidance is appropriate only in cooperative patients. As for any procedure, the patient that undergoes a LB should be able to understand and cooperate with the physician's instructions. An academic concern is that if the patient accidentally moves when the biopsy needle is in the liver, then a tear or laceration may occur (which would in turn greatly increase the risk of bleeding). Thus uncooperative patients who require LB should undergo the procedure under general anesthesia or via the transvenous route.

Coagulopathy is generally considered a contraindication to percutaneous LB, but the precise parameters that preclude LB are unsettled [47]. Generally, LB should be withdrawn when the prothrombin time (PT) is more than 3-4 seconds above the control value (International Normalized Ratio, INR>1.5) or when the platelet count is less than 60.000/mm3 [48]. Nevertheless, it is important to emphasize that the relationship of abnormal indices of peripheral coagulation to the occurrence of bleeding after LB in patients with acute as well as chronic liver disease is uncertain, as limited data are available [47,49]. In patients with mild to moderate prolongation of PT, administration of fresh frozen plasma or appropriate clotting factor concentrates may allow safe performance of a LB, as in hemophiliacs [50]. A low platelet count is probably less likely to result in bleeding in a cirrhotic patient with hypersplenism than in a leukemic patient with a comparable platelet count but platelet dysfunction. Probably, platelet dysfunction due to aspirin use is a major risk factor as well. Whether patients with renal insufficiency are at increased risk of bleeding complications after LB is also uncertain [28]. In summary, the decision to perform LB in the setting of abnormal hemostasis parameters should continue to be reached as the result of local practice because there is no specific INR and/or platelet count cut-off at or above which potentially adverse bleeding can be reliably predicted.

A LB is precluded by tense ascites, because the liver will bounce away from the needle, thereby preventing adequate sampling of tissue, and the ascites will provide insufficient tamponade in case of bleeding. In patients with tense ascites requiring a LB, a transvenous approach is commonly recommended. Acceptable options include total paracentesis performed immediately prior to percutaneous biopsy or transvenous or laparoscopic biopsy.

Relative contraindication is morbid obesity; in this case, transjugular biopsy is a logical alternative.

A standard LB is probably contraindicated by extrahepatic biliary obstruction, bacterial cholangitis, and the risk of bleeding after LB appears to be increased in patients with a known hematologic malignancy involving the liver [28].

Although LB in patients with mass lesions is usually safe, biopsy of known vascular lesions (ie hepatic hemangioma) should generally be avoided [51]. Patients who require LB and who have a large vascular lesion identified on imaging should undergo the procedure using real-time image guidance. Biopsy of potentially malignant lesions should be undertaken with care because it is believed that tumour vessels are more likely to bleed [51] and it can be also associated with a risk of tumour spread [52,53].

Biopsy of infectious lesions is generally safe. In the past, the presence of an echinococcal cyst was considered a contraindication to LB, because of the possibility of disseminating cysts throughout the abdomen and the risk of anaphylaxis. However, with recent advances in treatment, echinococcal cysts can be aspirated safely under ultrasound guidance [54].

5. Complications

When performing a LB, should be aware of multiple potential complications that may occur after biopsy.At the time that informed consent is obtained, it is reasonable to outline these complications clearly, warn the patient of the potential pain, and mention in a general statement that other complications, albeit rare, can occur.

Although the percutaneous biopsy is invasive, associated complications are rare, occurring in up to 6%, and 0.04% to 0.11% can be life threatening [33].

The different complication rates were attributed to variation in technique and to differences in the needles used, as well as differences in the severity of the liver disease and selection criteria in different centers.

The most common complication after percutaneous LB is pain [55]. Approximately 25% of patients have pain in the right upper quadrant or right shoulder; the pain is usually dull, mild and brief. Right upper-quadrant pain does not seems to be related to approach (i.e. subcostal vs. intercostal) [56]. The mechanism of pain following percutaneous biopsy is most likely a result of bleeding or possibly bile extravasation from the liver puncture wound, with subsequent capsular swelling, although the exact mechanism remains uncertain [57]. When present, pain can generally be managed with small amounts of narcotics. A decision about when to investigate with imaging and/or to hospitalize the patient for observation due to pain should be made on a case-by-case basis.

MAJOR
•Dearth
•Haemorrhage (intraperitoneal, intrahepatic, haemothorax)
•Perforation of the gallbladder or of the bowel
•Pneumothorax, haemothorax
•Biopsy of the right kidney or the pancreas
•Intrahepatic arteriovenous fistula
•Bile peritonitis
MINOR
•Pain (biopsy site, right upper quadrant and right shoulder pain)
•Transient hypotension (vasovagal response)
•Pneumoperitoneum
•Hemobilia
•Infection (bacterial sepsis, local abscess)
•Intrahepatic and subcapsular hematoma

Table 3. Complications of percutaneous liver biopsy

Transient hypotension, due to vasovagal reaction, can occur, particularly in patients who are frightened or emotional.

Major complications were defined as life threatening or those that required hospitalization, prolonged hospitalization or those that resulted in persistent or significant disability. Most serious complications occur within 24 hours of the procedure, and 60% happen within 2 hours; between 1% and 3% of patients require hospitalization [33].

The most common serious complication is bleeding because of transection of a vascular structure [26]; bleeding may occur in the absence of pain. Mild bleeding, defined as that sufficient to cause pain or reduced blood pressure or tachycardia, but not requiring intervention, occurs in about 1/500 biopsies [58]. Severe bleeding is defined clinically by a change in vital signs with imaging evidence of intraperitoneal bleeding. Such bleeding has been estimated to occur in between 1 in 2.500 to 1 in 10.000 biopsies after a percutaneous approach for diffuse liver disease [59]. Although very rare, clinically significant intraperitonealhemorrhage is the most serious bleeding complication of percutaneous LB; it usually becomes apparent within the first 2-3 hours after the procedure [26]. Free intraperitoneal blood may result from laceration of the liver capsule caused by deep inspiration during the biopsy or may be related to a penetrating injury of a branch of the hepatic artery or portal vein. The likelihood of hemorrhage increased with older age, presence of cirrhosis or liver cancer, and number of passes (≥ 3) with the needle during biopsy. The relationship between LB complications and the number of needle passes is well documented [51]. The frequency of complications increased with the number of passes performed at a rate of 26.4%, with one pass vs.

68% with two or more passes (P< 0.001) [38]. An additional factor in determining the risk of hemorrhage may be the type of needle used; cutting needles are more likely to result in hemorrhage than suction needles [26]. Severe bleeding requires hospitalization and is most often managed expectantly with placement of intravenous catheters, volume resuscitation by the administration of intravenous fluids and blood transfusion as necessary. If hemodynamic instability persists for a few hours despite the use of aggressive resuscitative measures, angiography with selective embolization of the bleeding artery or surgery (to ligate the right hepatic artery or resect a section) is required.

Subclinical bleeding leading to intrahepatic or subcapsular hematomas may be noted after LB even in asymptomatic patients. It is occurs in up to 23% of patients [60] and can be detectable by US. Large hematomas may cause pain associated with tachycardia, hypotension, and a delayed decrease in the hematocrit [33]. Conservative treatment of hematomas is generally sufficient.

After tranvenous biopsy bleeding is extremely rare because of the Glisson capsule is not breached except as a procedural complication from within the liver [61].

The least common of the hemorrhagic complications is hemobilia, which usually presents with the classic triad of gastrointestinal bleeding, biliary pain, and jaundice [26] approximately 5 days after the biopsy [62].

Transient bacteremia has been reported in 5.8 to 13.5 percent of patients after LB [63], and although such bacteremia is generally inconsequential, septicaemia and shock can rarely occur in patients with biliary obstruction and cholangitis.

Biliary peritonitis caused by puncture of the gallbladder is rare (0.00001% frequency) but can be fatal [64].

Pneumothorax, hemothorax, subcutaneous emphysema, perforation of any of several organs (lung, colon, and kidney), subphrenic abscess are other complications reported with LB. Pneumothorax may be self-limited but may require more aggressive intervention depending on the severity of symptoms. Visceral perforation is usually managed expectantly. In most situations, observation is all that is required, although surgical intervention may be needed in the case of gallbladder puncture and persistent bile leak, or in the case of secondary peritonitis.

Differences in complication rates, either minor or major, have been reported between the blind and US-guided LB. The use of US guidance can prevent inadvertent puncture of other organs or large intrahepatic vessels. US may also reduce the incidence of major complications such as haemorrhage, bile peritonitis, pneumothorax, etc.

With respect to the impact of the experience of the operator to the rate of complications, the evidences are controversial. A survey performed in Switzerland showed that the complication rate of percutaneous LB was mainly related to the experience and training of the operator, in particular a lower complication rate was reported for physicians who performed more than 50 biopsies a year [65]. Another study showed that the rate of complications in percutaneous LB was 3.2% if the operator had performed <20 biopsies, and only 1.1% if the operator had performed more than 100 biopsies [64] In contrast, Chevallier et al. showed that the operator's experience did not influence either the final histological diagnosis or the degree of pain suffered by patients [66].

In adult series, the rate of major complications associated with transjugular LB is low (0.5%; liver puncture-related, 0.2%; non-liver puncturerelated,0.3%), considering that it is currently performed in patients with coagulopathy [41]. Minor complications were significantly more frequent with Menghini needle, possibly related with the difficulty in controlling the depth of puncture increasing the risk of capsular penetration [46].

MINOR	
Pyrexia	Hypotension
Neck hematoma, bleeding	Abdominal pain
Neck pain	Subclinical capsular perforation
Carotide puncture	Small hepatic hematoma
Transient Horner's syndrome	Hepatic-portal vein fistula
Transient dysphonia	Hepatic artery aneurysm
Arm numbness/palsy	Biliary fistula
Supraventricular arrhythmia	Haemobilia
MAJOR	
Large hepatic hematoma	Ventricular arrythmia
Intraperitoneal haemorrhage	Pneumothorax
Inferior vena cava or renal vein perforation	Respiratory arrest

Table 4. Complications of transjugular liver biopsy

Factors associated with liver and non-liver puncture related complication rates included number of passes (liver puncture-related), young age, and number of transjugular biopsies.

The complications after laparoscopic LB include perforation of a viscus, bleeding, hemobilia, laceration of the spleen, leakage of ascitic fluid, hematoma in the abdominal wall, vasovagal reaction, prolonged abdominal pain, and seizures [67].

The most quoted mortality rate after percutaneous LB is less than or equal to 1/10.000 biopsies. Mortality is typically related to bleeding. Mortality is highest among patients who undergo biopsies of malignant lesions. Cirrhosis is another risk factor for fatal bleeding after LB. Mortality after transvenous biopsy was 0.09% [41] in adult series, but may reflect the selection of higher risk patients for this intervention. Indeed, mortality is significantly higher in children; smaller livers and horizontal hepatic veins may increase the technical difficulty and risk of capsular perforation, which might be minimized by combined fluoroscopic and US guidance [68].

6. Pathological considerations

Even though LB gives significant diagnostic and prognostic information and helps define treatment plans, it must be recognized that sampling variability and intra observer variability may restrain the diagnostic value of LB. The quality of LB is usually determined by length, width, fragmentation and complete portal tracts (CPTs) [33].

Sample size can affect the diagnostic accuracy of LB specimens [33]. s almost always means that size of the needle biopsy specimen should be of large enough size to accurately assess the degree of liver injury. Considering that a biopsy sample taken from an adult corresponds to a fraction of just 1/50,000th of the whole liver, a biopsy specimen would seem to be inadequate in the case of diffuse diseases, such as a chronic viral hepatitis, in which the liver changes may be unevenly distributed.

Several studies demonstrated that cirrhosis can be missed on a single blind percutaneous LB in 10%-30% of cases [69-71]. In a detailed study, Colloredo et al. [72] carefully evaluated the impact of sample size on correct stadiation of liver fibrosis in patients with chronic hepatitis C. By reducing progressively the dimensions of the same LB, they reported that the smaller the sample analyzed, the milder the diagnosis made by the pathologist with respect to the stage of fibrosis. The reduction in length (<2 cm) led to a significant decrease in number of complete portal tracts and underestimation of grading and staging. The study by Colloredo et al also introduced the concept of a "minimum number of CPTs." Since the number of portal tracts is proportional to biopsy size [73], there was evidence that with fewer than 11 to 15 CPTs grade and stage are significantly underestimated [72]. The lower number of complete portal tracts may explain the lower diagnostic accuracy obtained with smaller samples [73,74]. Guido and Rugge have suggested that a biopsy sample ≥20 mm containing at least 11 CPTs should be considered reliable for adequate staging [75]. Other authors have recommended even bigger samples, up to 25 mm in length [76]. Scheuer suggested that "bigger is better" [77]. Very recently, the American Association for the Study of Liver Diseases (AASLD) has recommended a biopsy sample of at least 20–30 mm in length, and containing at least 11 CPTs [48].

In summary, an adequate (although probably still imperfect) sample needs to be at least 2 cm long (1.4 mm width, 16G) and to contain no fewer than 11 CPTs. These criteria have been adopted rapidly as optimal standards.

Of equal importance to adequate specimen size is the necessity that a pathologist experienced in liver disease interprets the biopsy, ideally in partnership with the clinician who performed the biopsy and/or whom is caring for the patient. Rousselet et al. reported that the degree of experience of the pathologist (specialization, duration, and location of practice) may have a significant impact on the diagnostic interpretation of LB, even higher than that related to characteristics of the specimen (length, fibrosis class number, miscellaneous factors) [78].

Assessment of disease severity with liver histology is supported by a wide body of literature [79]. Complex scoring systems, such as the Knodell scoring system [80] and its revised form, the Ishak scoring system [81] have been developed for grading and staging of chronic viral hepatitis, and there is now a similar score for steatohepatitis [82]. Nevertheless, these are not highly reproducible and are only appropriate for statistical analysis of (large) cohorts of patients in clinical trials. In clinical practice, it was recommended to use the simple systems with three to four categories such as METAVIR [83] rather than complex (Ishak) scoring system [48].

7. Further research

Until a few years ago, LB was the only tool for the diagnosis of liver disease. However, the indications for performing a LB have undergone changes in the last decade. Given the invasive nature of LB, several simple and non-invasive methods (radiologic, immunologic, biochemical, genetic markers) have been studied and proposed as surrogates of liver histology. The main advantages of serum biomarkers vs. LB include being less invasive and the possibility to be easily repeated to monitor the status of liver disease. However, at this time, they are primarily useful for detecting advanced fibrosis or for excluding minimal or no fibrosis. They are not sufficiently accurate for assessing disease progression or the effect of therapy. Due to inadequate diagnostic accuracy or to lack of sufficient validation, current guidelines do not recommend serum biomarkers a substitute for LB that is still considered the reference standard. Notably, non-invasive serum biomarkers, when combined, may reduce by 50%-80% the number of liver biopsies needed for correctly classifying hepatic fibrosis. Serum biomarkers for liver fibrosis are particularly useful for the initial assessment as well as for long-term monitoring of particular subsets of patients (ie, chronic hepatitis C). In this view, combination algorithms of the most validated non-invasive methods for liver fibrosis and LB represent a rational approach to the diagnosis of liver fibrosis in chronic liver diseases. Novel imaging techniques, such as measuring the elasticity of the liver using transient elastography (Fibroscan) [84], may assess fibrosis more directly. However, the use of such techniques in routine clinical practice has not been well defined and require further investigation. LB cannot be avoided completely, but should be used in those cases in which non-invasive methods show poor accuracy. Nevertheless, large scale, prospective, independent studies are needed in other aetiologies of CLDs. Many questions about LB remain and they require much more research. For instance, it is not clear which biopsy devices or techniques are best. In addition, few if any studies have assessed the biopsy's long-term effects. Because the liver is cut and bleeds during procedure, there will be some subsequent scarring.

8. Conclusions

LB continues to play a central role in the evaluation of patients with suspected liver disease, but many aspects of the procedure remain controversial. For example, the precise degree of serum ALT elevations that should prompt a LB is debated, as is the need for LB in all patients with suspected NAFLD and chronic hepatitis C. The importance of LB in arriving at a diagnosis of diffuse parenchymal liver disease is being diminished by accurate blood testing strategies for chronic viral hepatitis, autoimmune hepatitis, and primary biliary cirrhosis. Further, imaging tests are superior to LB in the diagnosis of primary sclerosing cholangitis. However, many cases remain in which diagnostic confusion exists even after suitable laboratory testing and imaging studies. Diagnosing infiltrative disease (eg, amyloidosis, sarcoidosis), separating benign fatty liver disease from steatohepatitis, and evaluating liver parenchyma after liver transplantation are best accomplished by LB.

Percutaneous LB is contraindicated in patients with severe coagulopathy and ascites, but the degree of coagulopathy that contraindicates a LB is controversial. Also controversial are the technical aspects of LB, particularly the choice of needle (cutting vs. suction) and the use of US to mark or guide the biopsy site. Bleeding is the major complication of LB, with a risk of 0.3%; cutting needles are more likely to cause hemorrhage than are suction needles. While needle biopsy is still the mainstay in diagnosing hepatic fibrosis, its days of dominance seem limited as technology improves. When physical examination or standard laboratory tests reveal clear-cut signs of portal hypertension, LB will seldom add useful information. Similarly, when imaging studies provide compelling evidence of cirrhosis and portal hypertension, needle biopsy is not warranted. The combination algorithms warrant further evaluation in all chronic liver diseases, as they may help decrease the number of liver biopsies required. Moreover, transient elastography is playing an ever-increasing role in the assessment of hepatic fibrosis and will significantly reduce the need for biopsy in patients with liver disease.

Clearly, as our knowledge of various liver disorders advances and new especially non-invasive diagnostic tests are developed, the role of LB in medical practice will continue to evolve. Emergence of better imaging techniques, surrogate serological markers of liver fibrosis are among the many new and exciting developments that hold promise for the future.

Author details

Claudia Randazzo, Anna Licata and Piero Luigi Almasio

Department of Gastroenterology, University of Palermo, Italy

References

[1] Sherlock S. Aspiration liver biopsy: technique and diagnostic application. Lancet 1945;246:397-401.

[2] Hay JE, Czaja AJ, Rakela J, Ludwig J. The nature of unexplained chronic aminotransferase elevations of a mild to moderate degree in asymptomatic patients. Hepatology 1989;9:193-197.

[3] Sorbi D, McGill DB, Thistle JL, et al. An assessment of the role of liver biopsies in asymptomatic patients with chronic liver test abnormalities. Am J Gastroenterol 2000;95:3206-3210.

[4] Skelly MM, James PD, Ryder SD. Findings on liver biopsy to investigate abnormal liver function tests in the absence of diagnostic serology. J Hepatol 2001;35:195-199.

[5] Powell EE, Jonsson JR, Clouston AD. Steatosis: co-factor in other liver diseases. Hepatology 2005;42:5-13.

[6] Zein CO, Angulo P, Lindor KD. When is liver biopsy needed in the diagnosis of primary biliary cirrhosis? ClinGastroenterolHepatol 2003;1:89-95.

[7] Dahlin DC, Stauffer MH, Mann FD. Laboratory and biopsy diagnosis of amyloidosis. Med Clin North Am 1950;34:1171-1176.

[8] Polson J, LeeWM. AASLD position paper: the management of acute liver failure. Hepatology 2005;41:1179-1197.

[9] Takamori R, Wong LL, Dang C, et al. Needle-tract implantation from hepatocellular cancer: is needle biopsy of the liver always necessary? Liver Transplant 2000;6:67–72.

[10] European Association for the Study of the Liver. EASL Clinical Practice Guidelines: Management of hepatitis C virus infection. J Hepatol. 2011;55(2):245-64.

[11] Gleeson D, Heneghan MA; British Society of Gastroenterology. British Society of Gastroenterology (BSG) guidelines for management of autoimmune hepatitis. Gut 2011;60(12):1611-29.

[12] Verma S, Gunuwan B, Mendler M, et al. Factors predicting relapse and poor outcome in type I autoimmune hepatitis: role of cirrhosis development, patterns of transaminases during remission and plasma cell activity in the LB. Am J Gastroenterol 2004;99:1510-1516.

[13] European Association for the Study ofThe Liver. EASL Clinical Practice Guidelines: Management of chronic hepatitis B virus infection. J Hepatol 2012;57(1):167-85.

[14] European Association for the Study of the Liver. EASL Clinical Practice Guidelines for HFE hemochromatosis. J Hepatol 2010;53(1):3-22.

[15] European Association for the Study of the Liver. EASL Clinical Practice Guidelines: management of cholestatic liver diseases. J Hepatol 2009;51(2):237-67.

[16] European Association for Study of Liver. EASL Clinical Practice Guidelines: Wilson's disease. J Hepatol 2012;56(3):671-85.

[17] Pratt DS, Kaplan MM. Evaluation of abnormal liver-enzyme results in asymptomatic patients. N Engl J Med 2000;342:1266-71.

[18] Bianchi L: Liver biopsy in elevated liver function tests? An old question revisited. J Hepatol2001;35:290-294.

[19] Prati D, Taioli E, Zanella S, et al.Updated definitions of healthy ranges for serum alanine aminotransferase levels. Ann Intern Med 2002;137:1-9.

[20] Kaplan MM. Alanine aminotransferase levels: What's normal? Ann Intern Med 2002;137:49-51.

[21] Ruhl C, Everhart JE: Determinants of the association of overweight with elevated serum alanine aminotransferase activity in the United States. Gastroenterology 2003;124:71-79.

[22] Green RM, Flamm S: AGA technical review on the evaluation of liver chemistry tests. Gastroenterology 2002; 123:1367-1384.

[23] Chandok N, Hirschfield GM. Management of primary sclerosing cholangitis: conventions and controversies. Can J Gastroenterol 2012;26(5):261-8.

[24] Sebagh M, Rifai K, Féray C, et al.: All liver recipients benefit from the protocol 10-year liver biopsies. Hepatology2003;37:1293-1301.

[25] Spycher C, Zimmermann A, Relchen J: The diagnostic value of liver biopsy. BMC Gastroenterol2001;1:12.

[26] Piccinino F, Sagnelli E, Pasquale G, Giusti G. Complications following percutaneous liver biopsy. A multicentre retrospective study on 68,276 biopsies. J Hepatol 1986;2:165-173.

[27] Alexander JA, Smith BJ: Midazolam sedation for percutaneous liver biopsy. Dig Dis Sci1993;38:2209-2211.

[28] Grant A, Neuberger J: Guidelines on the use of liver biopsy in clinical practice. Gut 1999;45(Suppl IV):IV1-IV11.

[29] Sato S, Mishiro T, Miyake T, et al. Prophylactic administration of antibiotics unnecessary following ultrasound-guided biopsy and ablation therapy for liver tumors: Open-labeled randomized prospective study. Hepatol Res 2009;39(1):40-6.

[30] Hegarty JE, Williams R. Liver biopsy: techniques, clinical applications, and complications. Br Med J (Clin Res Ed) 1984;288:1254-6.

[31] Sherlock S, Dooley J. Diseases of the Liver and Biliary System. Oxford: Blackwell Science; 2002

[32] Crawford AR, Lin X-Z, Crawford JM: The normal adult human liver biopsy: a quantitative reference standard. Hepatology1998;28:323-331.

[33] Bravo AA, Sheth SG, Chopra S. Liver biopsy. N Engl J Med 2001;344:495-500.

[34] Vautier G, Scott B, Jenkins D. Liver biopsy: blind or guided? BMJ 1994;309:1455-1456.

[35] Caturelli E, Giacobbe A, Facciorusio D, et al.Percutaneous biopsy in diffuse liver disease: increasing diagnostic yield and decreasing complication rate by routine ultrasound assessment of puncture site. Am J Gastroenterol1996;91:1318-1321.

[36] Smith CI, Grau JE. The effect of ultrasonography on the performance of routine liver biopsy. Hepatology 1995; 22:384A.

[37] Riley TR. How often does ultrasound marking change the liver biopsy site? Am J Gastroenterol 1996;91:1292-1296.

[38] Cadranel JF, Rufat P, Degos F. Practices of liver biopsy in France: results of a prospective nationwide survey. For the group of Epidemiology of the French Association for the Study of the Liver (AFEF). Hepatology 2000; 32:477-481.

[39] Younossi ZM, Teran JC, Ganiats TG, Carey WD. Ultrasound-guided liver biopsy for parenchymal liver disease: an economic analysis. Dig Dis Sci 1998;43:46-50.

[40] Pasha T, Gabriel S, Therneau T, et al. Cost-effectiveness of ultrasound-guided liver biopsy. Hepatology 1998;27:1220-1226.

[41] Kalambokis G, Manousou P, Vibhakorn S, et al. Transjugular liver biopsy - indications, adequacy, quality of specimens, and complications - a systematic review. J Hepatol 2007;47(2):284-294.

[42] Lebrec D, Goldfarb G, Degott C, et al. Transvenous liver biopsy: an experience based on 1000 hepatic tissue samplings with this procedure. Gastroenterology 1982;83:338-340.

[43] Bull HJ, Gilmore IT, Bradley RD, et al. Experience with transjugular liver biopsy. Gut 1983;24:1057-1060.

[44] McAfee JH, Keeffe EB, Lee RG, Rosch J. Transjugular liver biopsy. Hepatology 1992;15:726-732.

[45] Lebrec D. Various approaches to obtaining liver tissue: choosing the biopsy technique. J Hepatol1996;25(suppl 1):20-24.

[46] Papatheodoridis DV, Patch D, Watkinson A, et al.Transjugularliver biopsy in the 1990s: a 2-year audit. Aliment PharmacolTher1999;13:603-608.

[47] Ewe K. Bleeding after liver biopsy does not correlate with indices of peripheral coagulation. Dig Dis Sci 1981; 26:388-393.

[48] Rockey DC, Caldwell SH, Goodman ZD, et al. Liver biopsy. Hepatology 2009;49:1017-44.

[49] Dillon JF, Simpson KJ, Hayes PC: Liver biopsy bleeding time: an unpredictable event. J GastroenterolHepatol1994;9:269-271.

[50] Venkataramani A, Behling C, Rond DR, et al.Liver biopsies in adult hemophiliacs with hepatitis C: a United States center's experience. Am J Gastroenterol 2000;95:2374-2376.

[51] McGill DB, Rakela J, Zinsmeister AR, Ott BJ. A 21-year experience with major hemorrhage after percutaneous liver biopsy. Gastroenterology 1990;99:1396-1400.

[52] Chang S, Kim SH, Lim HK, et al. Needle tract implantation after sonographically guided percutaneous biopsy of hepatocellular carcinoma: evaluation of doubling time, frequency, and features on CT. AJR Am J Roentgenol 2005;185:400-405.

[53] Liu YW, Chen CL, Chen YS, et al. Needle tract implantation of hepatocellular carcinoma after fine needle biopsy. Dig Dis Sci 2007;52:228-231.

[54] Schipper HG, Lameris JS, van Delden OM, et al.: Percutaneous evacuation (PEVAC) of multivesicularechinococcal cysts with or without cystobiliary fistulas which contain non-drainable material: first results of a modified PAIR method. Gut 2002;50:718-723.

[55] Eisenberg E, Konopniki M, Veitsman E, et al. Prevalence and characteristics of pain induced by percutaneous liver biopsy. AnesthAnalg 2003;96:1392-1396.

[56] Tan KT, Rajan DK, Kachura JR, et al. Pain after percutaneous liver biopsy for diffuse hepatic disease: a randomized trial comparing subcostal and intercostal approaches. J VascIntervRadiol 2005;16:1215-1219.

[57] Caldwell SH. Controlling pain in LB, or "we will probably need to repeat the biopsy in a year or two to assess the response". Am J Gastroenterol 2001;96:1327-1329.

[58] Myers RP, Fong A, Shaheen AA. Utilization rates, complications and costs of percutaneous liver biopsy: a population-based study including 4275 biopsies. Liver Int 2008;28:705-712.

[59] Firpi RJ, Soldevila-Pico C, Abdelmalek MF, et al. Short recovery time after percutaneous liver biopsy: should we change our current practices? ClinGastroenterolHepatol 2005;3:926-929.

[60] Minuk GY, Sutherland LR, Wiseman D, et al.Prospective study of the incidence of ultrasound-detected intrahepatic and subcapsular haematomas in patients randomized to 6 or 24 hours of bed rest after percutaneous liver biopsy. Gastroenterology 1987;92:290-293.

[61] Tobkes AI, Nord HJ. LB: review of methodology and complications. Dig Dis 1995;13:267-274.

[62] Lichtenstein DR, Kim D, Chopra S. Delayed massive hemobilia following percutaneous liver biopsy: treatment by embolotherapy. Am J Gastroenterol 1992;87:1833-1838.

[63] Reddy KR, Schiff ER. Complications of liver biopsy. In: Taylor MB (ed.) Gastrointestinal emergencies. 2nd ed. Baltimore: Williams & Wilkins;1997. p959-968.

[64] Gilmore IT, Burroughs A, Murray-Lyon IM, et al.Indications, methods, and outcomes of percutaneous liver biopsy in England and Wales: an audit by the British Society of Gastroenterology and the Royal College of Physicians of London. Gut 1995;36:437-441.

[65] Froehlich F, Lamy O, Fried M, Gonvers JJ. Practice and complications of liver biopsy. Results of a nationwide survey in Switzerland. Dig Dis Sci 1993;38(8):1480-1484.

[66] Chevallier P, Ruitort F, Denys A, et al. Influence of operator experience on performance of ultrasound-guided percutaneous liver biopsy. EurRadiol 2004;14:2086-2091.

[67] Vargas C, Jeffers LJ, Bernstein D, et al. Diagnostic laparoscopy: a 5-year experience in a hepatology training program. Am J Gastroenterol 1995;90:1258-1262.

[68] Hadbank K, Resterpo R, Ng V, et al. Combined sonographic and fluoroscopic guidance during transjugular hepatic biopsies performed in children: a retrospective study of 74 biopsies. Am J Roentgenol2003;180:1393-1398.

[69] Maharaj B, Maharaj RJ, Leary WP, et al. Sampling variability and its influence on the diagnostic yield of percutaneous needle biopsy of the liver. Lancet 1986;1:523-525.

[70] Pagliaro L, Rinaldi F, Craxi A, et al. Percutaneous blind biopsy versus laparoscopy with guided biopsy in diagnosis of cirrhosis. A prospective, randomized trial. Dig Dis Sci 1983;28:39-43.

[71] Poniachik J, Bernstein DE, Reddy KR, et al. The role of laparoscopy in the diagnosis of cirrhosis. GastrointestEndosc 1996;43:568-71.

[72] Colloredo G, Guido M, Sonzogni A, et al. Impact of liver biopsy size on histological evaluation of chronic viral hepatitis: the smaller the sample, the milder the disease. J Hepatol.2003;39:239-244.

[73] Rocken C, Meier H, Klauck S, et al. Large-needle biopsy versus thin-needle biopsy in diagnostic pathology of liver diseases. Liver 2001;21:391-397.

[74] Siddique I, El-Naga HA, Madda JP, et al. Sampling variability on percutaneous liver biopsy in patients with chronic hepatitis C virus infection. Scand J Gastroenterol 2003;38:427-432.

[75] Guido M, Rugge M. Liver biopsy sampling in chronic viral hepatitis. Semin Liver Dis 2004;24:89-97.

[76] Bedossa P, Dargere D, Paradis V. Sampling variability of liver fibrosis in chronic hepatitis C. Hepatology 2003;38:1449-1457.

[77] Scheuer PJ. LB size matters in chronic hepatitis: bigger is better. Hepatology 2003;38:1356-1358.

[78] Rousselet MC, Michalak S, Dupre F, et al. Sources of variability in histological scoring of chronic viral hepatitis. Hepatology 2005;41:257-264.

[79] Crawford JM. Evidence-based interpretation of liver biopsies. Lab Invest 2006;86:326-334.

[80] Knodell RG, Ishak KG, Black WC, et al. Formulation and application of a numerical scoring system for assessing histological activity in asymptomatic chronic active hepatitis. Hepatology 1981;1:431-435.

[81] Ishak K, Baptista A, Bianchi L, et al. Histological grading and staging of chronic hepatitis. J Hepatol 1995;22:696-699.

[82] Kleiner DE, Brunt EM, Van Natta M, et al. Design and validation of a histological scoring system for nonalcoholic fatty liver disease. Hepatology 2005;41:1313-1321.

[83] Bedossa P, Poynard T. An algorithm for the grading of activity in chronic hepatitis C. The METAVIR Cooperative Study Group. Hepatology 1996;24:289-293.

[84] Sandrin L, Fourquet B, Hasquenoph JM, et al. Transient elastography: a new noninvasive method for assessment of hepatic fibrosis. Ultrasound Med Biol2003;29(12): 1705-1713.

Chapter 2

Types of Liver Biopsy

Nobumi Tagaya, Nana Makino, Kazuyuki Saito,
Takashi Okuyama, Yoshitake Sugamata and
Masatoshi Oya

Additional information is available at the end of the chapter

http://dx.doi.org/10.5772/52914

1. Introduction

Liver biopsy (LB) is an important procedure in the diagnosis and treatment of liver diseases. However, procedures for performing LB vary amongst institutions, and no universal guidelines exist. LB is performed for two main reasons: diagnosis of a liver condition itself, and as an adjunct to an existing surgical procedure. Recently, it has become possible to employ both approaches with minimal invasiveness using the transjugular route or under the guidance of ultrasound, computed tomography, or laparoscopic and endoscopic ultrasound. Techniques for liver tissue sampling include percutaneous liver biopsy [1-6], transjugular liver biopsy [7-14], laparoscopic liver biopsy [15], and transgastric liver biopsy [16-20]. This chapter introduces these techniques and evaluates their outcomes.

2. Percutaneous Liver Biopsy (PLB)

PLB is performed either blind or under imaging guidance. In the latter context, ultrasound (US) or computed tomographic (CT) guidance is used. Although these results of US-guided PLB depend greatly on the skills of the gastroenterologist, hepatologist or radiologist and the technical capabilities and quality of the US instrument, the available data indicate that it has a lower complication rate, requires a lower number of passes, is associated with less pain and pain-related morbidity, has a lower likelihood of the need for a repeat procedure, affords better-quality tissue specimens, and has only a marginally increased cost in comparison with blind PLB [21].

PLB under image guidance essentially eliminates the risk of pneumothorax, or injury to the gallbladder or other viscera because the needle track is directly visualize of organ. Pain is the commonest complication, and up to 75% of patients suffer some discomfort after LB [21]. However, complications after PLB require careful observation. Piccinino et al. [22] reported that 61% of such complications appeared in the first 2 hours after the biopsy, 82% in the first 10 hours, and 96% in the first 24 hours. Strict observation is therefore required for the first 24 hours after PLB. Several large studies have shown rates of major complication after PLB ranging from 0.09% to 2.3%, severe complications in 0.57%, and mortality ranging from 0.03% to 0.11% [23-25]. Hardman et al. [4] reported one patient with graft vs. host disease and hypertension who died after PLB. This patient had multi-organ system failure at the time of biopsy and died within 24 hours of the biopsy. Furthermore, the complications of PLB seem to be related to the type of technique employed. In fact, the complications associated with US-guided PLB are significantly lower than those associated with blind PLB: 0.5% vs. 2.2% for severe complications [26], 2% vs. 4% [27] and 1.8% vs. 7.7% [28] for total complications. PLB under US guidance is recommended as a reasonable and cost-efficient procedure [1, 26, 28]. However, EI-Shabrawi et al. [5] have reported that blind PLB performed by the Menghini aspiration technique is safe even in infants and small children without mortality or major complications such as bile leakage, pneumothorax, and bleeding requiring blood transfusion. Szymczak et al. [6] also reported the safety and effectiveness of blind PLB based on an analysis of 1412 procedures, and showed that the rates of complications and failure were dependent on the experience of the operator. Moreover, the needle used was the Menghini-type suction needle, which carries a smaller risk of bleeding than cutting needles such as the widely employed Tru-cut needle. They concluded that the risk of complications and failure rate are low if the indications and contraindications are considered carefully and the biopsy is performed by a skilled and experienced operator.

Furthermore, with regard to bleeding after PLB, Alotaibi et al. [3] have reported that a positive color Doppler sign in US indicates bleeding along the biopsy tract, and that US-guided compression is effective for achieving appropriate hemostasis. Also, tract-plugging of the biopsy tract with Gelfoam or other thrombotic agents, is an important procedure for reducing the risk of bleeding and subcapsular hematoma in PLB [2]. Nevertheless, in patients with ascites or abnormal coagulation profiles, another procedure should be considered because of the high risk of possible bleeding complications.

3. Transjugular Liver Biopsy (TJLB)

TJLB was initially introduced in dogs as an experimental application by Dotter [29]. Rosch [7, 8] then reported its clinical application for transjugular cholangiography in 1973 and 1975. TJLB eliminates the need to traverse the peritoneal cavity and puncture the liver capsule. Furthermore, this technique is a safer biopsy option for patients with massive ascites, coagulopathy (prothrombin time greater than 3 seconds over the control value), thrombocytopenia (less then 60,000/cm^3), or those undergoing ancillary procedures such as measurement of pressures or opacification of the hepatic vein and inferior vena cava. It can also be applied for patients in whom PLB has failed, or those with morbid obesity, a small cirrhotic liver, suspected vascular tumor or peliosis hepatitis, or medical conditions associated with bleeding disorders such as hemophilia for whom PLB is contraindicated [11, 30, 31], as any bleeding is returned to the venous system rather than leaking into the abdomen.

However, there are several particular complications associated with TJLB, including hemorrhage, subcapsular or neck hematoma and ventricular arrhythmia. The rate of such complications ranges from 0% to 20% [11]. Hardman et al. [4] reported a large subcapsular hematoma caused by TJLB requiring embolization and prolonged admission. Lebrec et al. [9] also reported a fatal case of intraperitoneal hemorrhage due to perforation of the liver capsule caused by excessive of the needle. Therefore, such forward rotation must be avoided or carefully limited. Furthermore, there have been several direct instances of perforation of the liver capsule that resulted in aspiration of ascitic fluid, bile from the gallbladder, or renal tissue in patients with a small cirrhotic liver. In such patients, TJLB should be avoided or employed only with caution by advancing the needle into the liver parenchyma by only 1 cm instead of the usual 2 cm, or contrast medium should be injected after the biopsy to evaluate the integrity of liver capsule. The major drawback of TJLB is the size of the biopsy specimens obtained; they are generally smaller ($p < 0.001$) and more fragmented ($p < 0.01$) than those obtained by PLB [12]. Pathologically, in terms of the number of portal tracts ($p < 0.0001$) and the utility of specimens for histological evaluation ($p < 0.05$), the quality of TJLB samples appears to be significantly lower compared than those of PLB and LLB specimens [14]. With regard to technical success rate, that of TJLB (82%: 84/102) is significantly lower ($P = 0.005$) than PLB (100%: 100/100) or LLB (99%: 111/112) [14]. However, Bull et al. [10] reported a success rate of 97% (188/197) in 1983, and a recent meta-analysis including more than 7500 cases revealed a technical success rate of 96.8% [13]. These reports suggest that there is no significant difference between TJLB and others techniques in terms of success rate. The most common reason for failure was inability to catheterize the right hepatic vein. In actual practice, TJLB requires a longer procedure time (40 min) than PLB. A few deaths after TJLB have been reported, with a mortality rate of 0-0.5% [10, 32, 33]; mortality was due to hemorrhage from the liver or ventricular arrhythmia.

Therefore, TJLB should be attempted only by a skilled interventional radiologist or physician experienced in catheterization and cannulation of the internal jugular vein due to its more time-consuming nature, use of intravenous contrast, and the need for a dedicated fluoroscopy suite. In fact, TJLB can be valuable in cases for which PLB is hazardous, or when pressure measurement or venography is also required [34]. Despite the smaller biopsy samples obtained, the impact of TJLB on clinical decision-making appears to be comparable to that of PLB and LLB. In particular, it may help to determine the need for liver transplantation in patients with acute liver failure.

4. Laparoscopic Liver Biopsy (LLB)

There are several approaches for LLB, including PLB under laparoscopic observation, LB through an additional port under laparoscopic observation, or LB combined with another laparoscopic procedure. LLB allows direct observation of the biopsy site and yields with macroscopic information about the liver surface. This facilitates an adequate sample volume to be obtained, including wedge resection, without sampling error, and also allows laparoscopic confirmation of hemostasis. These are the advantages of LLB in comparison with PLB. If bleeding from the biopsy site persists, compression or coagulation can easily be applied using several types of special forceps.

However, LLB requires general anesthesia and specialized equipment, including insufflation devices and laparoscopic instruments. On the other hand, PLB under laparoscopic observation can be done under local anesthesia using pneumoperitoneum under sedation using midazolam and disoprivan, or under general anesthesia using an abdominal wall lift method [15]. For laparoscopy, pneumoperitoneum is created by N_2O insufflation via a Veress needle, generally inserted to the left of the umbilicus. A second port is added on the right side by inserting a trocar. A 16-gauge True-cut needle is inserted and biopsy samples of the liver can be taken from the left and right lobes under laparoscopic guidance. The biopsy sites can be prophylactically coagulated. Beckmann et al. [14] reported that the complications observed after LLB were bleeding and bile leakage, and that the complication rate (2.7%) was roughly equal to that of PLB (3%) and TJLB (2.9%).

In general, LLB requires a long set-up time for starting the procedure, gas insufflation to create an adequate operative field, preparation of several laparoscopic instruments, and an operating theater. LLB is the most appropriate method for patients who need both a pathological diagnosis of liver dysfunction or tumor and laparoscopic procedures for intra-abdominal diseases.

5. Transgastric Liver Biopsy (TGLB)

For TGLB, Hollerbach et al. [17] have reported an endoscopic ultrasound-guided fine-needle aspiration biopsy procedure for liver lesions. This method is one of several transgastric approaches and can be an alternative to PLB, particularly for patients with a risk of bleeding or small lesions in the liver, although targeting may be limited according to tumor location.

Recently, natural orifice translumenal endoscopic surgery (NOTES) has been introduced, creating no skin scars and involving only minimal invasiveness. NOTES has created a new access route (via the stomach) to the peritoneal cavity. TGLB using NOTES creates no damage to the outside of the body and allows direct observation of the biopsy site inside the body, unlike PLB or TJLB. In an experimental study, Mintz et al. [35, 36] reported successful LB using a hybrid technique that included standard laparoscope vision and surgical endoscopy. As outlined in a white paper from the American Society for Gastrointestinal Endoscopy and Society of American Gastrointestinal and Endoscopic Surgeons [37, 38], for clinical application of NOTES, it is necessary to establish safe access to the peritoneal cavity, complete closure of the access route, prevention of infection, correct intra-abdominal orientation, development of a multitasking platform, methods for management of accidental complications, awareness of unanticipated physiologic events, and training in the technique. In par-

http://dx.doi.org/10.5772/52914

ticular, infection or bacterial contamination in the abdomen due to opening of the digestive tract is a great concern in NOTES. However, no studies have quantified the bacteriological load to which the peritoneum is exposed during transgastric procedures [19]. Steele et al. [20] reported a pilot feasibility study of transgastric peritoneoscopy and liver biopsy during laparoscopic Roux-en-Y gastric bypass. LB was performed from segment II, III or IVb of the liver to obtain tissue samples adequate for histologic examination. None of patients exhibited any signs or symptoms of intra-abdominal or trocar wound infection after the procedure.

For TGLB [39], under general anesthesia a forward-viewing, double-channel endoscope is advanced into the stomach. Puncture of the gastric wall is performed with a 3-mm cutting-wire needle knife. The puncture site is enlarged to 8mm with a balloon dilator and then the endoscope is advanced into the peritoneal cavity. The peritoneal cavity is then inflated with air through the endoscope. The liver is easily visualized by retroflexion of the endoscope. LB is performed using routine biopsy forceps from the edge of the liver (segment III) (Fig. 1), and hemostasis of the biopsy site is achieved by electrocautery with biopsy forceps (Fig. 2). The gastric artificial orifice is then closed using endoscopic clips.

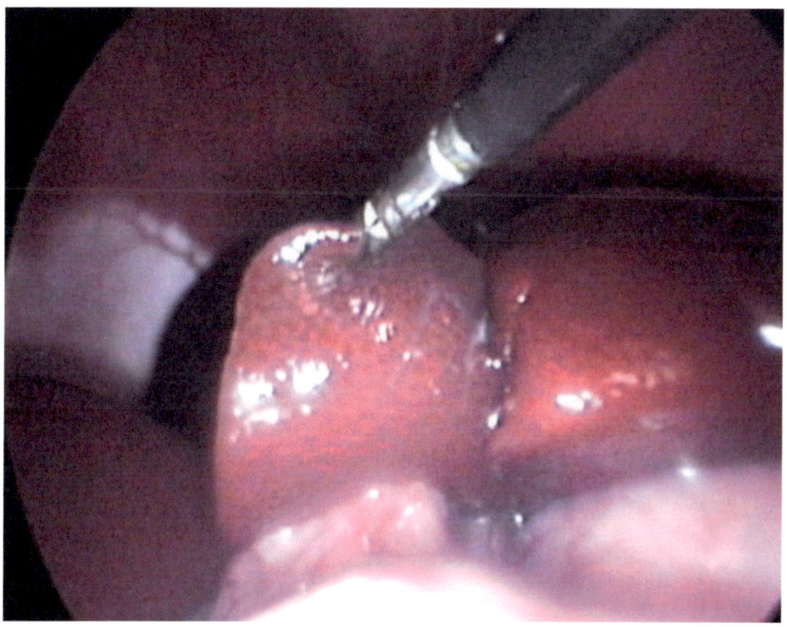

Figure 1. Liver biopsy was performed using routine biopsy forceps from the edge of the liver.

Transgastric peritoneoscopy developed by Kalloo et al. [16, 18] showed no association with serious infection or other complications in the peritoneal cavity during long- term observation. Furthermore, Hazey et al. [40] reported that although contamination of the peritoneal cavity was observed during laparoscopic Roux-en-Y gastric bypass, no clinically significant episode, such as abscess formation or infectious complications, occurred. From these findings, although peroral TGLB requires the creation of an artificial injury in a normal organ, it will likely become a widely used alternative to other LB methods.

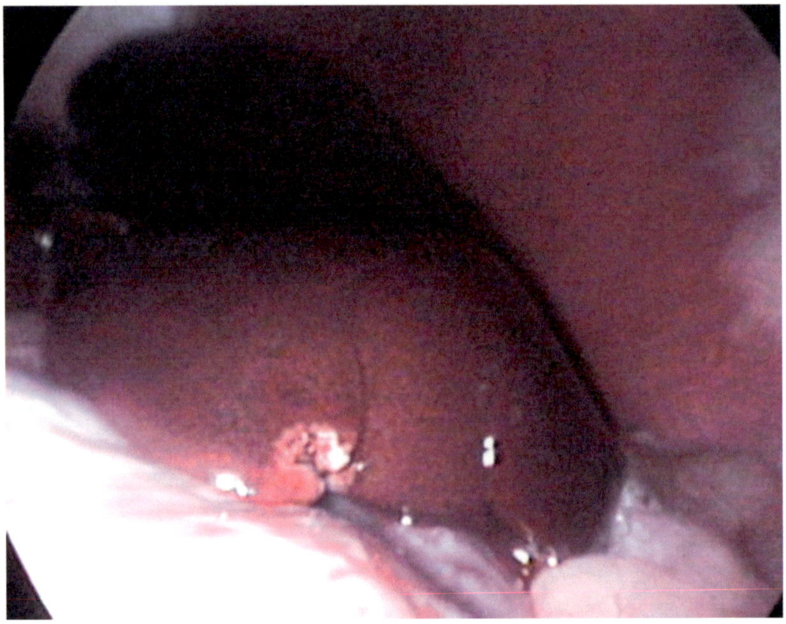

Figure 2. Hemostasis was confirmed at the site of liver biopsy.

6. Conclusion

In conclusion, TGLB is technically feasible and has the potential to become an alternative to routine liver biopsy. The transgastric endoscopic approach has a wide range of diagnostic and therapeutic applications.

Author details

Nobumi Tagaya*, Nana Makino, Kazuyuki Saito, Takashi Okuyama, Yoshitake Sugamata and Masatoshi Oya

*Address all correspondence to: tagaya@dokkyomed.ac.jp

Department of Surgery, Dokkyo Medical University Koshigaya Hospital, Koshigaya, Saitama, Japan

References

[1] Lindor KD et al. (1996). The role of ultrasonography and automatic-needle biopsy in outpatient percutaneous liver biopsy. Hepatology 23: 1079-1983.

[2] Sporea I et al. (2008). Why, who and how should perform liver biopsy in chronic liver disease. World J Gastroenterol 14: 3396-3402.

[3] Alotaibi M et al. (2010). The positive color Doppler sign post biopsy: effectiveness of US-directed compression in achieving hemostasis. Pediatr Radiol [DOI 10.1007/s00247-010-1848-7].

[4] Hardman RL et al. (2010). Single-institution results of image-guided nonplugged percutaneous versus transjugular liver biopsy. Cardiovasc Intervent Radiol [DOI 10.1007/s00270-010-9924-9].

[5] El-Shabrawi et al. (2012). Outpatient blind percutaneous liver biopsy in infants and children: Is it safe? Saudi J Gastroenterol 18 (1): 26-33.

[6] Szymczak A et al. (2012). Safety and effectiveness of blind percutaneous liver biopsy: Analysis of 1412 procedures. Hepat Mon 2012: 32-37. [DOI: 10.5812/kowsar.1735143X.810].

[7] Rosch J et al. (1973). Transjugular approach to liver biopsy and transhepatic cholangiography. N Engl J Med 289: 227-231.

[8] Rosch J et al. (1975). Transjugular approach to the liver, biliary system, and portal circulation. Am J Roentgenol Radium Ther Nucl Med 125 (3): 602-608.

[9] Lebrec D et al. (1987). Transvenous (transjugular) liver biopsy. An experience based on 100 biopsies. Am J Dig Dis 23 (4): 302-304.

[10] Bull HJM, et al. (1983). Experience with transjugular liver biopsy. Gut 24: 1057-1060.

[11] McAfee JH et al. (1992). Transjugular liver biopsy. Hepatology 15 (4): 726-732.

[12] Meng HC et al. (1994). Transjugular liver biopsy: comparison with percutaneous liver biopsy. J Gastroenterol Hepatol 9 (5): 457-461.

[13] Keshava SN, et al. (2008) Transjugular liver biopsy: What to do and what not to do. Ind J Radiol Imaging 18: 245-248.

[14] Beckmann MG, et al. (2009). Clinical relevance of transjugular liver biopsy in comparison with percutaneous and laparoscopic liver biopsy. Gastroenterol Res Pract [DOI: 10.1155/2009/947014].

[15] Chiesa OA, et al. (2009). Isobaric (gasless) laparoscopic liver and kidney biopsy in standing steers. Can J Vet Res 73 (1): 42-48.

[16] Kalloo AN et al. (2000). Flexible transgastric peritoneoscopy: a novel approach to diagnostic and therapeutic interventions in the peritoneal cavity [abstract]. Gastroenterology, 118, pp.A1039.

[17] Hollerbach S, et al. (2003). Endoscopic ultrasound-guided fine–needle aspiration biopsy of the liver: histological and cytological assessment. Endoscopy 35 (9): 743-749.

[18] Kalloo AN et al. (2004). Flexible transgastric peritoneoscopy: a novel approach to diagnostic and therapeutic interventions in the peritoneal cavity. Gastrointest Endosc 60 (1): 114-117.

[19] Babatin MA et al. (2007). NOTES: Evolving trends in endoscopic surgery. Saudi J Gastroenterol 13 (4): 207-210.

[20] Steele K et al. (2008). Flexible transgastric peritoneoscopy and liver biopsy: a feasibility study in human beings (with video). Gastrointest Endosc 68 (1): 61-66.

[21] Vijayaraghavan GR et al. (2011). Imaging-guided parenchymal liver biopsy: How we do it. J Clin Imaging Sci [DOI: 10.4103/2156-7514.82082].

[22] Piccinino F et al. (1986). Complications following percutaneous liver biopsy. A multicentre retrospective study on 68,276 biopsies. J Hepatol 2: 165-173.

[23] Poynard T et al. (2000). Appropriateness of liver biopsy. Can J Gastroenterol 14: 543–548.

[24] McGill DB et al. (1990). A 21-year experience with major hemorrhage after percutaneous liver biopsy. Gastroenterology 99: 1396–1400.

[25] Cadranel JF et al. (2000). Practices of liver biopsy in France: results of a prospective nationwide survey. For the Group of Epidemiology of the French Association for the Study of the Liver (AFEF). Hepatology 32: 477-481.

[26] Pasha T et al. (1998). Cost-effectiveness of ultrasound-guided liver biopsy. Hepatology 27: 1220-1226.

[27] Younossi ZM et al. (1998). Ultrasound-guided liver biopsy for parenchymal liver disease: an economic analysis. Dig Dis Sci 43: 46-50.

[28] Farrell RJ et al. (1999). Guided versus blind liver biopsy for chronic hepatitis C; clinical benefits and costs. J Hepatol 30: 580-587.

[29] Dotter CT. (1964) Catheter biopsy: experimental technique for transvenous liver biopsy. Radiology 82: 312-314.

[30] Bravo AA et al. (2001). Liver biopsy. N Engl J Med 344: 495-500.

[31] Rockey D et al. (2009). American Association for the Study of Liver Diseases. Liver biopsy. Hepatology 49: 1017-1044.

[32] Colapinto RF. (1985). Transjugular biopsy of the liver. Clin Gastroenterol 14 (2): 451-467.

[33] Kalambokis G et al. (2007). Transjugular liver biopsy-indications, adequacy, quality of specimens, and complications: A systematic review. J Hepatol 47: 284-294.

[34] Gilmore IT, et al. (1977). Transjugular liver biopsy. Br Med J 9: 100-101.

[35] Mintz Y et al. (2007). NOTES: The hybrid technique. J Laparoendosc Adv Surg Tech 17: 402-406.

[36] Mintz Y et al. (2008). NOTES: A review of the technical problems encountered and their solutions. J Laparoendosc Adv Surg Tech18: 583-587.

[37] ASGE & SAGES. (2006). ASGE/SAGES working group on natural orifice translumenal endoscopic surgery: White paper October 2005. Gastrointest Endosc 63: 199-203.

[38] Rattner D & Kalloo A: ASGE/SAGES Working Group. (2006). ASGE/SAGES working group on natural orifice translumenal endoscopic surgery. October 2005. Surg Endosc 20: 329-33.

[39] Tagaya N, et al. (2010). Transgastric liver biopsy using the NOTES technique: an animal study. In Tech-Open Access Publisher, Inc., Liver Biopsy. Part 1, Chapter 11, pp 171-178.

[40] Hazey JW et al. (2008). Natural-orifice transgastric endoscopic peritoneoscopy in humans: Initial clinical trial. Surg Endosc 22: 16-20.

Chapter 3

Rethinking the Role of Liver Biopsy in the Era of Personalized Medicine

Teresa Casanovas Taltavull

Additional information is available at the end of the chapter

http://dx.doi.org/10.5772/53120

1. Introduction

Indications and methods of liver biopsy have changed over the past few years [1]. However, an histological diagnosis may be needed for optimal management of a patient [2, 3].

Although modern biochemical, immunological, and radiographic techniques have facilitated the diagnosis and management of liver diseases they have not made liver biopsy obsolete. Clinicians rely on information derived from the liver biopsy to inform patients and to make their therapeutic options [4].

There are, however, many controversies surrounding liver biopsy resulting potential limitations, such as sampling errors and interobserver variations [5], which can lead to misclassification therefore, P. Bedossa et al. consider that when it comes to liver biopsy the term "best" standard is more appropriate than "gold" standard [6].

It is essential, when analysing the indications, contraindications, complications and other aspects of the liver biopsy, to consider present hepatology and personalized medicine.

Practiced since the late 19th century, liver biopsy remains the criterion standard in the evaluation of the etiology and extent of disease of the liver. Paul Ehrlich performed a percutaneous liver biopsy in Germany in 1883. [7]. Since then, this method has been improved with the introduction of different needle types for cutting and aspiration. But, until the 1950s, when Menghini developed an aspiration technique which led to a wider use of the procedure and broadened its applications, it was not common. While in the early 1960 and 1970s the liver biopsy was used for making a diagnosis in cases of suspected medical liver disease, today it is more often performed to assess the prognosis or evaluate therapeutic strategies [1].

With regards to the technique used to carry out the liver biopsy there has also been a major change, it used to be performed blindly by clinicians, specialists in gastroenterology or hepatology at the patient's bed whereas at present, percutaneous biopsies are performed primarily by radiologists.

Currently, a liver biopsy can be obtained either transvenously or transcutaneously, or by combining imaging modalities such as ultrasound, computed tomography, and laparoscopy. The choice of one technique over another is based on availability, personal preference, and the clinical situation.

Liver biopsy techniques: Percutaneous, transjugular or laparoscopic

- Percutaneous liver biopsy can be transthoracic, with an intercostal liver access or subcostal, when the patient has an enlarged liver extending below the costal margin. Clinicians have now discarded blind liver biopsies in favour of ultrasound-guided biopsies.
- Transjugular or transvenous liver biopsy was first described in 1964. It is a technique used in order to avoid percutaneous liver biopsy in patients who are at a higher risk of bleeding. However, it has its limitations and is considered an inferior biopsy due to the fragmentation of the obtained specimen, which may reduce the accuracy of the diagnosis. It is performed in a vascular catheterisation laboratory by a radiologist with special training in interventional radiology. Videofluoroscopy equipment and cardiac monitoring are mandatory due to the risk of cardiac arrhythmia as the catheter passes through the right atrium. With this method, hepatic venography, wedged hepatic venous pressure, caval pressure and atrial pressure measurements can also be obtained during the procedure. The most frequent indications for the transjugular route are: severe coagulopathy, ascites, obesity, suspected vascular tumour or peliosis hepatis.
- Laparoscopic liver biopsy. This technique is well established and its use varies between centers. It is indicated in centers where access to transvenous liver biopsy is not available, and in patients with focal liver lesions and coagulopathy for whom obtaining histology is essential for their management.

The decision to use a particular technique is based on the risk profile of the patient. If he or she has advanced liver failure with coagulopathy and ascites, liver biopsy is unnecessary, but the diagnosis of the underlying disease is crucial in specific circumstances in order to determine a therapy, for example in cases of liver transplant. Before a liver biopsy it is necessary to carry out an ultrasound to quantify vascular permeability and because it may rule out anatomical abnormalities and can identify mass lesions that are clinically silent. When cirrhosis is suspected on clinical grounds, or by non-invasive methods liver biopsy is usually avoided.

2. Contraindications to percutaneous liver biopsy

Absolute contraindications: the main contraindication to percutaneous liver biopsy is significant coagulopathy, others are: uncooperative patient, history of unexplained bleed-

http://dx.doi.org/10.5772/53120

ing, prothrombin time 3–5 seconds more than control, platelet count less than 50,000/ mm^3, the use of a non-steroidal anti-inflammatory drugs, (unless discontinued 7 to 10 days previously), blood for transfusion unavailable, suspected hemangioma, another vascular tumor or echinococcal cysts in the liver, and the inability to identify an appropriate site for biopsy.

Relative contraindications: Morbid obesity, ascites, hemophilia, infection in the right pleural cavity or below the right hemidiaphragm.

Accepted indications: Given the new developments that have proved the efficacy of liver biopsy, its role in the management of patients with chronic liver diseases has much evolved in recent years and will continue to evolve as new non invasive technologies are developed.

• Diagnosis
1. Many parenchimal liver diseases 2. Abnormal liver tests 3. Fever of unknown origin 4. Focal or diffuse abnormalities on imaging studies
• Prognosis-Staging of known parenchimal disease
• Management –Developing treatment plans based on histologic analysis
Contraindications for percutaneous liver biopsy
• Absolute: uncooperative patient, severe coagulopathy, infection of the hepatic bed, extrahepatic biliary obstruction.
• Relative: ascites, morbid obesity, possible vascular lesions, amyloidosis, hydatid disease.

Table 1. Indications and contraindications for liver biopsy

Its importance in diagnosis, staging and prognosis largely depends on the indication and the clinical question relying on an answer from the histological result.

2.1. Is liver biopsy always necessary?

The utility of routine liver biopsy has been the subject of debate in recent years. Due to liver biopsy being associated with a small but definite risk, a biopsy should only be performed when the findings contribute to a better management of the patient. It is argued that for the purposes of management, liver biopsy is neither needed in cases with advanced fibrosis nor those diagnosed with cirrhosis by other methods, nor in patients with mild disease, for whom a therapeutic decision is not urgent. Until recently, liver biopsy played a key role in the evaluation of chronic liver disease, but now in the presence of better diagnostic tests on disease etiologies and treatments its role has to be re-evaluated. Recognition and confirmation of the pattern of injury (chronic hepatitic, chronic cholestatic, steatohepatitic, etc.) is the pathologist's priority when evaluating the liver biopsy.

Moreover, liver biopsy provides information on the severity and distribution of lesions (codified in the staging and grading of chronic liver disease), the presence of confounding patterns of injury (such as steatohepatitis coexisting with chronic viral hepatitis), and the presence of additional findings such as steatosis or iron accumulation that may have prognostic or therapeutic relevance.

2.2. Who should be biopsied?

As a rule patients with standard clinical and radiological features are not biopsied. However, in the presence of non concordant or atypical results, a biopsy may be recommended. The decision whether to perform a liver biopsy in some patients is clear, however in cases with a suspected concomitant diagnosis or when results from other methods are non conclusive confirmation is needed [8,9].

Type of Injury	Causes
Fatty change	Ethanol, fatty liver disease, obesity, diabetes, drugs
Councilman bodies	Viral hepatitis, drugs, toxins, ischemia (acidophilic bodies)
Mallory bodies * (hyaline) (see pages: 13, 15, 17 and 18)	Ethanol, obesity, diabetes, drugs, Wilson disease, biliary tract disease, hepatocellular carcinoma
Hydropic change (ballooning degeneration)	Viral hepatitis, drugs, cholestasis, fatty liver disease
Cholestasis	Duct obstruction or injury, drugs, viral hepatitis
Interlobular duct injury	Primary biliary cirrhosis, primary sclerosing cholangitis, hepatitis C
Piecemeal necrosis	Viral hepatitis, primary biliary cirrhosis, drugs, Wilson disease
Increased iron stores	Hemochromatosis, transfusions, hemolysis
Granulomas** (see pages: 19, 20 and 21)	Sarcoid, infections (tuberculosis, fungi), drugs

Table 2. Patterns of liver cell injury found in liver biopsies and clinical differential diagnosis

3. The generally accepted indications of liver biopsy are the following

- Diagnosis for a better scoring of grading and staging of chronic viral hepatitis C or hepatitis B, alcoholic liver disease, non-alcoholic steato-hepatitis, or autoimmune hepatitis.
- In patients with raised ferritine for the diagnosis of hemochromatosis
- If there are suspected disorders of cupper metabolism for the diagnosis of Wilson's disease, with quantitative estimation of copper in liver tissue.
- Evaluation of possible autoimmune hepatitis

- In cholestatic liver diseases: primary biliary cirrhosis, primary sclerosing cholangitis and overlap syndromes.
- Evaluation of abnormal results of biochemical tests of the liver in association with a serologic workup that is negative or inconclusive
- Evaluation of the efficacy or the adverse effects of treatment regimens (e.g.,methotrexate therapy for psoriasis).
- Alcohol related disease. Non-alcoholic fatty liver disease (NAFLD) or Non-alcoholic steatohepatitis (NASH).
- Diagnosis of a liver mass, in selected cases, when image tests are inconclusive.
- Evaluation of fever of unknown origin, with an eventual culture of liver tissue.
- Evaluation of the status of the liver post transplantation or of the donor liver pre transplantation.

4. Methods: How to handle a liver biopsy

Liver samples should be fixed in 10% neutral buffered formalin because this enables all routine histochemical and immunohistochemical staining to be carried out. A small portion of the sample could be snap-frozen for adjunctive molecular studies for diagnostic or research purposes, particularly when multiple etiologies are clinically suspected.

As for stains, a good collagen stain to assess fibrosis is mandatory. Perls' stain for iron is recommended and the Periodic Acid-Schiff (PAS) stain with and without diastase digestion is useful for assessing hepatocyte cytoplasm glucogen content.

Special stains for special circumstances are ordered if indicated by the clinical situation. For instance, the Ziehl-Nielsen is ordered for mycobacteria, and Grocott's silver methanamine stain is used when granulomas are observed or when fungi infection is suspected. The Congo Red stain is requested when amyloid is suspected to be present Rhodamine stain, Victoria blue or orcein stain is used to detect copper deposition when there is clinical suspicion of Wilson's disease. Immunohistochemistry is used to confirm the presence of Hepatitis B surface antigen and Hepatitis B core antigen [10].

Cultures could be indicated in selected cases such as Mycobacterias [11].

5. Histologic diagnosis and clinical correlation

The pathological report that used to be too descriptive now has to include etiology, aspects related to prognosis and possible therapy [12,13].

In order to promote the clinico-pathological diagnostic correlation with the intention of improving communication and clarifying individual cases, regular meetings between clinicians and pathologists are necessary. It is not only important to hold formal conferences but also to increase daily exchanges. To facilitate the communication between pathologists, radiologists, surgeons and clinicians it is desirable, when feasible, for the same teams to work together.

6. Writing the histology report

In order to produce a clinically relevant liver histology report pathologists should follow the internationally accepted guidelines.

1. The adequacy of the biopsy should be assessed by measuring the length of the specimen and counting the number of portal tracts. The data should be written up in the final report to make clinicians aware of any potential sampling error in the grading and staging. To reduce sampling error the amount of tissue required is usually 1 to 4 cm long and needs to include at least four portal tracts.

2. The type and severity of necroinflammation and fibrosis should be described in words. By only using numbers to report the presence or not of bridging necrosis for example, some clinically useful information might be omitted. A validated scoring system should be used for grade of activity and stage of fibrosis.

3. As well as being described, the existence of adjunt data should be scored subjectively, such as steatosis graded on a scale of 0-3 and siderosis graded on a scale of 0-4.

4. Other diagnostic criteria may be useful in differential diagnoses:

   - Differentiating viral hepatitis from other chronic disorders, such as cell dysplasia and thus separately reporting the presence of cell changes.

   - Using immunostaining when appropriate, for example Hepatitis B Virus antigens [14].

   - Searching for any concomitant diseases.

5. Chronic viral hepatitis, primary biliary cirrhosis and autoimmune hepatitis have typical histological lesions and it is advisable to consider the characteristics of: portal tract inflammation, interface hepatitis, lobular necrosis and bile duct damage, separately [15].

6. Concomitant histological features in liver specimens of hepatitis C cases: auto-immunity, co-infections, steatosis, hemosiderosis, malignancy –related changes, hepatitis due to drugs and/or vascular problems. Furthermore, biopsy frequently detects associated lesions such as steatosis or steatohepatitis providing information related to management and prognosis of patients with chronic hepatitis C.

7. Finally the conclusions should be written in order to make the histological diagnosis, stating whether the pathological findings are consistent with chronic hepatitis or not, whether a specific viral etiology may be suspected or whether there are changes related to concomitant diseases, specifying which.

http://dx.doi.org/10.5772/53120

	Chronic viral hepatitis	Primary Biliary Cirrhosis (PBC)	Autoimmune Hepatitis
Portal tract inflammation	Mononuclear cells	Mononuclear cells; eosinophils	Mononuclear cells; plasma cells
Interface hepatitis	Common	Common;ductular reaction (i.e. biliary piecemeal necrosis)	Present
Lobular necrosis	Variable degree usually focal	Variable; usually mild and focal	Severe, may be confluent
Bile duct damage	Common in hepatitis C (usually mild)	Duct destruction present	May be present

Table 3. Specific features in liver biopsy differential diagnosis and pathological findings

7. Use of liver biopsy in clinical practice

Here we will discuss some of the most prominent findings of liver biopsy in the following clinical settings:

a. Viral Hepatitis : Hepatitis B, Hepatitis C.

b. Metabolic diseases: Hemochromatosis, Porphyria, Wilson disease, Alpha 1- anti-trypsin disease.

c. Autoimmune and cholestatic diseases: Auto-Immune Hepatitis, Primary Biliary Cirrhosis (PBC), Primary Sclerosing Cholangitis (PSC), Overlap Syndrome.

d. Alcoholic liver disease

e. Non-alcoholic Fatty Liver Diseases and Non-Alcoholic Steato-Hepatitis (NAFLD and NASH). Liver steatosis.

f. Drug-Induced Liver Injury (DILI).

g. Infections and pyrexia of unknown origin.

h. Cirrhosis. Fibrosis progression.

i. Hepatocellular Carcinoma (HCC) and other benign or malignant focal lesions. The role of the fine neddle aspiration biopsy (FNAB) and other imaging diagnostic tools.

j. New evolving fields for liver biopsy: Liver transplantation and living donors. Bone marrow transplantation. Morbid obesity

7.1. Chronic viral hepatitis C and B

In the past the majority of liver biopsies were performed in chronic hepatitis C patients. However, recently this has changed, due to a better understanding of the etiology, pathogenesis, the natural history of the disease and available therapies.

As the ability to treat hepatitis C effectively improves, the value of information gained from a liver biopsy decreases. The most effective therapy currently available, a combination of pegylated interferon α and ribavirin, can induce sustained viral clearance, implying a definitive cure and improved long term prognosis. This occurs, after anti-viral treatment in up to 80% of patients infected with genotypes 2 and 3. In patients with genotype 1 receiving recently approved telaprevir and boceprevir, triple therapy constituents, an average of 70-75% can achieve sustained viral clearance. Due to the high percentage of positive response in persons with genotypes 2 and 3, the need for a liver biopsy in such cases has been questioned.

The terminology used to assess the appearance of liver biopsies with chronic viral hepatitis has also evolved.

The first classification of chronic hepatitis based on histological criteria was published in 1968. At that time, only three diseases causing chronic hepatitis could be diagnosed, hepatitis B, non A-non B (hepatitis C, since 1989) and autoimmune hepatitis. This classification which also had prognostic implications only had two categories, namely "chronic persistent hepatitis" and "chronic active hepatitis". Three years later, the term chronic lobular hepatitis was added to represent findings similar to those observed in acute hepatitis.

During the 1990s, there were great changes in the understanding of chronic viral hepatitis by pathologists and hepatologists. The new concepts recognized that the traditional categorization of pathologic changes (chronic persistent hepatitis, chronic lobular hepatitis, and chronic active hepatitis) was inadequate for assessing histological changes during clinical trials. Pathologic processes were separated rather than considered as part of a continuum of pathologic changes that occur in chronic hepatitis C. Pathologists introduced the idea of staging for fibrosis and grading for the inflammatory component to the pathological evaluation of chronic hepatitis C.

7.1.1. Grading and staging of chronic hepatitis C Scoring Systems (Table 4) [16-20]

Grading is the assessment of the activity of a disease, which may increase and decrease as a disease flares and subsides, or may remain static throughout the disease.

Grade and stage evaluation is a standard part of the pathologic assessment of liver biopsies in chronic hepatitis. Pathological staging has focused on the assessment of fibrosis as the best surrogate marker of the disease process. Staging divides the fibrotic continuum into discrete categories and all of the existing staging systems have cirrhosis as their highest stage. Several systems exist for grading and staging of chronic hepatitis and all have been used effectively to assess changes in pathology following therapeutic intervention. These systems include the methods of Scheuer, Desmet, Batts and Ludwig,and the METAVIR system used to score individual features of inflammation and fibrosis semi-quantitatively in clinical studies [14-20].

Steatosis and Steatohepatitis in chronic hepatitis C Steatosis in hepatitis C is mainly macrovesicular and a common finding in genotype 3 [21] it is also related to a high body mass index and older age. More recently, steatosis has been recognized as a feature worthy of study, from an etiologic standpoint and especially in terms of its clinical significance. Estimation of the degree of steatosis has been hampered by the lack of standard definitions and

http://dx.doi.org/10.5772/53120

breakpoints between grades. Although the intrinsic mechanism and involved factors for accelerated fibrosis are unclear, steatosis has been associated with increased inflammation, hepatocellular apoptosis and the presence of perisinusoidal fibrosis [22].

Utility of biopsy in hepatitis C. Nowadays, the majority of Hepatitis C patients can be managed without having to undergo a liver biopsy since liver biopsy rarely identifies unsuspected etiology and hepatitis C diagnosis relies on blood antibody and HCV RNA determinations. However, a biopsy allows to identify patients most in need of therapy or to find clinically unsuspected cirrhosis, which when found it is necessary to screen for varices and hepatocellular carcinoma.

Moreover clinical and laboratory surrogates for biopsy may be useful in identifying cirrhosis and biopsy is not necessary if clinical, image and analytical data concur. Post-treatment biopsy is not needed, nevertheless a new liver biopsy, could be performed if new treatments or clinical trials arrive in order to stratify patients by prognosis.

Fibrosis stage	Knodell et al. 1981 [16]	Scheuer, 1991 [17]	METAVIR, 1994 [18]	Batts and Ludwig, 1995 [19]	Ishak et al. 1995 [20]
0	No Fibrosis	No Fibrosis	No Fibrosis	No Fibrosis	No Fibrosis
1	Fibrous portal expansion	Enlarged fibrotic portal tracts		Portal fibrosis	Fibrous expansion of some portal areas, with or without short fibrous septa
2		Periportal or portal-portal septa but intact architecture	Enlargement of portal tracts	Periportal fibrosis	Fibrous expansion of most portal areas, with or without short septa
3	Bridging Fibrosis (portal-portal or portal-central linkage	Fibrosis with architectural distortion but no obvious cirrhosis		Septal fibrosis	Fibrous expansion of most portal areas with occasional portal to portal bridging
4	Cirrhosis	Probable or definite cirrhosis		Cirrhosis	Fibrous expansion of portal areas with marked bridging (portal to portal as well as portal to central)
5					Marked bridging with occasional nodules (incomplete cirrhosis)
6					Cirrhosis probable or definite

Table 4. Comparison of commonly used scoring systems for fibrosis staging in chronic Hepatitis C

7.1.2. Natural history

The degree of inflammation, fibrosis stage, and steatosis seen on liver biopsy are key histological predictors of progression to cirrhosis. (Table 5) (see page 28).

Based on retrospective data, it has been shown that most patients with moderate inflammation on initial liver biopsy developed cirrhosis after 20 years, and nearly all patients with severe inflammation or bridging fibrosis developed cirrhosis in 10 years. Patients with mild inflammation and/or minimal fibrosis have a low risk of progression to cirrhosis. Hepatic steatosis is also an emerging risk factor for fibrosis progression in hepatitis C [22]. Clinical information may help to refine prognosis, but cannot substitute the valuable information obtained from a liver biopsy. Poynard's group showed three clinical factors which are independently associated with faster progression of fibrosis: male, aged over 40 at the time of infection, and having a daily alcohol consumption of 50 grams or more [23]. Other factors predicting progression to cirrhosis include immunosuppression and co-infection with hepatitis B or HIV [24].

Utility of biopsy in hepatitis B Liver biopsy is not mandatory but may show moderate or severe inflammation which is why before starting antivirals, usually for a long period, our protocol is to perform a liver biopsy and to individualize the therapeutic decision [25]. It has been proved that long-term therapy may improve histology but the role of serial liver biopsies has yet to be established outside of clinical trials. Fibroscan has yet to be validated for patients with chronic hepatitis B but research on this is ongoing [26].

It is important to identify cirrhosis to indicate anti-hepatitis B therapy and hepatocellular carcinoma screening is also recommended for all hepatitis B surface antigen-positive (HBsAg+) patients, cirrhotic or not. New guidelines on anti-HBV treatment say that it is advisable to treat patients with elevated DNA-HBV and minimally elevated or fluctuating alanine aminotransferase (ALT), [27, 28].

Features typical of chronic viral hepatitis inflammation, like fibrosis, is considered to be one of the key characteristics of chronic viral hepatitis. It is a chronic necroinflammatory process in which hepatocytes are preferentially injured compared with bile ducts. The grade of inflammation is a stratification of the overall necroinflammatory changes into mild, moderate, and marked categories. Unlike the fibrosis systems, which are based on distinctive architectural changes that can be highlighted with special stains, assessment of inflammation is more subjective and hence shows more interobserver variations. Usually varying degrees of portal and periportal inflammation(with lymphocytes, plasma cells, and macrophages), lobulillar hepatitis, and fibrosis are to be individually considered and scored.

Interface hepatitis occurs when the inflammatory infiltrate crosses the limiting plate; it is usually associated with local hepatocyte damage, piecemeal necrosis, and inflammation.

Lobular inflammation is accompanied by some hepatocellular necrosis (acidophilic or Councilman bodies). Chronic hepatitis leads to progressive fibrosis and, without treatment, to cirrhosis. The fibrosis begins in portal areas, extends to periportal areas, bridging also other portal tracts and central veins. Histopathological findings in the liver

http://dx.doi.org/10.5772/53120

biopsy that help to predict etiology chronic hepatitis B may show some of the changes described previously, as well as a ground-glass change to the cell cytoplasm. This change reflects accumulation of hepatitis B surface antigen within the endoplasmic reticulum of the hepatocytes [29].

Chronic hepatitis C may be associated with prominent lymphoid aggregates within portal tracts, sometimes including germinal centers and, occasionally, bile duct damage, although not to the degree seen in line primary biliary disorders. In addition, biopsies may show focal, nonzonal macrovesicular steatosis [30].

Patterns of liver cell injury found in liver biopsy and differential diagnosis. Chronic viral hepatitis have no unique histopathologic features, it is therefore necessary to consider various causes. In addition to viral infection, chronic hepatitis may be autoimmune or drug related. Histological features of chronic cholestatic disease, including PBC, primary sclerosing cholangitis (PSC), autoimmune cholangitis, as well as metabolic diseases including Wilson disease and α_1-antitrypsin deficiency, may overlap with some of the findings with "so called" chronic hepatitis.

7.2. Metabolic liver diseases

Many rare diseases originate in the liver, either affecting the liver directly or causing extrahepatic disease [31]. For example, liver histology is usually normal in primary hyperoxaluria while the kidneys and other organs may be irreparably damaged; however, cure is only possible with a liver transplant. In other inherited disorders, the liver disease may remain asymptomatic until precipitous acute liver failure develops; the classic example is Wilson disease. Here we present the diseases most frequently observed in adult patients.

7.2.1. Hematochromatosis: The role of liver biopsy in the diagnosis of hepatic iron overload in the era of genetic testing [32]

Hemochromatosis is an autosomal recessive disorder that leads to massive deposits of iron in many organs, including liver, pancreas, heart, joints, and skin. The gene responsible for hereditary hemochromatosis, HFE, is located on chromosome 6. The two most common mutations are C282Y (present in up to 80% of cases) and H63D. The defining characteristic of this disease is the failure to prevent unneeded iron from entering the circulatory pool as a result of genetic changes compromising the synthesis or activity of hepcidin, the iron hormone.Hemochromatosis results from the interaction between genetic and acquired factors. Depending on the underlying mutation, the coinheritance of modifier genes, the presence of nongenetic hepcidin inhibitors, and other host-related factors, clinical manifestation may vary from simple biochemical abnormalities to severe multiorgan disease [33]. The indication of a liver biopsy in the era of genetic testing is being questioned. But, in our opinion, liver biopsy continues to play an important role in the diagnosis, prognosis and management of patients with elevated serum ferritin and abnormal liver function test results in general hepatology practice. Genetic tests for HFE mutations (C282Y, H63D) and liver biopsies are complementary in the workup of these patients.

Liver biopsy allows a quantitative iron concentration study and the identification of the grade of hepatic iron overload, localization pattern and associated liver pathology for diagnosis and management of patients [34].

Liver biopsies may be relatively normal or show bridging fibrosis or even micronodular cirrhosis. Untreated, hemochromatosis leads to the development of micronodular cirrhosis. Prior to the availability of genetic testing, the diagnosis of hemochromatosis was always determined with liver biopsy and quantitation of tissue iron. With the availability of genetic testing for the C282Y and/or H63D mutations, liver biopsy is more often reserved for evaluation of clinical status or complications (i.e. degree of fibrosis, development of hepatocellular carcinoma) rather than for primary diagnosis [35]. A biopsy can also help determine if other disease processes are present, such as hepatitis C or fatty liver disease [36].

We suggest that patients with suspected hemochromatosis undergo genetic testing for the C282Y and H63D mutations, especially if they have a family history of hemochromatosis,in order to establish the genotype of the patient and permit genetic counseling. A liver biopsy may not be necessary in young C282Y homozygotes or in heterozygotes without evidence of liver disease.

Disorders that have to be considered in the clinical differential diagnosis of hemochromatosis

The list of disorders associated with increased hepatic iron is long. The majority of patients with hepatic iron accumulation from any cause do not have hepatic iron concentration (HIC) that is above the upper limit of normal (approximately 1100 mg/μg dry liver weight). Furthermore the pattern of distribution of the iron in the liver may be of some help in establishing the diagnosis [37]:

- predominantly hepatocellular distribution of iron leads to a diagnosis of genetic hemochromatosis, alcoholic liver disease and/or porphyria cutanea tarda.
- predominant presence of iron in Kupffer cells, may be the result of multiple transfusions and/or hemolytic anemias.
- a mixed distribution of iron may be a sign of megaloblastic anemia or anemia secondary to chronic infection.

7.2.2. Porphyria Cutanea Tarda (PCT)

It is the most common form of porphyria across the world. PCT is usually an acquired liver disease caused by exogenous factors, such as excess alcohol intake, iron overload, chronic hepatitis C and oestrogen therapy.

The pathogenesis of PCT is varied; it may be hereditary or acquired, leading to hepatic iron loading and to an increase of oxidative stress. Iron loading is usually only mild or moderate in degree. However, in patients with excessive alcohol intake and/or chronic hepatitis C infection, hepcidin production by hepatocytes decreases. This decrease is responsible for increased iron absorption from the gut. The important role that PCT often plays in the hepatitis C virus setting has recently been emphasized [38].

7.2.3. *The role of liver biopsy in determining the diagnosis of Wilson disease*

Wilson disease is an autosomal recessive disorder of copper metabolism, characterized by excessive accumulation of copper in the liver and other organs. Genetic evaluation is difficult because most patients are compound heterozygotes. For patients with Wilson disease the norm is to perform a liver biopsy with a quantitative copper testing of the liver; levels are typically greater than 250 mg/g dry weight liver (normal level, 38 mg/g) [39].When the diagnosis of Wilson disease is considered prior to liver biopsy other tests are undertaken. - Serum ceruloplasmin (less than 20 mg/dL in patients with Wilson disease; normal levels, 23 to 50 mg/dL). - 24-hour urinary copper (greater than 100 mg/dL; normal, less than 30 mg/dL). -Kayser-Flescher ring has to be studied by ophthalmologic testing. The liver biopsy in this disease can present differently, depending on the patient's age. In children and young adolescents, the most common finding may be fatty change. In older adolescents and young adults, a liver biopsy may show chronic hepatitis with piecemeal necrosis. Adults tend to show cirrhosis, and Mallory bodies*. In adolescents or adults, confluent necrosis may lead to a severe hepatic failure that may require an urgent liver transplant [40].

7.2.4. *Alfa$_1$ -antitrypsin (A_1-AT) deficiency on liver biopsy*

A_1-AT is the major circulating inhibitor of serine proteases (Pi). Its primary target is the potent elastase found in polymorphonuclear cells (PMNs). It is a glycoprotein synthesized in the liver. Many of the Pi variants are associated with fairly normal serum concentrations and function and thus are of little clinical significance. However, a few, result in low circulating levels of α1-AT (i.e., PiZZ) and are of pathologic significance. Liver biopsies from affected patients demonstrate classic PAS-positive, diastase-resistant globules within periportal hepatocytes. Portal fibrosis and chronic hepatitis may also be present. Liver cell dysplasia may be seen, and patients older than 50, especially men, are at risk of developing hepatocellular carcinoma. The presence of PAS-positive, diastase-resistant globules is not always diagnostic for A1-AT deficiency because various inflammatory conditions may be associated with overproduction of the enzyme, as is the case in cardiac congestion or hypoxia. For this reason clinical correlation is required [41].

7.3. Autoimmune Hepatitis (AIH)

Autoimmune hepatitis (AIH) is an inflammatory condition of the liver that can affect patients of all ages, sexes, and races [42].

Timely diagnosis and immunosuppressive therapy may control disease activity in almost all affected patients and various case series have reported near normal or normal life expectancy in patients diagnosed and treated adequately [43]. Untreated AIH, however, has 5-year mortality above 50%.

It was first described as a form of chronic hepatitis in young women, showing jaundice, elevated gammaglobulins and amenorrhea, which eventually leads to cirrhosis. There is not a single test to diagnose AIH but a set of diagnostic criteria has been suggested in order to classify patients as having probable or definite AIH depending on a score.

Clinical appearance ranges from an absence of symptoms to a severe fulminant presentation. It is usually clinically associated with other autoimmune diseases such as rheumatoid arthritis, ulcerative colitis, autoimmune thyroiditis, or diabetes mellitus. A family history has been reported [44].

A liver biopsy should be obtained at first diagnosis before therapy for grading, staging and confirmation of the diagnosis. Histological appearance is not characteristic, although typical features such as periportal hepatitis with lymphocytic infiltrates, plasma cells and piecemeal necrosis, with more advanced disease bridging necrosis, are frequent. Variable degrees of portal fibrosis are present [45]. In non treated patients or in non-responsive to corticosteroid therapy cirrhosis eventually occurs.

Differential diagnosis which has been revisited recently by the International Autoimmune Hepatitis Group comprises: chronic hepatitis not caused by other etiologies (viral, drug-induced), acute hepatitis alone or acute hepatitis superimposed on underlying chronic liver disease and autoimmune diseases with associated duct damage and duct loss [47].

Early diagnosis may be difficult because the clinical picture is heterogeneous and the liver histology sometimes shows atypical features.

A simple and accurate diagnostic scoring system for AIH has been established but not totally validated yet. In 1993, the International Autoimmune Hepatitis Group (IAIHG) proposed specific diagnostic criteria, which were revised in 1999. These criteria were made by expert consensus and introduced to allow comparison of studies from different centers [46]. Some of the items were of questionable value which is why in 2008 the IAIHG published a new simplified scoring system for wider applicability in routine clinical practice, based on the data of patients with well-established diagnoses and validated in another group of patients [47].The new score includes autoantibodies, immunoglobulin G, histology, and exclusion of viral hepatitis, allowing a reliable diagnosis of AIH applying simple scores.

7.3.1. Primary Biliary Cirrhosis (PBC)

PBC is a chronic progressive cholestatic liver disease that occurs in middle-aged patients, usually women, and is often associated with other autoimmune diseases. Patients may present with jaundice and pruritus in advanced cases. Laboratory testing reveals serum anti–mitochondrial antibody (AMA) as well as increased alkaline phosphatase, bilirubin, and γ-glutamyl transpeptidase [48]. The histological staging of PBC considers the degree of bile duct damage and fibrosis [49].

- **Stage 1** early disease is characterized by damage to septal and larger interlobular bile ducts, reflected by biliary epithelial damage with infiltration of the duct by lymphocytes, plasma cells, eosinophils, and rare polymorphs. The inflammatory infiltrate confined within the portal tract, may include granulomas and lymphoid follicles (florid duct lesion).

- **Stage 2** the inflammatory process extends beyond the portal tract, and changes of interface hepatitis (piecemeal necrosis) may be seen. Bile ducts begin to disappear and proliferation of bile ductules (cholangioles) may also be present along the edges of the portal tracts. These changes are associated with features of chronic cholestasis, including feathery degeneration within the cytoplasm of hepatocytes, accumulation of bile pigment, periportal accumulation of copper (not generalized as in Wilson disease), and, occasionally, Mallory bodies*.

- **Stage 3** is associated with increasing fibrosis and bridging between portal areas, with decreased amounts of inflammation.

- **Stage 4** represents biliary cirrhosis, usually micronodular. In the past the diagnosis was done in very advanced disease, biliary cirrhosis, hence its name.

7.3.2. Primary Sclerosing Cholangitis (PSC)

Primary sclerosing cholangitis (PSC) is a disease with a variable clinical course, with obliteration of the biliary tree that leads to biliary cirrhosis and its complications such as portal hypertension and liver failure. The term "primary" is used to distinguish this condition from the bile duct strictures that are secondary to bile duct injury, cholelithiasis or ischaemia [50].

Patients may present with increased alkaline phosphatase and positive perinuclear antineutrophil cytoplasmic antibodies (pANCAs). In this disease, liver biopsy does not have a crucial role in the diagnosis. Ultrasound is used for the initial investigation and may show bile duct dilatation and liver and splenic changes; however, it is unspecific for PSC. [51,52]. The classic lesion of PSC in the histological study is onionskin or concentric periductular fibrosis, with damage to the ductal epithelium, but it is rarely seen on percutaneous biopsy. The most common findings on a biopsy in early-stage disease are nonspecific [46], fibrosis with inflammation of portal tracts and paucity of normal bile ducts. In addition, in patients with extrahepatic obstruction, proliferation and dilatation of interlobular ducts and an increased number of periportal PMNs can be observed. Endoscopic retrograde cholangiopancreatography (ERCP) is the next choice test for diagnosis, but it is invasive, for this reason its role is under debate [53]. Transhepatic cholangiography can be used if ERCP is unsuccessful, but again is invasive. Non-invasive alternatives to ERCP are: magnetic resonance cholangiopancreatography (MRCP), which is increasingly used and is useful for excluding other disease and evaluating the biliary system [54]. Transient elastography (FibroScan®) has potential as a non-invasive method for detection of cirrhosis in patients with more advanced liver disease [55].

PSC shares many clinical biochemical and pathologic features with primary biliary cirrhosis, although PSC, can affect both intrahepatic and extrahepatic ducts. PSC is strongly associated with inflammatory bowel disease, particularly ulcerative colitis. Due to its major morbidity and mortality the diagnosis has to be confirmed. At the time of diagnosis, PSC typically involves both intra and extrahepatic bile ducts in the majority of cases. The most dismal sequel of PSC is the development of colangio carcinoma (CC) in 14% of patients (which may not be demonstrable radiographically with the usual diagnostic methods) [56].

A wide spectrum of disease severity exists, ranging from patients who present with advanced liver disease requiring liver transplantation within a short time to those who remain asymptomatic for decades. The natural course of PSC is determined by interindividual variability, the rate of progression and the development of CC, which can occur at any time.

The differential diagnosis has to be established among : autoimmune hepatitis, overlap syndromes, infectious hepatitis, other bile duct diseases presenting as acute or chronic cholangitis, and biliary strictures, cholangiocarcinoma, gallstones, hepatomegaly and primary biliary cirrhosis.

Liver biopsy in PSC is only needed to diagnose small-duct PSC or to exclude other diseases that may be associated with PSC or with similar features and confounding aspects. Liver biopsy also may be useful for staging the disease. However, serial liver biopsy in monitoring the disease is not indicated [57].

Recently some authors have developed the Mayo clinic risk score, a multivariate statistical survival model, on the basis of the long-term course of the disease in 486 PSC patients seen at three centers in United States. In this score, the need for liver biopsy has been eliminated. This scoring system has its advantages; it is non-invasive and was found to be well correlated to actual survival. It also performs better than the Child-Pugh classification for cirrhosis, which does not predict survival with PSC [58].

7.3.3. Autoimmune Hepatitis (AIH) with overlap variants

Overlap syndromes of AIH are not uncommon but are not well defined. Histology, clinical and serological indicators imply more than one liver disease at the same time.

The diagnosis of an overlap syndrome relies on the biochemical profile, either cholestatic or hepatitic in addition to the auto-antibodies pattern and elevated gamma globulins. The histopathology can show portal inflammation with or without involvement of bile ducts [59].

In adult patients with an overlap of PBC and AIH, which is the the most common, antinuclear as well as antimitochondrial antibodies are present. Chronic hepatitis C may trigger autoimmune activation, with concomitant positive autoimmune antibodies. AIH may be associated with Ig G4 autoimmune cholangitis (IAC). In contrast to PSC, IAC-IgG4, has no associated intestinal bowel disease and pancreatitis [60].

The value of a biopsy in liver diseases such as PSC or suspected metastatic disease, which is characterized by a zonal affection of the liver has to be dealt with individually and completed with other imaging techniques.

Liver biopsy is advisable if diagnostic tests show abnormal liver function results which may be indicative of many etiologies e.g. nonalcoholic steatohepatitis with strongly elevated antinuclear antibodies and abnormal iron studies, or co-infection with HIV and hepatitis C in a patient with abnormal liver function tests taking hepatotoxic drugs etc.

7.4. Alcohol: Fibrous progression related to alcohol injury

Many patients with ethanol injury show initial scarring around central veins with delicate fibrosis along the sinusoids [61]. Eventually, bridging fibrosis connects central veins and portal tracts. When cirrhosis is fully developed, most of the native central veins have been obliterated. Alcoholic cirrhosis is micronodular and the scarring is relatively uniform throughout the liver. With complete alcohol abstinence, the nodules can regenerate to a larger size, but the central veins are decreased in number and the nodules may lack some portal tracts [62].

7.5. Non-Alcoholic Fatty Liver Disease, (NAFLD) and Non-Alcoholic Steatohepatitis, (NASH)

The histological appearance in these disorders may be very similar to the injury related to alcohol. In non-alcoholic steatohepatitis, the liver exhibits fat and perivenular sinusoidal collagen deposition and may be indistinguishable from alcoholic perivenular fibrosis on histological grounds alone. Clinical correlations are basic for its diagnosis [63].

Sometimes a biopsy shows a pattern which looks like alcoholic hepatitis, but the patient denies alcohol use. A differential diagnosis for alcoholic hepatitis has to be done, and non-alcoholic fatty liver disease, (NALDF) and non-alcoholic steatohepatitis, (NASH) should be considered [63].

For many decades, typical "alcoholic hepatitis" was often diagnosed with liver biopsy, and in some patients' medical records were completed with somewhat judgmental comments about their persistent denial of alcohol intake. Now, there are other known causes for Mallory bodies (*) and steatosis found in liver biopsies which, in the past, were classified as alcohol related liver injury. In retrospect, we now know that many patients with "alcoholic hepatitis" were treated unfairly [64].

It is clear that similar patterns of injury can be seen in non-alcoholics, especially in the setting of diabetes and obesity, referred to as nonalcoholic steatohepatitis (NASH) or nonalcoholic fatty liver disease (NAFLD). This represents a significant form of chronic liver disease in both adults and children, with a spectrum ranging from indolent to end-stage liver disease. It may be an underlying cause of cryptogenic cirrhosis and has been reported to recur after a liver transplant. Other conditions associated with NASH include acute starvation, accelerated weight loss, intestinal bypass, disorders of lipid metabolism, and various drugs. Careful clinicopathologic correlation is required to determine the cause. Liver biopsy evaluation allows us to establish the degree of steatosis, inflammation, and fibrosis stage [65].

Liver steatosis

The diagnosis of liver steatosis has several implications in chronic liver diseases.

- Liver steatosis is associated with liver fibrosis progression and a decreased rate of sustained viral response in chronic hepatitis C.
- Donor liver macrovesicular steatosis is independently associated with graft failure at one year after liver transplantation.
- After major hepatic resection, liver steatosis induces an increased risk of post-operative complications and elevated risk of death.

- Finally, liver steatosis is the main lesion observed in non-alcoholic fatty liver disease (NAFLD) which, as a consequence of the worldwide burden of visceral obesity, is now an important cause of chronic liver disease in western countries.

At present, the histological examination of a liver biopsy continues to be the reference for evaluating liver steatosis despite its limitations. The procedure is invasive and impaired by sampling bias, which results in imperfect reproducibility and only allows for a semi-quantitative grading of steatosis [66]. The non-invasive diagnosis of liver steatosis is done by imaging techniques and blood tests, but diagnostic accuracy remains to be validated and their use in clinical practice has yet to be recommended. Ultrasonography is considered the imaging technique of choice for steatosis screening, but its sensitivity in detecting fatty liver is only 60–94% and is operator dependent. Other techniques, such as computed tomography, proton magnetic resonance spectroscopy and magnetic resonance imaging offer high accuracy for quantification of liver fat but have low availability, high cost and lack standardization [67].

The diagnosis of hepatic steatosis and steatohepatitis or non-alcoholic steatohepatitis (NASH) is not yet possible without liver biopsy. Therapeutic targets of drug development are in early stages. As regards the study of factors most likely associated with disease progression, the National Institute of Diabetes and Digestive and Kidney Diseases (NIDDK) has sponsored the NASH Clinical Research Network (CRN) who has developed a histological scoring system, which is used for clinical trials for NASH [68].

The histological lesions for the diagnosis of NASH are: zone 3 macrosteatosis, hepatocyte ballooning and mixed lobular inflammation. Other findings that are common include mild-moderate portal inflammation, acidophil bodies, glycogenated nuclei, lipogranulomas and perisinusoidal fibrosis. In addition, the following may be present: Mallory's hyaline (*) in hepatocytes, megamitochondria and mild siderosis.

(*) Mallory bodies or Mallory's hyaline are irregular, rope-like eosinophilic intracytoplasmic strings that represent aggregates of cytokeratin filaments. The cytokeratins form a filamentous support network within the hepatocytes. Cellular damage is due, for example, to etanol producing hepatocyte ballooning degeneration, which can cause the keratins to misfold and aggregate. Mallory bodies may be found in alcoholic, nonalcoholic steatohepatitis, and Wilson disease, cholestatic conditions such as primary biliary cirrhosis (PBC) and with certain drugs, such as amiodarone. Although the fat and neutrophils can resolve relatively quickly after alcohol abstinence, hyaline can take up to 6 weeks to disappear [69].

The histological severity of NAFLD is determined by the Non-alcoholic fatty liver disease Activity Score (NAS) and the Fibrosis Score, developed and validated by the CRN [68]. This scoring system is very useful for assessing change in clinical trials but it is not meant to replace a full interpretation of histological findings by a pathologist [70].

Some investigators have observed that there is significant sampling variability and that the histological lesions of NASH are unevenly distributed throughout the liver parenchyma and can lead to substantial misdiagnosis and staging inaccuracies. For example, Ratziu et al. reported that on 51 patients with NAFLD who underwent paired biopsies, the discordance rate for steatosis would have been missed in 24% of cases if only one biopsy had been done and a difference of one stage of fibrosis or more was seen in 41% of paired biopsies [71].

7.6. Liver injury caused by drugs

Drug and toxin induced liver injury is a common cause for abnormal liver tests in humans [72]. Liver injury related to drugs can be subdivided into intrinsic and idiosyncratic injury. Intrinsic injury is produced through direct or indirect mechanisms and idiosyncratic injury may be mediated by hypersensitivity or by metabolic toxic metabolites [73].

Drug induced liver cell injuries have different morphological patterns such as, hepatocellular injury, cholestatic injury, bile duct injury, vascular injury, portal fibrosis, neoplasia or miscellaneous (pigments and inclusions).

The list of implicated products is very long and in some cases mixed lesions can be found. Drug "signature" is a well-known concept which implies that the drugs responsible for the injury can be identified from the different lesions it causes to the liver. For example, diclofenac and minocyline produce a chronic hepatitis pattern, steatohepatitis can be induced by amiodarone and tamoxifen, vascular toxicity may be associated with azathioprine etc. [74].

Histological changes that suggest drug- or toxin-related liver injury are atypical therefore, in some cases, depending on the findings, it is worth the pathologist asking the clinician specific questions in order to do a differential diagnosis and to identify the drug [75]:

Is the patient's blood analysis compatible with hepatitis? Has viral injury been excluded?

- What are the patient's toxic exposures at work, home, or play?
- Has every drug been sought and disclosed?
- Granulomas (**) may also be part of the inflammatory reaction in drug injury [76].

If granulomas have been found, have other causes of granulomas been excluded? (see below) [77]

If significant fatty change is found is there any possibility that it could be related to toxic ethanol injury?

If an abundance of eosinophils is observed in a liver biopsy, a hypersensitivity reaction is suspected which may resemble viral hepatitis. Eosinophils may also be present nonspecifically in viral hepatitis, in connective tissue disorders, and in some neoplasms (usually in Hodgkin's disease infiltrates). However, when eosinophils are a striking feature, it is advisable that the clinician search for a drug, a toxin, or even a nutritional supplement ("natural medicines").

If numerous liver cell mitotic figures show up in the liver biopsy, this may suggest that a short episode of drug exposure is to blame.

7.6.1. Drug Induced Liver Injury (DILI) examples

The American Association of Reumatology has provided guidelines for monitoring patients receiving Methotrexate therapy as there is a known relation between this treatment and hepatotoxicity [78].

A few years ago methotrexate was used for treating reumathoid arthritis. Now patients with psoriasis are also treated with this drug, albeit at a lower dose. Many potentially hepatotoxic medications, used in such cases are worth investigating [78].

Amoxi-clavulanic acid is one of the examples of a broadly used antibiotic which has been implicated in liver toxicity. Typically the patient with this toxicity presents with jaundice. After excluding other causes, such as viral hepatitis, autoimmunity, or other etiologies, and in presence of a normal biliary tree, a liver biopsy is recommended, which may show a cholestatic hepatitis pattern. After discontinuation of the drug the evolution is usually favourable [79].

7.6.2. Granulomas in liver biopsies

Granuloma is defined as an aggregate of histiocytes and can only be diagnosed through histopathological examination.

Causes of granulomas in the liver: most systemic granulomatous diseases involve the liver to some extent; tuberculosis and sarcoidosis are the most common causes [80]. Other infectious agents include bacteria (brucellosis, nocardiosis, tularemia, Q fever [*Coxiella burnetii*], spirochetes), various fungi, protozoa, and viruses (cytomegalovirus, Epstein-Barr virus). Noninfectious causes in addition to sarcoidosis include PBC, drug reaction, extrahepatic inflammatory disease, such as chronic inflammatory bowel disease, rheumatoid arthritis), neoplasms (Hodgkin disease) and foreign substances (talc, mineral oil) .

7.6.3. Can negative stains for fungi and acid-fast bacilli exclude infection in patients with fever of unknown origin?

Definitely not. Cultures for these organisms are more sensitive than special histological stains. If infection is a possibility, a core of liver should be submitted with sterile precautions and without fixative to the microbiology laboratory. In addition, tissue in formalin should be sent to the pathology laboratory for microscopic sections. A tissue sample may also be sent for molecular analysis to determine whether an infectious agent is present, depending on the possibilities [82, 83].

7.6.4. Different types of granulomas useful in determining specific diagnosis

- Epithelioid granulomas are nodular aggregates of plump macrophages, often associated with multinucleated giant cells, lymphocytes, and plasma cells. They are typically seen in sarcoidosis. The presence of central caseating necrosis suggests tuberculosis.
- Fibrin-ring granulomas are formed by a fibrin band encircling a lipid droplet, with associated inflammation. They were first described with Q fever but may also be seen after in-

fection with cytomegalovirus or Epstein-Barr virus as well as with drug (allopurinol) toxicity and in association with systemic lupus erythematosus.

- Lipogranulomas are composed of lipid deposits and vacuolated macrophages. They are formed in the presence of exogenous or endogenous fat accumulation.
- Microgranulomas may be a nonspecific finding, they are usually subtle and composed of small, round clusters of plump Kupffer cells.

There are many causes of hepatic granulomas, including local irritants, infections, infestations and hypersensitivity to drugs. The constituents of these lesions, depending on the etiology and inflammatory cytokines produced include large epithelioid cells, multinucleated giant cells, varied numbers of mononuclear cells and eosinophils. The causes vary in frequency from one country to another. Although the etiology may be determined from the histological features, from special stains for micro-organisms, from culture of part of the biopsy specimen or polymerase chain reaction of the paraffin-embedded specimen, or from clinical and serological data, the cause of hepatic granulomas remains unknown in one third of cases. It is likely that approximately one third of granulomatous liver reactions are caused by drugs, including allopurinol, carbamazepine, procainamide, diphenylhydantoin, quinidine, isoniazid, and sulphanilamide.

7.7. The role of liver biopsy in infections and pyrexia of unknown origin

Although the usefulness of liver biopsy in the diagnosis of fever of unknown origin is still controversial, a review of the literature shows that liver biopsy can be effective in confirming histopathological diagnosis and microbiological analysis [83].

Based on the findings of a liver biopsy evaluating Fever of Unknown Origin (FUO), we can conclude that abnormal liver biopsy is helpful in determining the cause of the FUO. The most common cause of fever was of an infectious origin. Other causes were neoplastic disorders or inflammatory [87].

Liver biopsy was performed after routine studies were negative. Therefore results such as histoplasmosis and tuberculosis indicate that, despite advances in diagnostic technology, liver biopsy continues to be useful in the diagnosis of FUO. In endemic areas, histoplasmosis and tuberculosis should be considered in the differential diagnosis of FUO [85].

7.8. Cirrhosis

Cirrhosis is pathologically defined as a diffuse process in which the normal anatomical lobules are replaced by architecturally abnormal nodules separated by fibrous tissue. Therefore, focal scarring, even if significant and associated with nodules, is not cirrhosis because the process is not diffuse [86]. In the past the description of a liver as "cirrhotic" implied an ominous prognosis in a patient with liver disease. In chronic hepatitis, the most important goal is to delay or to stop the development of cirrhosis. Nowadays, treatments to prevent its progression are available. At present there are many known stages as opposed to before when there only one was considered, G Garcia-Tsao in the article "In search of a pathophysiological classification of cirrhosis." [86].

7.8.1. Fibrosis progression

One of the most crucial developments is the reformulation of the concept of cirrhosis from a static to a dynamic process. This concept is likely to be even better defined in the future.

As fibrotic scars advance and extend the normal architecture changes and nodules are formed [88]. Moreover, the angiogenic process that naturally accompanies scar formation permits the creation of abnormal channels between central hepatic veins and portal vessels, resulting in the shunting of blood around the regenerating parenchyma. Normal vascular structures, along with sinusoidal channels, may be obliterated, leading to portal hypertension. Some authors describe cirrhosis as a vascular disease [89]. Clinical consequences of cirrhosis result from the decreased ability of the parenchyma to synthesize clotting factors and other substances combined with the complications related to portal hypertension [90].

Knowledge on the level of fibrotic progression between normal histology to cirrhosis has considerable prognostic weight. Patients with bridging fibrosis on biopsy are much closer to end-stage liver disease than those with minimal or no fibrosis. Fibrosis is not an autonomous feature, but rather a tissue progressive lesion resulting from other pathologic mechanisms such as inflammatory, degenerative or dystrophic processes [91].

The first transition in this process occurs between the normal, non-fibrotic state and the expansion of the portal area by fibrosis, to the extension of short, incomplete septations around the portal area, change that gives to the portal areas an irregular stellate shape.

In the next transition, development of bridges between vascular structures, portal-portal bridging fibrosis and portal-central bridging, occur. Gradually, more and more bridges are formed, accompanied by distortion of the architecture due to hepatocellular regeneration and contraction of fibrotic scars. When these changes diffusely involve the biopsy, it is classified as cirrhosis [92].

Progressive fibrosis leads to cirrhosis and it is now known that cirrhosis can be reversible. There was a lot of controversy surrounding this issue a few years ago [93]. For patients in a precirrhotic stage of fibrosis, liver biopsy remains the gold standard of assessment. Prior to 1995, there was no published system which subdivided advanced stages of cirrhosis. Only the Ishak modification of the Histologic Activity Index (HAI) subdivided cirrhosis into three categories [94].

Nowadays, since Garcia-Tsao et al.reported compensated and decompensated phases in the clinical evolution of liver cirrhosis, many prophylactic measures and controls have been implemented in order to improve survival and quality of life [87]. Cirrhosis is usually clinically evident. Once the pathologic stage of cirrhosis has been reached, clinical scales such as the Child-Pugh score have to be used because they represent the prognosis and the staging of the liver disease better [95]. The present debate questioning the need for liver biopsy versus non invasive tests will be discussed below.

7.8.2. A needle biopsy specimen does not always permit the diagnosis of cirrhosis

Micronodular cirrhosis (nodules of 3 mm or less), which may develop as a result of ethanol injury, biliary tract disease, or hemochromatosis, is usually uniform throughout the liver, and nodules may be identified on a needle specimen. However, macronodular cirrhosis (nodules greater than 3 mm), due most commonly to chronic viral hepatitis, constitutes a less uniform pattern [96].

7.9. Hepatocellular Carcinoma (HCC) and other benign or malignant focal lesions: The role of Fine Needle Aspiration Biopsy (FNAB) [97]

Indications of liver biopsy with regards to diffused or local lesions

Liver biopsy is useful for diagnosis of a diffused disease and guided liver biopsy remains essential for the diagnosis of localized lesions.

7.9.1. Fine needle aspiration biopsy (FNAB)

This technique has a crucial role in the evaluation of focal liver lesions or localized lesions. Liver tumors appear as nodular or localized lesions which can be malignant or non-malignant and can be either primary from the liver or metastasic. If clinical, biochemical and radiologic findings are inconclusive, some phases of the diagnostic process may require a liver biopsy in order to establish the diagnosis and their staging and management [99].

Malignant lesions. Hepatocellular carcinoma (HCC), the most frequent malignant liver cancer, is usually discovered during screening programs in cirrhotic patients. Regarding treatment, the only curative option is surgery, both limited hepatectomy of the tumor or liver transplant in very select cases [100].

In liver lesions with typically recognized features of HCC, defined by using advanced radiological methods, liver biopsy has no place. However, a liver biopsy will be performed in patients with atypical liver tumors suggestive of a possible colangiocarcinoma. These cases require another form of therapy and the prognosis is worse [99].

Besides, when surgery is indicated in a patient with suspected liver cirrhosis, a liver biopsy has to be performed in the non-neoplasic liver. Pathological diagnosis may help to asses the functional capacity, specific prognosis and whether surgery could be performed.

Metastasis of the liver with an unknown primary tumor should be biopsied to obtain information of the primary tumor in order to determine therapy.

Concern has been expressed about the risk of spreading malignant cells via the needle tract, but this rarely occurs when using needles with a diameter of less than 1.3 mm, which also minimizes the risk of bleeding. The procedure is simple, safe and painless [101].

7.9.2. Non-malignant lesions

In cases of Hemangioma or Focal Nodular Hyperplasia (FNH), diagnosed and confirmed by radiology, biopsy is usually not necessary.

FNH and hepatic adenoma are benign tumors and are less frequently observed than HCC. Their diagnosis is done using imaging techniques (ultrasound or helicoidal scanner). However, differential diagnosis is necessary because, although FNH only requires radiological follow-up, in some cases, higher risk circumstances have been recognized and surgery is recommended [102].

7.9.3. Most prevalent mass lesions [102, 103]

- Benign: cysts, hemangioma, adenoma, liver abscess (amebic or pyogenic), focal nodular hyperplasia, fatty infiltration, rare primary liver neoplasms.
- Malignant: hepatocellular carcinoma, cholangiocarcinoma, metastatic, rare primary liver neoplasms, rare primary bile duct neoplasms.

7.10. New evolving fields for liver biopsy: Liver transplantation, Bone marrow transplantation, Living donors and Morbid obesity

7.10.1. Liver transplantation

With regards to liver transplantation, liver biopsy remains very useful in the management of transplanted patients. In this clinical situation, if a rejection is suspected and other complications have been ruled out, a guided biopsy will be performed. This procedure can be of great value in order to confirm the specific diagnosis and to indicate treatment [104].

In the first few weeks and months after transplantation, the major causes of abnormal liver tests include preservation injury, acute rejection, opportunistic infections (e.g., cytomegalovirus, hepatitis), vascular compromise, and/or biliary stricture. Of these, acute allograft rejection is the most common and results from direct alloantigenic stimulation of recipient T cells by donor dendritic cells (antigen-presenting cells). The effector T cells can then preferentially injure biliary epithelial cells of both interlobular and septal bile ducts as well as endothelial cells of intrahepatic arteries and veins.

The main histological features of acute rejection Acute rejection is characterized by an infiltration of mixed, predominantly mononuclear cells within portal tracts. The inflammatory infiltrates include lymphocytes, macrophages, plasma cells, polymorphonuclear neutrophils and eosinophils. The inflammatory cells typically infiltrate the bile duct epithelium and are associated with bile duct damage. Subendothelial inflammation (endothelialitis), which may involve both portal and central veins, is also a typical feature. The most common grading system is the Banff schema, a consensus document proposed by an international panel of pathologists and liver transplant physicians [105]. Criteria helping to distinguish recurrent hepatitis C after transplantation from allograft rejection; Hepatitis C (HCV) recurs in virtually all patients transplanted for that disease.

Distinguishing recurrent hepatitis from acute allograft rejection, which can overlap, is difficult. There are usually three main phases to recurrent HCV:

- Graft reinfection (from 0 to 3 months post-transplant). HCV-related inflammation is rarely seen at this time. Liver biopsies may show mild lobular disarray, few necrotic hepatocytes (acidophil bodies), and fatty change.
- Established graft infection (from 3 to 6 months), acute hepatitis including ballooning degeneration of hepatocytes, acidophil bodes, and Kupffer cell prominence can be observed. Varying degrees of portal tract inflammation may also be present.
- Progressive liver damage (after 6 months), features related to chronic HCV infection such as, mononuclear portal infiltrates and interface hepatitis are observed. Bile duct damage, although mild, may occur, and granulomas may be detected. Up to half of patients will have histological evidence after 1 year.

The role of liver biopsy in the evaluation of abnormal liver tests after the first year post transplantation Common causes after the first year include acute rejection, opportunistic infection, recurrent viral hepatitis, chronic rejection, steatohepatitis, or recurrent diseases. Chronic rejection occurs as a consequence of repeated episodes of acute rejection that are unresponsive to immunosuppression. The main histological abnormalities are loss of small bile ducts (ductopenic rejection) and/or obliterative vasculopathy (affecting large and medium-sized arteries). Unlike acute allograft rejection, the degree of bile duct damage is typically out of proportion to the degree of inflammation.

Complications of liver transplantation are not limited to acute and chronic rejection and recurrence of original disease, but include surgical complications, most commonly hepatic artery occlusion, infections, and development of de novo malignancies. In the early post transplantation period preservation injury, damage to the graft during harvesting and implantation, may lead to significant graft dysfunction. In post-perfusion biopsies, heavy neutrophilic infiltrate and hepatocyte necrosis may be predictive of initial poor graft function.

Ischemic complications, such as hepatic artery thrombosis, are one of the most serious complications and may lead to early graft loss or biliary stricture. In these patients liver biopsy is usually not performed.

Infectious complications that generally occur after transplantation, cytomegalovirus(CMV) for example, remains common and is frequently associated with parenchymal microabscesses which are found in the liver biopsy of CMV patients.

7.10.2. Bone marrow transplantation

A liver biopsy is effective in the evaluation of a bone marrow transplant recipient with elevated liver tests [106]. Known complications of bone marrow transplantation include veno-occlusive disease (VOD) and graft-versus-host disease (GVHD). A biopsy is necessary to diagnose VOD. It develops within 1 to 4 weeks after transplantation and is characterized by occlusion of central veins, sinusoidal fibrosis, and pericentral hepatocyte necrosis. Acute GVHD develops within 6 weeks after transplantation and affects the skin, gastrointestinal tract, and liver. It is characterized by degenerative bile duct lesions with some degree of mononuclear inflammation. Cholestasis may be present. Chronic GVHD is a multiorgan process that develops 80 to 400 days after transplantation and is often preceded by acute GVHD. The changes in the liver are similar to those in acute disease, but the ducts show more prominent changes and are likely to be reduced in number or destroyed. A prominent periportal mononuclear infiltrate, or even piecemeal necrosis, may be seen.

7.10.3. Liver transplant living donor

Liver biopsies detect silent donor disease in potential living liver donors, especially patients suffering subclinical non-alcoholic fatty liver disease (NAFLD). The contribution of liver biopsy or even the need to perform this, when a potential donor is being evaluated is a controversial issue [107]. In the University of Pittsburgh Medical Center a retrospective study of the histopathologic examination and diagnoses of 284 patients, who were evaluated as living donors from 2001 to 2005 was carried out. Hepatic histology was correlated with liver injury tests and with demographic characteristics in an otherwise normal healthy population. A minority (n=119; 42%) of biopsies from this population of 143 males/141 females (average age=36.8years; mean BMI=26.6) were completely normal. The remainder showed steatosis (n=107; 37%), steatohepatitis (n=44; 15%), or unexplained low-grade/early stage chronic hepatitis, primary biliary cirrhosis, or nodular regenerative hyperplasia (n=16; 6%). Biopsy findings disqualified 29/56 donors, negative factors were: obesity, age and liver iron content, contributing to NAFLD pathogenesis. The conclusion was that liver biopsy provides valuable information about otherwise undetectable liver disease in potential liver donors.

7.10.4. Morbid obesity

About 90 per cent of morbidly obese patients show histological abnormalities of the liver. Morbid obesity may lead to severe disease showing steatosis, ballooning degeneration, lobular inflammation and fibrosis in the study of liver biopsy. These features are similar to the lesions observed in alcoholic hepatitis and may end in cirrhosis and liver failure. Many factors such as, alcohol, drugs, diabetes, viruses, can contribute to progressive liver damage. The development of severe fatty liver disease may be asymptomatic showing a poor correlation with liver function tests. It has been reported that after bypass surgery, weight loss is accompanied by improvement in fatty change and the liver function tests are normal.

Histopathologic findings in the liver of 160 patients who were undergoing laparoscopic gastric bypass or gastric banding for morbid obesity, were recorded, also clinical data (gender, age, BMI and associated diseases) and laboratory evaluation were obtained [108].The diagnosis obtained were : 63 non-nonalcoholic steatohepatitis (non-NASH), 54 NASH, 26 chronic hepatitis B (CHB), 15 alcoholic steatohepatitis and NASH, and 2 chronic hepatitis C (CHC).The coexistence of clinical and histological features of steatohepatitis with another chronic liver disease may reflect the biological significance of the chronic inflammatory condition in the obese population, which requires further investigation.

8. Non-invasive tests for liver disease and assessment of fibrosis and cirrhosis

Limitations of biopsy have led clinical investigators to study alternative methods to investigate liver disease especially for the assessment of liver fibrosis. Since fibrosis is of sufficient importance in chronic liver disease and because it progresses to cirrhosis it is frequently used as the outcome and prognostic variable in clinical studies. Hepatic fibrosis is currently viewed as a dynamic process that may regress after successful treatment of chronic liver diseases. Serum markers, such as non-invasive markers, offer an attractive alternative. They are objective, allowing a dynamic calibration of fibrosis, can be performed repeatedly, are more cost effective and many of them are performed as a routine analysis [109].

Indirect markers of liver fibrosis: among them, the AST to Platelet Ratio Index (APRI), combines aspartate amiotransferase (AST) with platelet count. It was used in several studies conducted in cohorts of patients with hepatitis C and showed a rather good diagnostic performance and reproducibility, [110] particularly for cirrhosis. Forns and colleagues reported a fibrosis index (Forns' index) based on platelet count, γ-glutamyl transferase (GGT), and cholesterol levels [111]. It is rather good for excluding significant fibrosis, but only average for diagnosing significant fibrosis. However, one important limit of both APRI and Forns' indexes are that they leave almost half of the patients unclassified.

Another widely investigated combination set of noninvasive markers of liver fibrosis is the Fibrotest; a combination of five blood tests based on a mathematical formula: GGT, bilirubin, haptoglobin, apolipoprotein A1, alfa2 macroglobulin adjusted for gender and age. According to the investigators, it could exclude cases with significant fibrosis (METAVIR > F2), having 100% of negative predictive value, and more than 90% positive predictive value, using liver biopsy as a reference [112].

8.1. Elastography (FibroScan)

Another noninvasive method for the assessment of liver fibrosis is elastography (FibroScan) [113].

FibroScan device (EchoSens, Paris, France) uses a mild-amplitude, low frequency vibration transmitted through the liver. It induces an elastic shear wave that is detected by pulse-echo ultrasonography as the wave propagates through the organ. The velocity of the wave correlates with tissue stiffness which correlates well with the degree of fibrosis.

This device is in widespread use in many parts of the world, but is not yet approved in the United States.

Most of the studies have been conducted on patients with chronic hepatitis C but a few studies have also covered fibrosis and cirrhosis due to other etiologies.

This technique, however, has its limitations: it uses expensive equipment, and has decreased accuracy in obese patients and in patients with ascites. Elastography results are not valid in presence of hepatic steatosis, cholestasis, necroinflammation, or portal hypertension. The patient's age and levels of aminotransferases need to be taken into account when interpreting results of liver stiffness [114].

	IN FAVOUR of LIVER BIOPSY	**AGAINST OF LIVER BIOPSY**
Chronic HCV hepatitis	In selected indications for grading and staging	Not necessary for diagnosis. Possible use of non-invasive methods in follow-up controls
Chronic HBV hepatitis	Grading and staging advisable before starting treatment	Not necessary for diagnosis. Possible use of non-invasive methods in follow-up controls
Non-alcoholic steatohepatitis (NASH)	NASH is a always an histopathological diagnosis	Assessment of fibrosis possible with non-invasive methods
Alcoholic steatohepatitis (ASH)	ASH is a histopathological diagnosis. But in alcoholic acute hepatitis liver biopsy usually is not performed	Assessment of fibrosis possible with non-invasive methods,(in abstinent patients)
Autoimmune Hepatitis	For diagnosis and staging liver biopsy is needed	Non validated methods yet for non-invasive assessment of fibrosis
Primary Biliary Cirrhosis (PBC)	Not needed in typical mild cases without biliary duct damage	Possible non-invasive assessment of fibrosis
Hemochromatosis	In general, liver biopsy performed for diagnosis and staging, and iron content in the liver	Non validated methods for non-invasive assessment of fibrosis
Wilson disease	For diagnosis and staging and copper content in the liver	Non other options

Table 5. Indication for liver biopsy in different chronic liver diseases in the era of non-invasive methods

In spite of that, elastography is complementary as the combination of noninvasive markers and elastography improves the overall accuracy. In one of the metanalysis, for significant fibrosis, the area under the ROC for Fibrotest and FibroScan were 0.81 (95% CI 0.78-84) and 0.83 (0.03-1.00), respectively [115].

http://dx.doi.org/10.5772/53120

Fibrotest, and elastography (Fibroscan) as first line estimates of fibrosis in patients with chronic hepatitis C are recommended and liver biopsy will probably be indicated only as a second line diagnosis and reserved for cases of discordance or non-interpretability [112].

Some authors conclude that elastography appears reliable to detect significant fibrosis and cirrhosis in patients with chronic hepatitis C, besides it may turn out to be a valuable diagnostic procedure and follow-up of patients with chronic liver diseases of different causes [115].

8.2. Liver biopsy: Consensus among pathologists?

It is crucial that biopsy interpretation be done by experienced liver pathologists. Pathologists have tried to define the features (including length and number of complete portal tracts) of an adequate liver biopsy sample able to correctly assess the classification of liver fibrosis. Some authors have recommended big samples of 1 to 4 cm in length containing at least 11 complete portal tracts, which could be more reliable for adequate grading and staging [116, 117]

Feature	Effect on response to therapy	Effect on natural history
Fibrosis	Reduces response	Presence implies progression
Inflammation	No effect	Related to increased amount of current fibrosis and increased rate of progression
Steatosis	Reduces response	Related to increased amount of current fibrosis, unclear effect on progression
Iron accumulation	Unclear effect	Related to increased amount of current fibrosis, unclear effect on prospective rate
(adapt from Semin Liver Dis 2005)		

Table 6. Relevance of histological features of chronic hepatitis C to disease progression and therapeutic response

Many intraobserver and interobserver variations have been estimated in the assessment of features, classification, and scoring of liver biopsy assessment. One study reported differences in the evaluation of liver biopsies in chronic viral hepatitis C among 10 pathologists specializing in liver diseases. These pathologists independently reviewed 30 liver biopsy specimens of viral hepatitis C and completed a histological form for each of the specimens. Five pairs of pathologists were then randomly designated and they independently reviewed the biopsy specimens and filled out a new coding form. The interobserver variation was calculated for each item among the 10 individuals and then among the five pairs. Five features showed an almost perfect or a substantial degree of concordance among the 10 observers (cirrhosis, fibrosis, fibrosis grading by Knodell index, steatosis and portal lymphoid aggregates). The 17 other indicators showed a weaker concordance. Five items had a higher concordance when viewed by a pair of pathologists than when studied by only one pathologist (steatosis, periportal necrosis grading by Knodell index, lobular necrosis grading by Knodell index, centrilobular fibrosis, and ductular proliferation). This study reveals that certain features of major importance in assessing disease activity show significant observer variation. The acceptable degree of concordance was related mainly to the fibrosis score, whereas other numerical items displayed substantial observer variations. Simultaneous observation by two pathologists increased the reproducibility of numerical scoring and of certain viral hepatitis C lesions. A classification of chronic hepatitis C based on dissociated semiquantitative assessment of necroinflammatory lesions and fibrosis offers more reproducibility than the use of a global numerical index [107].

As a single percutaneous liver biopsy yields only a minute percentage (1 / 50 000 or 0.002%) of the total hepatic tissue, paired biopsies have been evaluated in several published studies, especially for assessing steatosis and NASH. For quantification, better references are required, such as imaging techniques or morphometry, which determines the area of steatosis on liver biopsy.

In fact, as liver steatosis is not homogeneous, classical optical examination of a liver biopsy by a pathologist for measuring liver steatosis by the determination of the percentage of hepatocytes containing lipid vesicles is highly subjective, and steatosis grading corresponds only to a semiquantitative scale [68].

The role of the liver biopsy in disease management is evolving nowadays and has to be reconsidered given the modern pathologic assessment of liver biopsy. Pathologists have made progress in the interpretation of liver biopsies and in processing the information in a concise and scientific way available to clinicians. After evaluating the disease state and interpreting the tests results, the clinician in charge of the patient should consider the individual patient when making recommendations with regards to treatment.

Role of the liver biopsy in personalized medicine

The liver biopsy specimen aims to obtain a valuable material for the assessment of fibrosis and cirrhosis. Despite limitations related to sampling and interpretation, histological examination remains the best standard for staging and diagnosing chronic liver diseases. Its indications are decreasing because new therapeutical options for chronic viral hepatitis have improved [118]. Moreover, new non-invasive tests have been developed and their use may increase in the future, especially for long term management [119] (Table 7).

All invasive procedures involve risks, consequently the benefits of obtaining liver for histology should always be weighed against the possible morbidity of the procedure. The decision to indicate a liver biopsy has to be taken depending on the center's facilities and the availability of experienced liver pathologists to interpret the biopsy.

http://dx.doi.org/10.5772/53120

Ethics related to liver biopsy mainly include issues on the indications, information on potential risks and benefits and validity of available alternative options. Patients should be adequately informed and participate in the decisions for liver biopsy and treatment [120].

	Liver biopsy	**Transient elastography**
Advantages	- Direct measure of liver fibrosis - Well established staging system - Assessment of architectural disturbances related to liver fibrosis - Evaluation of associated lesions (inflammation, steatosis, iron, alcohol)	- Non-invasive - Easy to repeat - No risk to patient - Performed in the outpatient clinic - Results available immediately - Reproducible - Highly performance for detecting cirrhosis
Disadvantages	- Invasive and painful - Difficult to repeat - Potentially severe complications - Contraindicated if ascites, coagulopathy etc. - Sampling and interobserver variability	- Unable to discriminate between intermediate stages of fibrosis - False positive in case of acute hepatitis, extrahepatic cholestasis and congestive heart failure
(adapt L Castera & M Pinzani, Gut 2010)		

Table 7. Use of liver biopsy in clinical practice. Respective advantages and disadvantages of liver biopsy and transient elastography for assessing fibrosis in chronic liver disease

12. Conclusions

What will be the real impact of Liver Biopsy now and in the near future in the era of personalized medicine?

1. The practice of liver biopsy will remain as an important component in the evaluation of liver disease. However, the value of liver biopsy should be contemplated as a complementary tool in modern medicine because of the presence of new non-invasive diagnostic measures, better prognostication methods and more advances in imaging techniques.

2. Non invasive tests such as Fibroscan, or similar, adding serum markers will be increasingly used to identify the amount of fibrosis, and will spare, in most patients, the performance of a liver biopsy.

3. Liver biopsy provides information that is used in conjunction with other data to inform and to guide therapy. The team that joins pathologists, clinicians, radiologists and other specialists meets in order to make clinico-pathological correlations. New classifications incorporating clinical data in the histological dictamen will be implemented.

4. Therapies, etiology, pathogenesis, cellular and molecular mechanisms, changes in tissue architecture and invasive (HVPG) and noninvasive diagnostic approaches, should be added to the liver biopsy information.

5. In the liver transplant field, liver biopsy has allowed many scientific advances and in most of these patients liver biopsy will continue to be mandatory for their management.

6. Patients seeking a second opinion or who are referred to a tertiary care center, will require a deep review of previous obtained specimens in order to confirm and to plan their management.

7. Since chronic viral hepatitis is a prevalent disease in the general population, the number of liver biopsies will be limited in the next years because it is costly and aggressive so validated non-invasive methods will be favoured.

8. Nevertheless, some questions surrounding non-invasive markers will remain. Non-invasive markers have been validated against the biopsy, and the overall accuracy of biopsy is only 80%, it is probably statistically impossible for a marker to perform any better than a biopsy.

9. Increasing research on hepatic fibrosis, diagnoses and therapy, is ongoing so valuable results of predicting changes in fibrosis content over time have to be followed by histological liver assessment. Moreover, considering the possible regression of cirrhosis, now clinicians and pathologists have become more interested in studying histological features of tissue repair and fibrosis regression in the liver.

10. The number of liver biopsy will be sparing in common patients but it will play a crucial role in research; for example studying rare diseases, stem cells and genetic disorders. Moreover, its role is evolving in many research fields such as obesity, bone marrow transplant, and oncology.

Acknowledgements

I would like to thank Aisling Dowd, for her help while preparing the manuscript

Author details

Teresa Casanovas Taltavull

Chronic Hepatitis Coordinator Program, Liver Transplant Unit, Hospital Universitari de Bellvitge, L'Hospitalet de Llobregat, Barcelona, Spain

References

[1] Rockey DC, Caldwell SH, Goodman ZD et al.; American Association for the Study of Liver Diseases. Liver biopsy. Hepatology. 2009; 49(3):1017-1044.

[2] Colloredo G, Guido M, Sonzogni A, Leandro G. Impact of liver biopsy size on histological evaluation of chronic viral hepatitis: the smaller the sample, the milder the disease. J Hepatol 2003; 39(2):239–244.

[3] Udell JA, Wang CS, Tinmouth J, et al. Does this patient with liver disease have cirrhosis? JAMA. 2012; 307(8):832-842.

[4] Bedossa P, Dargère D, Paradis V. Sampling variability of liver fibrosis in chronic hepatitis C. Hepatology 2003; 38(6): 1449–1457.

[5] Scheuer PJ. Liver biopsy size matters in chronic hepatitis: bigger is better. Hepatology 2003; 38(6):1356–1358.

[6] Bateman AC. Patterns of histological change in liver disease: my approach to 'medical' liver biopsy reporting. Histopathology. 2007; 51(5):585-596.

[7] Pinzani M. Exploring beyond cirrhosis.Hepatology. 2012; 56(2):778-780.

[8] Poynard T, Ratziu V, Bedossa P. Appropriateness of liver biopsy. Can J Gastroenterol 2000; 14:543-548.

[9] Czaja AJ, Carpenter HA.Optimizing diagnosis from the medical liver biopsy.Clin Gastroenterol Hepatol 2007; 5(8):898-907.

[10] Crawford JM. Evidence-based interpretation of liver biopsies. Lab Invest 2006; 86(4): 326–334.

[11] Campbell MS, Reddy KR. Review article: the evolving role of liver biopsy. Aliment Pharmacol Ther 2004; 20(3):249-59.

[12] Schiano TD, Azeem S, Bodian CA, et al. Importance of specimen size in accurate needle liver biopsy evaluation of patients with chronic hepatitis C. Clin Gastroenterol Hepatol 2005; 3(9):930–935.

[13] Bravo AA, Sheth SG, Chopra S. Liver biopsy. N Engl J Med 2001; 344 (7): 495–500.

[14] Lefkowitch JH.Special stains in diagnostic liver pathology.Semin Diagn Pathol. 2006; 23(3-4):190-8. Review.

[15] Batts KP, Ludwig J. Chronic hepatitis. An update on terminology and reporting. Am J Surg Pathol 1995; 19: 1409-1417.

[16] Knodell RG, Ishak KG, Black WC, et al. Formulation and application of a numerical scoring system for assessing histological activity in asymptomatic chronic active hepatitis. Hepatology 1981; 1(5):431–435.

[17] Scheuer PJ. Classification of chronic viral hepatitis: a need for reassessment. J Hepatol 1991; 13(3):372–374

[18] Bedossa P, Poynard T. An algorithm for the grading of activity in chronic hepatitis C. The METAVIR Cooperative Study Group. Hepatology 1996; 24:289–293.

[19] Ishak K, Baptista A, Bianchi L, et al. Histological grading and staging of chronic hepatitis.J Hepatol 1995; 22(6):696–699.

[20] Desmet VJ, Gerber M, Hoofnagle JH, Manns M, Scheuer PJ. Classification of chronic hepatitis: diagnosis, grading and staging. Hepatology 1994; 19(6):1513–1520.

[21] Kumar D, Farrell GC, Fung C, et al. Hepatitis C virus genotype 3 is cytopathic to hepatocytes: Reversal of hepatic steatosis after sustained therapeutic response. Hepatology 2002; 36:1266-1272.

[22] Bressler BL, Guindi M, Tomlinson G, et al. High body mass index is an independent risk factor for nonresponse to antiviral treatment in chronic hepatitis C. Hepatology 2003; 38:639-644.

[23] Poynard T, Bedossa P,& Opolon P Natural history of liver fibrosis progression in patients with chronic hepatitis C. The OBSVIRC, METAVIR, CLINIVIR, and DOSVIRC groups. Lancet1997; 349(9055):825-832.

[24] Mohsen AH, Easterbrook PJ, Taylor C, et al. Impact of human immunodeficiency virus (HIV) infection on the progression of liver fibrosis in hepatitis C virus infected patients.Gut 2003;; 52(7):1035-1040.

[25] Papatheodoridis GV, Manolakopoulos S, Liaw YF, & Lok A. Follow-up and indications for liver biopsy in HBeAg-negative chronic hepatitis B virus infection with persistently normal ALT: A systematic review. J Hepatol 2012; 57(1):196-202.

[26] Castera L. Noninvasive methods to assess liver disease in patients with hepatitis B or C. Gastroenterology 2012; 142(6):1293-1302.

[27] European Association For The Study Of The Liver. Clinical Practice Guidelines: Management of chronic hepatitis B virus infection.J Hepatol 2012; 57(1):167-185.

[28] Grattagliano I, Ubaldi E, Bonfrate L, & Portincasa P. Management of liver cirrhosis between primary care and specialists.World J Gastroenterol 2011; 17(18):2273-2282.

[29] Shao J, Wei L, Wang H, Sun Y et al. Relationship between hepatitis B virus DNA levels and liver histology in patients with chronic hepatitis B. World J Gastroenterol 2007; 13(14):2104-7.

[30] Gebo KA, Herlong HF, Torbenson MS, et al. Role of liver biopsy in management of chronic hepatitis C: a systematic review. Hepatology 2002; 36:S161-S172.

[31] Arroyo M, & Crawford JM. Hepatitic inherited metabolic disorders.Semin Diagn Pathol. 2006; 23(3-4):182-189.

[32] Nash S, Marconi S, Sikorska K, et al. Role of liver biopsy in the diagnosis of hepatic iron overload in the era of genetic testing. Am J Clin Pathol 2002; 118(1):73-81.

[33] Ioannou GN, Tung BY, & Kowdley KV. Iron in hepatitis C: villain or innocent bystander? Semin Gastrointest Dis. 2002; 13(2):95-108.

[34] Falize L, Guillygomarc'h A, Perrin M, et al. Reversibility of hepatic fibrosis in treated genetic hemochromatosis: a study of 36 cases. Hepatology 2006; 44(2):472–477

[35] Bonkovsky HL, Poh-Fitzpatrick M, Pimstone N, et al. Porphyria cutanea tarda, hepatitis C, and HFE gene mutations in North America. Hepatology 1998; 27(6):1661-1669.

[36] Ryan Caballes F, Sendi H, & Bonkovsky HL. Hepatitis C, porphyria cutanea tarda and liver iron: an update.Liver Int 2012; 32(6):880-93.

[37] Brunt EM, Olynyk JK, Britton RS, et al. Histological evaluation of iron in liver biopsies: relationship to HFE mutations. Am J Gastroenterol 2000; 95(7):1788-93.

[38] Cribier B, Chiaverini C, Dali-Youcef N, et al. Porphyria cutanea tarda, hepatitis C, uroporphyrinogen decarboxylase and mutations of HFE gene. A case-control study. Dermatology 2009; 218(1):15-21.

[39] Merle U, Schaefer M, Ferenci P, Stremmel W. Clinical presentation, diagnosis and long-term outcome of Wilson's disease: a cohort study. Gut 2007; 56(1):115-20.

[40] Ferenci P, Steindl-Munda P, Vogel W, et al. Diagnostic value of quantitative hepatic copper determination in patients with Wilson's Disease. Clin Gastroenterol Hepatol. 2005; 3(8):811-818.

[41] Clark VC, Dhanasekaran R, Brantly M, et al. Liver Test Results Do Not Identify Liver Disease in Adults with α-1 Antitrypsin Deficiency. Clin Gastroenterol Hepatol 2012 Jul 23. [Epub ahead of print]

[42] Yeoman AD, Westbrook RH, Al-Chalabi T, et al. Diagnostic value and utility of the simplified International Autoimmune Hepatitis Group (IAIHG) criteria in acute and chronic liver disease. Hepatology 2009; 50(2):538-545.

[43] Czaja AJ, Carpenter HA. Decreased fibrosis during cortico-steroid therapy of autoimmune hepatitis. J Hepatol 2004; 40(4):646–652

[44] Chandok N, Silveira MG,& Lindor KD.Comparing the simplified and international autoimmune hepatitis group criteria in primary sclerosing cholangitis. Gastroenterol Hepatol (N Y) 2010; 6(2):108-112.

[45] Sherlock S.Primary biliary cirrhosis, primary sclerosing cholangitis, and autoimmune cholangitis. Clin Liver Dis 2000; 4(1):97-113.

[46] Neuhauser M, Bjornsson E, Treeprasertsuk S, et al. Autoimmune hepatitis-PBC overlap syndrome: a simplified scoring system may assist in the diagnosis. Am J Gastroenterol 2010; 105(2):345-353.

[47] Hennes E M, Zeniya M, Czaja AJ et al. and The International Autoimmune Hepatitis Group. Simplified Criteria for the Diagnosis of Autoimmune Hepatitis. Hepatology 2008; 48:169-176.

[48] Boberg KM, Chapman RW, Hirschfield GM, et al.; International Autoimmune Hepatitis Group.Overlap syndromes: The International Autoimmune Hepatitis Group (IAIHG) position statement on a controversial issue. J Hepatol 2011; 54(2):374-385.

[49] Nakanuma Y, Zen Y, Harada K, et al. Application of a new histological staging and grading system for primary biliary cirrhosis to liver biopsy specimens: Interobserver agreement. Pathol Int 2010; 60(3):167-174.

[50] Levy C & Lindor KD. Primary sclerosing cholangitis: epidemiology, natural history, and prognosis. Semin Liver Dis 2006; 26(1):22-30.

[51] Burak KW, Angulo P, & Lindor KD. Is there a role for liver biopsy in primary sclerosing cholangitis? Am J Gastroenterol 2003; 98(5):1155-1158.

[52] Olsson R, Hägerstrand I, Broomé U, et al. Sampling variability of percutaneous liver biopsy in primary sclerosing cholangitis. J Clin Pathol 1995; 48(10):933-935.

[53] Dave M, Elmunzer BJ, Dwamena BA, & Higgins PD. Primary sclerosing cholangitis: meta-analysis of diagnostic performance of MR cholangiopancreatography..Radiology 2010; 256(2):387-396.

[54] Tischendorf JJW, Andreas Geier A, & Trautwein C. Current Diagnosis and Management of Primary Sclerosing Cholangitis. Liver Transplantation 2008; 14:735-746.

[55] Klibansky DA, Mehta SH, Curry M, et al. Transient elastography for predicting clinical outcomes in patients with chronic liver disease.J Viral Hepat 2012; 19(2):e184-193.

[56] Burak K, Angulo P, Pasha TM, et al; Incidence and risk factors for cholangiocarcinoma in primary sclerosing cholangitis. Am J Gastroenterol 2004; 99(3):523-526.

[57] Bjornsson E, Olsson R, Bergquist A, et al. The natural history of small-duct primary sclerosing cholangitis. Gastroenterology 2008; 134(4):975-980.

[58] Wiesner RH, Porayko MK, Hay JE, et al. Liver transplantation for primary sclerosing cholangitis: impact of risk factors on outcome.Liver Transpl Surg 1996; 2(5 Suppl 1): 99-108.

[59] Poupon R. Autoimmune overlapping syndromes. Clin Liver Dis 2003; 7:865–878.

[60] Deshpande V, Sainani NI, Chung RT, et al.IgG4-associated cholangitis: a comparative histological and immunophenotypic study with primary sclerosing cholangitis on liver biopsy material. Mod Pathol 2009; 22(10):1287-1295.

[61] Tiniakos DG Liver biopsy in alcoholic and non-alcoholic steatohepatitis patients. Gastroenterol Clin Biol 2009; 33(10-11):930-939.

[62] Talley NJ, Roth A, Woods J,& Hench V. Diagnostic value of liver biopsy in alcoholic liver disease. J Clin Gastroenterol 1988; 10(6):647-650.

[63] Hezode C, Lonjon I, Roudot-Thoraval F, et al. Impact of moderate alcohol consumption on histological activity and fibrosis in patients with chronic hepatitis C, and specific influence of steatosis: a prospective study. Aliment Pharmacol Ther 2003; 17:1031-1037.

[64] Yoshioka Y, Hashimoto E, Yatsuji S, et al. Nonalcoholic steatohepatitis: cirrhosis, hepatocellular carcinoma, and burnt-out NASH. J Gastroenterol 2004; 39(12): 1215-1218.

[65] Brunt EM, Ramrakhiani S, Cordes BG, et al. Concurrence of histologic features of steatohepatitis with other forms of chronic liver disease. Mod Pathol 2003; 16:49-56.

[66] Brunt EM. Nonalcoholic steatohepatitis: definition and pathology. Semin Liver Dis 2001; 21(1):3-16. Review.

[67] Yoneda M, Yoneda M, Mawatari H, et al. Noninvasive assessment of liver fibrosis by measurement of stiffness in patients with nonalcoholic fatty liver disease (NAFLD). Dig Liver Dis 2008; 40(5):371-378.

[68] Brunt EM, Janney CG, Di Bisceglie AM, Neuschwander-Tetri BA, Bacon BR. Nonalcoholic steatohepatitis: a proposal for grading and staging the histological lesions. Am J Gastroenterol 1999; 94(9):2467–2474.

[69] Kanel GC. Hepatic lesions resembling alcoholic liver disease. Pathology (Phila) 1994; 3(1):77-104.70.

[70] Strnad P, Paschke S, Jang KH,& Ku NO. Keratins: markers and modulators of liver disease. Curr Opin Gastroenterol 2012; 28(3):209-16. Review.

[71] Ratziu V, Giral P, Charlotte F, et al. Liver fibrosis in overweight patients. Gastroenterology 2000; 118: 1117–1123.

[72] Navarro VJ, Senior JR. Drug-related hepatotoxicity. N Eng J Med 2006; 354: 731–739.

[73] Ghabril M, Chalasani N, & Björnsson E. Drug-induced liver injury: a clinical update. Curr Opin Gastroenterol 2010; 26(3):222-226.

[74] Rockey DC, Seeff LB, Rochon J, et al. US Drug-Induced Liver Injury Network. Causality assessment in drug-induced liver injury using a structured expert opinion process: comparison to the Roussel-Uclaf causality assessment method. Hepatology 2010; 51(6):2117-26.

[75] Goodman ZD. Drug hepatotoxicity. Clin Liver Dis 2002; 6:381–397.

[76] Lagana SM, Moreira RK, & Lefkowitch JH. Hepatic granulomas: pathogenesis and differential diagnosis. Clin Liver Dis 2010; 14(4):605-617.

[77] Ishak KG, Zimmerman HJ. Drug-induced and toxic granulomatous hepatitis. Baillieres Clin Gastroenterol 1988; 2(2):463-480.

[78] Nohlgård C, Rubio CA, Kock Y, Hammar H. Liver fibrosis quantified by image analysis in methotrexate-treated patients with psoriasis. J Am Acad Dermatol 1993; 28(1): 40–45.

[79] Chang CY,& Schiano TD. Review article: drug hepatotoxicity. Aliment Pharmacol Ther 2007 15; 25(10):1135-1151.

[80] Valla DC, Benhamou HP. Hepatic granulomas and hepatic sarcoidosis. Clin Liver Dis 2000; 4:269–285.

[81] Snyder N, Martinez JG, & Xiao SY..Chronic hepatitis C is a common associated with hepatic granulomas.World J Gastroenterol 2008 7; 14(41):6366-6369.

[82] Scheuer PJ. Classification of chronic viral hepatitis: a need for reassessment. J Hepatol 1991; 13:372-374.

[83] Holtz T, Moseley RH, Scheiman JM. Liver biopsy in fever of unknown origin: a reappraisal. J Clin Gastroenterol 1993; 17:29–32.

[84] Knockaert DC, Vanneste LJ, Vannester SB, et al. Fever of unknown origin in the 1980s: an update of the diagnostic spectrum. Arch Intern Med 1992; 152:51–55.

[85] Lamps LW. Hepatic granulomas, with an emphasis on infectious causes. Adv Anat Pathol 2008; 15(6):309-18. Review.

[86] Schuppan D, & Afdhal NH.Liver cirrhosis. Lancet 2008 Mar 8; 371(9615):838-851.

[87] Garcia-Tsao G, Friedman S, Iredale J, Pinzani M. Now there are many (stages) where before there was one: In search of a pathophysiological classification of cirrhosis. Hepatology 2010; 51(4):1445–1449.

[88] Germani G, Dhillon A, Andreana L, et al. Histological subclassification of cirrhosis. Hepatology 2010; 52(2): 804–805.

[89] Kumar M, Sakhuja P, Kumar A, et al. Histological subclassification of cirrhosis based on histological-haemodynamic correlation. Aliment Pharmacol Ther 2008; 27(9): 771–779.

[90] Sethasine S, Jain D, Groszmann RJ, & Garcia-Tsao G. Quantitative histological-hemodynamic correlations in cirrhosis. Hepatology 2012; 55(4):1146-53.

[91] Standish RA, Cholongitas E, Dhillon A, Burroughs AK, Dhillon AP. An appraisal of the histopathological assessment of liver fibrosis. Gut 2006; 55(4):569–578.

[92] Germani G, Dhillon A, Andreana L, et al. Histological subclassification of cirrhosis. Hepatology 2010; 52(2): 804–805.

[93] Serpaggi J, Carnot F, Nalpas B, et al. Direct and indirect evidence for the reversibility of cirrhosis. Hum Pathol 2006; 37(12):1519–1526.

[94] Goodman ZD, & Ishak KG. Histopathology of hepatitis C virus infection. Semin Liver Dis 1995; 15(1):70-81.

[95] Cholongitas E, Papatheodoridis GV, Vangeli M, et al. Systematic review: The model for end-stage liver disease--should it replace Child-Pugh's classification for assessing prognosis in cirrhosis? Aliment Pharmacol Ther 2005; 22(11-12):1079-1089. Review.

[96] Hytiroglou P, Snover DC, Alves V, et al. Beyond "cirrhosis": a proposal from the International Liver Pathology Study Group. Am J Clin Pathol 2012; 137(1):5-9.

[97] Varadarajulu S, Fockens P, & Hawes RH. Best practices in endoscopic ultrasoundguided fine-needle aspiration. Clin Gastroenterol Hepatol 2012; 10(7):697-703.

[98] Laurent V, Corby S, Antunes L, et al. Liver and focal liver contrast: radiologic-pathologic correlation. J Radiol 2007; 88(7-8 Pt 2):1036-47.

[99] Adam R, Azoulay D, Castaing D,et al. Liver resection as a bridge to transplantation for hepatocellular carcinoma on cirrhosis: a reasonable strategy? Ann Surg 2003; 238 (4): 508-18; discussion 518-519.

[100] Kitao A, Zen Y, Matsui O, et al. Hepatocellular carcinoma: signal intensity at gadoxetic acid-enhanced MR Imaging--correlation with molecular transporters and histopathologic features. Radiology 2010; 256(3):817-826.

[101] Robertson EG, & Baxter G. Tumour seeding following percutaneous needle biopsy: the real story! Clin Radiol 2011; 66(11):1007-1014.

[102] Closset J, Veys I, Peny MO, et al. Retrospective analysis of 29 patients surgically treated for hepatocellular adenoma or focal nodular hyperplasia. Hepatogastroenterology. 2000; 47(35):1382-1384.

[103] Shortell CK,& Schwartz SI.Hepatic adenoma and focal nodular hyperplasia.Surg Gynecol Obstet 1991; 173(5):426-431.

[104] Longerich T, & Schirmacher P.General aspects and pitfalls in liver transplant pathology. Clin Transplant 2006; 20 Suppl 17:60-68.

[105] Demetris AJ, Adams D, Bellamy C, et al. Update of the International Banff Schema for Liver Allograft Rejection: Working recommendations for the histopathologic staging and reporting of chronic rejection. An international panel. Hepatology 2000; 31:792–799.

[106] Chahal P, Levy C, Litzow MR, et al. Utility of liver biopsy in bone marrow transplant patient. J Gastroenterol Hepatol 2008; 123:222–225.

[107] Sugawara Y & Makuuchi M. Living donor liver transplantation: present status and recent advances.Br Med Bull 2006; 10; 75-76:15-28.

[108] Liew PL, Lee WJ, Lee YC, et al. Hepatic histopathology of morbid obesity: concurrence of other forms of chronic liver disease.Obes Surg 2006; 16(12):1584-1593.

[109] Imbert-Bismut F, Ratziu V, Pieroni L, et al. Biochemical markers of liver fibrosis in patients with hepatitis C virus infection: a prospective study. Lancet 2001; 357:1069-1075.

[110] Jin W, Lin Z, Xin Y, et al. Diagnostic accuracy of the aspartate amino transferase-toplatelet ratio index for the prediction of hepatitis B-related fibrosis: a leading metaanalysis. BMC Gastroenterol 2012; 14; 12:14. Review.

[111] Forns X, Ampurdanès S, Llovet JM, et al. Identification of chronic hepatitis C patients without hepatic fibrosis by a simple predictive model. Hepatology. 2002; 36(4 Pt 1): 986-992.

[112] Poynard T, de Ledinghen V, Zarski JP, et al. Fibrosis-TAGS group. Relative performances of FibroTest, Fibroscan, and biopsy for the assessment of the stage of liver fibrosis in patients with chronic hepatitis C: a step toward the truth in the absence of a gold standard. J Hepatol 2012; 56(3):541-548.

[113] Castera L, Forns X, Alberti A. Non-invasive evaluation of liver fibrosis using transient elastography. J Hepatol 2008; 48(5):835–847.

[114] Cardoso AC, Carvalho-Filho RJ, Stern C, et al. Direct comparison of diagnostic performance of transient elastography in patients with chronic hepatitis B and chronic hepatitis C. Liver Int 2012; 32(4):612-621.

[115] Cross TJ, Calvaruso V, Maimone S, et al. Prospective comparison of Fibroscan, King's score and liver biopsy for the assessment of cirrhosis in chronic hepatitis C infection. J Viral Hepat 2010; 17(8):546-54.

[116] Guido M, Rugge M. Liver biopsy sampling in chronic viral hepatitis. Semin Liver Dis 2004; 24:89-97.

[117] Intraobserver and interobserver variations in liver biopsy interpretation in patients with chronic hepatitis C. The French METAVIR Cooperative Study Group. Hepatology 1994 Jul; 20(1 Pt 1):15-20.

[118] Sebastiani G, & Alberti A. How far is noninvasive assessment of liver fibrosis from replacing liver biopsy in hepatitis C? J Viral Hepat 2012; 19 Suppl 1:18-32.

[119] Carey E, Carey WD. Noninvasive tests for liver disease, fibrosis, and cirrhosis: Is liver biopsy obsolete? Cleve Clin J Med 2010; 77(8):519-527.

[120] Papatheodoridis GV. Ethics related to liver biopsies and antiviral therapies in chronic viral hepatitis. Dig Dis Sci 2008; 26(1):59-65.

Section 2

Clinical Practice of Liver Biopsy

Chapter 4

Safety and Reliability Percutaneous Liver Biopsy Procedure in Children with Chronic Liver Diseases

Anna Mania, Paweł Kemnitz,
Magdalena Figlerowicz, Aldona Woźniak and
Wojciech Służewski

Additional information is available at the end of the chapter

http://dx.doi.org/10.5772/52619

1. Introduction

Liver biopsy remains a golden standard in the evaluation of various liver diseases. It is one of the most specific test allowing to assess the severity of various liver diseases. Clinical evaluation may be inadequate as chronic liver diseases could be asymptomatic for a long period of time. The routinely used laboratory test may be irrelevant, as diffuse changes may possibly be present in the liver in spite of liver function test being within reference values. Percutaneous biopsy allows to obtain a tissue specimen suitable for pathological assessment. Liver biopsy is an important procedure in diagnosing liver diseases in infants and children as it often provides diagnostic information not possible to obtain by other methods. Therefore, liver biopsy is considered to be a golden standard in the diagnostics and follow-up of the patients with chronic diffuse hepatopathies. The role of the liver biopsy is to confirm the diagnosis of chronic hepatitis, assess the necroinflamatory activity (grading) and the severity of fibrosis (staging), confirm the presence of cirrhosis. Other hepatopathies may be excluded as well as associated diseases using this method [1].

The size of liver sample varies from 1 to 4 cm in length and 1.2 to 1.8 mm in diameter. Biopsy specimen represents 1/50,000 of the total mass of the liver, therefore the procedure carries the risk of sampling error. The specimen should be sufficient in length (2-2.5 cm) and number of portal spaces (at least 11). The fragmentation of the specimen should be avoided [2]. Liver assessment is also affected by an interpretative error and intraobserver variability of histological interpretation. Moreover, liver biopsy is an invasive procedure carrying the risk of certain complications including pain, bleeding, pneumothorax, puncture of bile ducts or the gall bladder.

Repeating samples in different time intervals are useful in monitoring the efficacy of treatments. Many patients are, however, reluctant to experience repeated biopsies, which limits the ability to monitor disease progression and treatment effects. [3].

Due to the limitations of the procedure many non-invasive techniques were developed such as single serological markers, panels of different markers, imaging techniques and elastography [4]. None of the non-invasive methods is suitable and reliable enough to entirely substitute the liver biopsy. Non-invasive techniques are very helpful in the detection of severe lesions. However, results obtained from patients with intermediate lesions very often overlap between different categories of staging. Nevertheless non-invasive methods are useful in situations where contraindications to liver biopsy do not allow to perform the procedure.

Liver biopsy can be percutaneous, transjugular or laparoscopic. Percutaneous liver biopsy can be blind, ultrasound- guided or ultrasound assisted. Various approaches differ in the number of potential complications and require various equipment. Ultrasound guidance allows safer intercostal approach and may be useful in the evaluation of relative position of the liver, gall bladder, kidneys and lungs. The technique reduces the risk of hemothorax and pneumothorax and puncture of the gall bladder.

The aim of this study was to evaluate safety and reliability of the liver biopsy in children in relation to obtained results and potential complications.

2. Material and methods

Seventy five cases of percutaneous liver biopsies carried between 2005-2012 were analyzed. The biopsies were performed in children aged 4-17 years (mean 15.30±2.35 years). Study group included 26 girls, 49 boys. Procedures were done due to chronic hepatitis C (CHC) – 44 cases, chronic hepatitis B (CHB) – 16 cases, autoimmune hepatitis (AIH) – 3 cases, hepatitis/hepatomegaly of unknown origin (HUO)– 12 cases, non-alcoholic fatty liver disease (NAFLD) – 2 cases. Number of the procedures performed in the following years has been presented in Figure 1.

Written informed consent was obtained from the parents and patients aged 16 years and over according to Polish law regulations. Before the procedure children were clinically evaluated and blood samples were taken for standard hematological and clinical chemistry analysis. Children with coagulopathies and thrombocytopenia below 80,000/mm^3 were excluded from the procedure. All children underwent abdominal ultrasound performed the day before the procedure to exclude potential hemangiomas and malposition of the organs. All children were managed by Menghini procedure in sedation. Children aged less than 5 years received general anesthesia. 36 biopsies were ultrasound guided directly prior to the procedure (performed by the operator), 39 biopsies were blind. The ultrasound prior to the biopsy was performed to identify the intercostal space and to avoid accidental puncture of the gall bladder, the lung, right kidney and large vessels. Immediately after the procedure ultrasound examination was performed searching for potential complications such as accidental puncture or bleeding. In the case of blind biopsied ultrasound examination was performed by radiologists in situations where complications were suspected basing on clinical symptoms. All patients were monitored 24 hours after the procedure in the department for vital signs, pain and other consequences.

Histological evaluation was performed using Ishak scoring system for grading and staging.

Categorical variables were compared using Fisher's exact test or chi-square test were appropriate. Result with p value <0.05 were considered statistically significant.

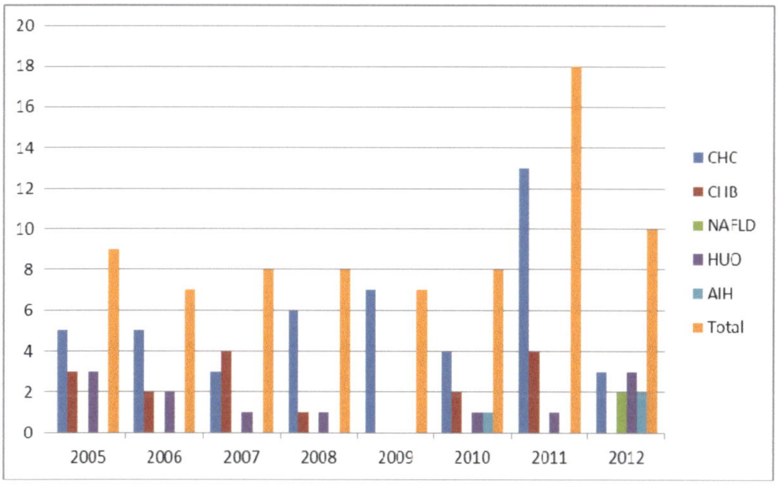

Figure 1. Number of liver biopsy performed in the Department of Infectious Diseases and Child Neurology due to various reasons in years 2005-2012 (until July) CHC- chronic hepatitis C, CHB – chronic hepatitis B, NAFLD – non-alcoholic fatty liver disease, HUO – hepatitis/hepatomegaly of unknown origin, AIH – autoimmune hepatitis

3. Results

Liver samples were obtained in all children. Adequate sample size was not obtained in the case of 5 children - 2 samples were to short and did not contain the adequate number of portal spaces, one sample was fragmented. Four inadequate samples resulted from the blind liver biopsy and 1 was obtained by the ultrasound guided procedure (p=0.21). No significant adverse events were observed. No clinical signs of hemorrhage, no cases of pneumothorax, puncture of the gallbladder nor severe infections were observed. Larger bile ducts were punctured in 4 cases – all undergoing blind procedure (p=0.07). 12 patient were complaining on pain in the right upper quadrant of the abdomen following the procedure that required more intensive analgesics – 3 undergoing ultrasound guided procedure, 9 having blind liver biopsy done (p=0.07). Pain was mild to moderate and resolved after analgesics. There were no deaths following the procedure in both groups of children.

Results from pathological assessment were presented in Table 1. The majority of children underwent liver biopsy due to CHC. Remaining indications were CHB, AIH, NAFLD, HUO. In patients with viral hepatitis grading and staging assessed according to Ishak scoring system was usually mild to moderate. Nevertheless, severe lesions were also present in some patients. Figure 2 and Figure 3.show examples of inflammatory changes and portal fibrosis in various patients with CHC. In patients with AIH and NAFLD diagnosis was confirmed by pathological assessment. Ten of HUO patients gained diagnosis either of metabolic disorders or NAFLD thanks to pathological evaluation. Normal liver histology was described in 2 patients.

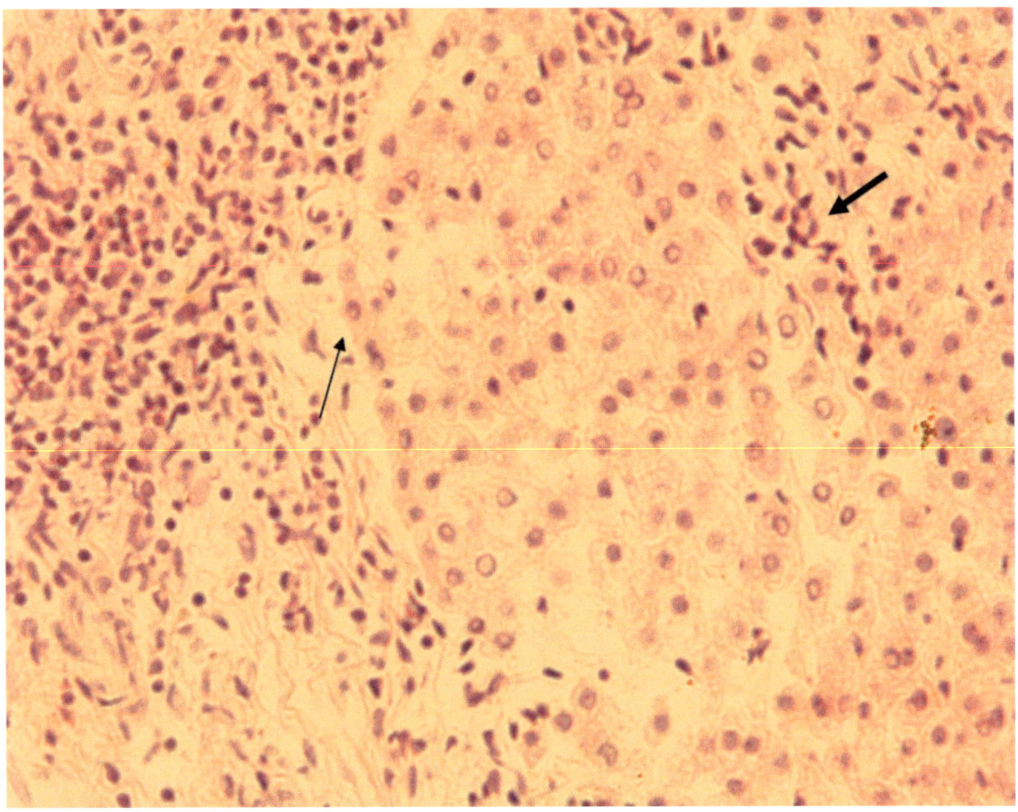

Figure 2. Liver biopsy specimen of the patient with CHC where inflammatory infiltrates cross lamina basalis of the lobuli (thin arrows) and intralobular focus of inflammatory infiltrate (thick arrow).Staining: hematoxylin+eosine. Magnification 40x

Fifteen children with viral hepatitis underwent repeated procedures allowing to assess the progression of lesions in time. In 9 of them the progression of lesions was described, 6 had similar results in both biopsies.

http://dx.doi.org/10.5772/52619

Indication for the biopsy	Result	Number of children
CHC - 44	Grading	
	1	23
	2	11
	3	5
	4	5
	Staging	
	0	1
	1	19
	2	17
	3	5
	4	2
CHB - 16	Grading	
	1	3
	2	8
	3	3
	4	2
	Staging	
	1	3
	2	7
	3	5
	4	1
NAFLD - 2	Steatosis	1
	Steatohepatitis	1
HUO - 12	Metabolic disorders	3
	Nonalcoholic steatohepatitis	6
	Wilson disease	1
	Normal liver histology	2
AIH - 3	Autoimmune hepatitis	3

Table 1. Histological assessment of the liver biopsy specimens performed in 75 children. CHC- chronic hepatitis C, CHB – chronic hepatitis B, NAFLD – non-alcoholic fatty liver disease, HUO – hepatitis/hepatomegaly of unknown origin, AIH – autoimmune hepatitis

4. Discussion

Studies describing the safety of liver biopsy performed on larger cohorts of patients seem to prove that the procedure results in more complications in children than in adults [5]. Nevertheless, Lebensztejn et al. described the group of 250 pediatric patients undergoing blind procedure with serious complications as internal hemorrhage and puncture of the gallbladder occurring in 3 children [6].

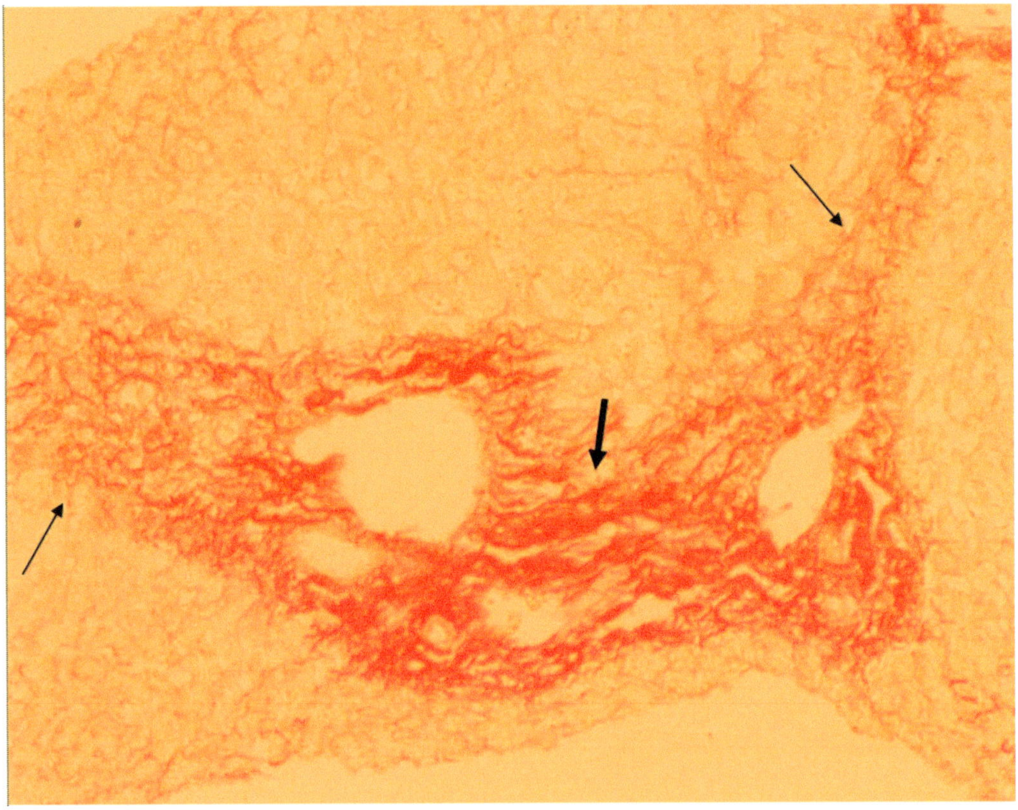

Figure 3. Syrius red staining of the liver specimen of CHC patient with present fibrosis in dilated portal space (thick arrow) and porto-portal bridging. Magnification 40x.

Number of biopsies in the current study was lower, however even the number of mild complications was relatively low. Moreover, no serious adverse events were noted among children from the study group. Noted complications included puncture of larger bile ducts and pain after the procedure. Although the results were not statistically significant, both problems were more frequent in children undergoing blind liver biopsy. Ultrasound assistance during the whole procedure was found to reduce the number of potential consequences [7]. Thus, ultrasound guidance even performed right before and after the biopsy makes the whole procedure safer. Since the majority of complications occur within first hours after the liver biopsy all children were monitored for 24 hours after the procedure as inpatients. Although hospitalization increases the costs of the procedure, monitoring enables quick response to encountered complications and prompt treatment, if necessary. Another issue is general anesthesia performed in small children in order to obtain liver sample. Although costly, general anesthesia decreases fear, pain and enables to perform the procedure in safe circumstances, reducing the risk of hemorrhage caused by lack of cooperation from the patient side.

The majority of children underwent the liver biopsy due to chronic viral hepatitis – mostly CHC. Histological assessment was not necessary to establish diagnosis since it is usually based on blood tests. However, information regarding grading and staging was essential for treatment decisions since the length of treatment may vary depending on the severity of lesions. In patients with CHB decisions regarding the initiation of the treatment may depend on the presence of lesions in the liver tissue [8]. In both types of chronic viral hepatitis patient with liver cirrhosis requires different approach than the child with mild lesions in the liver. In children with AIH the diagnosis was confirmed by the detection of specific inflammatory cells in the liver tissue. Although the number of NAFLD was small, the procedure distinguished between simple steatosis and steatohepatitis. Patients who underwent the procedure due to HUO benefited from diagnosis in 10/12 children. Metabolic disorders were detected in 3 patients and steatosis was detected in 6 children, 1 child was found to have Wilson's disease. Normal liver histology found in the specimens from the following 2 children with HOU raises questions regarding indications to the liver biopsy. The decision concerning the procedure was always carefully made basing on clinical and laboratory findings. Obtained results may be a consequence of the limitations of the procedure regarding sample size and sample error related to the site of the biopsy. Diffuse liver diseases are hardly ever evenly distributed in the organ.

Another problem with pathological assessment is an intraobserver variety. Except for skillful operator, an experienced pathologist is essential for proper evaluation of the samples. However, differences in the assessment between to various pathologists are difficult to avoid even with the use of validated scoring systems.

In recent years many non-invasive methods of liver assessment were developed. Imaging techniques allow to describesteatosis, focal changes, malformations, inflammatory processes of bile ducts and advanced fibrosis. Mild changes are, however, still difficult to detect. Elastography has been developed to evaluate liver stiffness being a useful tool to assess liver fibrosis [9]. Fibrosis is also evaluated by different serological markers and panels of direct and indirect markers or combination of both. Various cut-offs of the markers to detect advanced fibrosis and cirrhosis were validated in numerous studies [4]. Nevertheless, problem with intermediate stages of fibrosis still exist, since in such cases serological markers overlap.

Attempts to completely replace the biopsy with other non-invasive methods are not effective as the collection of adequate liver sample and proper histological evaluation allows to determine the extent ofthe liver damage and helps to establish the diagnosis.

5. Conclusions

Percutaneous liver biopsy is safe even in small children. Although severe complications are rare, patients require frequent monitoring. Ultrasound guidance seem to reduce the number of complications. Remaining a golden standard, the liver biopsy has certain limitations and drawbacks that influence the results.

Acknowledgements

This paper was supported by a grant from The Ministry of Science and Higher Education No –NN407 012036 to A. Mania

Abbreviations

AIH – autoimmune hepatitis, CHB – chronic hepatitis B,CHC – chronic hepatitis C, NAFLD – non-alcoholic fatty liver disease, HUO – hepatitis/hepatomegaly of unknown origin,

Author details

Anna Mania[1], Paweł Kemnitz[1], Magdalena Figlerowicz[1], Aldona Woźniak[2] and Wojciech Służewski[1]

1 Department of Infectious Diseases and Child Neurology, Faculty of Medicine, University of Medical Sciences in Poznan, Poland

2 Chair of Clinical Pathology, Faculty of Medicine, University of Medical Sciences in Poznan, Poland

References

[1] Sporea I, Popescu A, Sirli R. Why, who and how should perform liver biopsy in chronic liver diseases. World J Gastroenterol2008; 14(21): 3396-3402

[2] Cholongitas E, Senzolo M, Standish RA, Marelli L, Quaglia A, Patch D, Dhillon AP & Burroughs AK. A systemic review of the quality of liver biopsy specimens. Am J ClinPathol 2006; 125: 710–21

[3] El-ShabrawiMH El-Karaksy HM, Okahsa SH, Kamal NM, El-Batran G, Badr KA. Outpatient blind percutaneous liver biopsy in infants and children: is it safe? Saudi J Gastroenterol. 2012;18:26-33.

[4] Mania A, Kemnitz P, Mazur-Melewska K, Figlerowicz M, Służewski W. Non-invasive assessment of liver – serum markers and imaging techniques. In: Takanashi H. (ed.)Liver biopsy. Rijeka: InTech; 2011. p265-282.

[5] Potter C, Hogan MJ, Henry-Kendjorsky K, Balint J, Barnard JA. Safety of pediatric percutaneous liver biopsy performed by interventional radiologists.J PediatrGastroenterolNutr. 2011;53:202-6.

[6] Lebensztejn DM, Kaczmarski M, Sobaniec-Lotowska M, et al (2000). Blind liver biopsy in children—diagnostic significance and complications in authors' own material. Med SciMonit 6:1155–1158.

[7] Nobili V, Comparcola D, Sartonelli MR, Natali G, Monti F, Falappa P, Marcelini M. Blind and ultrasound-guided percutaneous liver biopsy in children. PediatrRadiol 2003; 33:772-775.

[8] Kemnitz P, Mozer-LisewskaI,Mania A, Michalak M, Wozniak A, Kowala-Piaskowska A, Figlerowicz M, Pohland J, Służewski W. Clinical importance of transcutaneous needle biopsy of the liver in children with chronic hepatitis B. Exp. ClinHepatol 2009; 5;38-43.

[9] Castera L, Vergniol J, Foucher J, Le Bail B, Chanteloup E, Haaser M, Darriet M, Couzigou P & De Ledinghen V. Prospective comparison of transient elastography, Fibrotest, APRI, and liver biopsy for the assessment of fibrosis in chronic hepatitis C. Gastroenterology 2005; 128: 343-350.

Chapter 5

Risks and Benefits of Liver Biopsy in Focal Liver Disease

Letiția Adela Maria Streba,
Eugen Florin Georgescu and Costin Teodor Streba

Additional information is available at the end of the chapter

http://dx.doi.org/10.5772/52620

1. Introduction

Even with the recent evolution of imaging techniques, and with the ever-increasing role of serum markers, direct analysis of tissue samples maintains its role in modern medicine. This is especially true for the diagnosis and assessment of the prognosis and evolution of a series of viral, tumoral and inflammatory liver diseases. Thus, liver biopsy and histological assessment of the liver parenchyma can still be called by many the "gold standard" in diagnosis and staging of associated disease. However, liver biopsy in itself implies a series of risks and inherent discomfort for the patient. With the increasing availability of other non-invasive methods routinely used in diagnosis and staging of liver-related diseases, many debate the necessity and ethical implications of tissue sampling.

In the following pages, we will try and synthetize the historical evolution of liver biopsy, describe the techniques used over the years and present its current recommendations and their alternatives, with focus on the so-called "virtual liver biopsy" techniques currently employed.

2. Historical landmarks and recent developments in liver biopsy

The first written documented report of a successful liver biopsy was made by Paul Ehrlich in the book "On diabetes" published in 1884. He published an account of the procedure performed in 1880 in Berlin, along with graphical illustrations of the instruments and the liver samples collected. This came detailed account was based on previous theoretical advantages of this technique discussed by the French physician AGM Vernois in 1844, who in turn based his assumption on successful procedures performed for puncturing purulent echinococcus, as early as 1825 (Récamier) and 1833 (Stanley). Cytology was reported as a diagnosis method for liver disease by L. Lucatello (in Rome) in 1895, while F. Schupfer performed liver and spleen biopsies with a thicker needle twelve years later, in 1907. This new approach provided cylindrical-shaped tissue samples which could be histologically prepared and analyzed [1].

Other scarce accounts of successful procedures followed in the next couple of decades (Olivet, 1926; Huard 1935; Silverman, 1938; Baron, 1939; Kofler, 1940; Dible, 1943), using different aspiration techniques performed with different modified biopsy needles [1].

A new stage in modern liver biopsy techniques was reached when, in 1957 and repeated in the following year, Menghini performed and reported on the first "one-second needle biopsy" performed with a special small caliber needle with no trocar and a sharp bevel. This was the first time needle liver biopsy was introduced worldwide as a praised diagnostic technique capable of providing enough histological material for an accurate interpretation of the pathological changes present in the parenchyma [1].

Following this radical advancement, liver biopsy became more spread and the technique evolved once modern imagistic methods allowed for better and safer puncturing of the liver parenchyma. Thus, the technique entered the image-guided age of investigation performed under computed tomography (CT) or ultrasound (US) real-time screening. Reports from Denmark, China, the United Kingdom, France or the United States of America populated the 1960–1980 literature, once the technique became widespread and fully acknowledged by the academic community. Its utility in diagnosing liver diseases and later on in staging hepatitis or malignancies was undisputed for entire decades of the 20th century [1].

Recent advancements, based on the advent of new imagistic high-accuracy techniques based on both US and CT/RM approaches, highly diminished the role played by this invasive investigation. The term "virtual biopsy" became more and more present in recent literature, once both doctors and patients alike became more confident and were introduced to these high-yield methods, such as Transient or Acoustic Radiation Force Elastography. Moreover, advanced serum markers (such as, for example, the Fibrotest-Actitest battery of tests) allow for an accurate non-invasive staging in hepatitis. The introduction of arterial uptake contrast-enhanced US and CT/RM techniques substantially decreased the role of biopsy in diagnosing liver biopsy [2–4].

However, histology remains one of the most accurate methods for evaluating liver parenchymal changes, and is always used in malignancies when the diagnosis is uncertain or when other non-invasive methods fail to provide an accurate staging for hepatitis. Along with these non-invasive techniques came a revolution in in-situ biopsy methods. Such is probe-based confocal laser endoscopy (pCLE), which uses miniaturized probes connected to a laser source through fiber optics, small enough to fit inside a biopsy needle, thus providing rapid live assessment of liver architecture [5].

3. Modern liver biopsy techniques and sampling adequacy

3.1. Percutaneous biopsy

All modern percutaneous liver biopsy techniques have rapidity as a common denominator. Either cutting or suction needles can be used for transthoracic or subcostal biopsy, either after palpation or imaging assessment of the puncturing zone, or, preferably, under continuous image guidance. The transthoracic approach is the preferred method used, under real-time US or (more rarely) CT guidance and after a thorough imaging investigation of the liver and puncture route. All percutaneous methods imply two phases, one extra-hepatic corresponding to the needle puncturing the skin and reaching the needle, and a hepatic stage in which the needle passes the liver capsule, collects the parenchyma material, and is swiftly extracted. It is considered a relatively safe procedure, complication rates varying between studies, from 0.75% up to 13.6% [6].

Trucut needles and their modified versions driven by spring-loaded biopsy guns are increasingly used and are the instruments of choice in many centers worldwide, especially in Europe [7]. Needle diameters vary between 1.20 mm to 1.60 mm, smaller calibers being used when a high risk of complications is suspected.

Suction needles are less expensive and their operation allows for rapid intra-hepatic handling, thus being easier to use and possibly imply less bleeding-related complications. The most widespread types are the Menghini, Jamshidi and Klatskin needles, which remained virtually unchanged since their introduction in the second half of the last century. The maximum required time for a complete syringe suction of the cytological material and the consecutive needle retraction is 0.5 seconds. The intrahepatic phase is reduced to as low as 0.1 seconds when the needle is operated by an expert practitioner [8].

Image guidance has become mandatory in centers where the gastroenterologist can perform his or her own US exam. Real-time surveillance of the procedure greatly decreases the risk of complications (such as bleeding) and minimizes post-procedural complaints such as pain or hypotension. Hepatologists in the United States usually prefer to have a radiologist performing the procedure under CT or US guidance [8].

3.2. Transjugular (transvenous) biopsy

The transjugular route is preferred when the risk for complications is high and therefore a percutaneous approach is not considered safe enough for the patient. Patients with clinical ascites, known hemostatic defect, cirrhotic liver with clinical signs of organ deficiency (smaller size and increased palpatory stiffness) or morbid obesity are usually prime candidates for this approach. Another situation when the transvenous approach is preferred is when additional pressure measurements in the hepatic vein are required [8].

The resources needed for this procedure are higher than percutaneous approaches; however, complication rates are lower (2.5% up to 6.5%) according to some authors [9], with mortality rates of approximately 0.09% in high-risk patient groups [10]. The expertise of the performing physician also plays a crucial role in the success rate of this procedure, and should be considered along with the higher resource costs when choosing this access route for a lower-risk patient [1].

Another very important aspect is the lower quality of the tissue specimens collected through the transjugular approach. The tissue cylinders are thinner and more fragmented than those obtained through percutaneous biopsy, and usually represent only 1-2 cm of the liver parenchyma, containing fewer portal fields [11].

3.3. Surgical or laparoscopic biopsy: Novel approaches for liver biopsy

This approach is preferred in patients with peritoneal involvement when an abdominal cancer is present, with associated ascites or peritoneal disease with ascites of suspected hepatic origin. Also, focal hepatic lesions can be targeted for biopsy through the laparoscopic channel.

Biopsy can thus be performed with either normal needle systems, or by wedge resection. However, the later approach may overestimate the level of fibrosis, as the resection is performed too close to the fibrotic capsule that envelops the liver. The procedure is always conducted under general anesthesia and requires controlled pneumoperitoneum by infusion of nitrous oxide, always performed by trained physicians, allowing for a good control of bleeding and a minimum set of complications due to the large working area created. In direct comparison with percutaneous biopsy, the laparoscopic approach provides a higher level of accuracy as it allows the evaluation of the surrounding peritoneum [12]. The main complications are related to the general anesthesia used for the procedure, the local abdominal and intra-peritoneal traumas associated, as well as the risk of bleeding, which is also present in the other types of biopsy.

Advancements to surgical techniques led to the development of the natural orifice transluminal endoscopic surgery (NOTES), a new surgically-derived endoscopic technique that uses a transgastric or transanal route to facilitate the access to the abdominal cavity. One recent study presented a liver biopsy performed through a transgastric flexible endoscopic device which permitted the inspection of the liver and surrounding intraperitoneal space. The technique can be applied to morbidly obese patients or to patients at high risk of complications [13]. This approach remains however limited at the present time to a few highly selected patients, and is performed only by trained surgeons and gastroenterologists, at moderate to high costs and in selected centers.

Recent studies also focused on evaluating the liver capsule in cirrhotic patients through pCLE inserted through a laparoscopic channel, this being a promising field in the advancement of minimally invasive biopsy techniques [14]. Another study describes the use of pCLE in a routine minilaparoscopy setting, performed under conscious sedation. The authors could describe subsurface serial images in real time, allowing for an in vivo analysis of the liver parenchyma [5]. This approach may lead the way to targeted biopsy through live assessment of the liver parenchyma, as well as immediate morphological and dynamic evaluation of intrahepatic structures.

3.4. Adequacy of liver biopsy samples

Analysis of the biopsy material under ultraviolet fluorescent light may be required in order to identify porphyria. Liver tissue obtained through biopsy is then quickly transferred into a buffer solution, usually 4% or 10% neutral formalin, to avoid the alterations it may sustain due to hepatic enzymes autolysis. It can then be subjected to various preparation techniques, in accordance to what diagnostic tests will follow with that specific sample (frozen section, RNA detection etc.) [1].

An adequate biopsy fragment is between 1 and 4 cm long, weighting between 10 to 50 mg, with a minimal diameter of 1 mm. Fragmented samples from Menghini needles are acceptable, as their added size is somewhere in the vicinity of 2 cm (usually range from 1 to 2.5 cm in length). In order to properly represent the parenchymal architecture, at least 10–11 portal tracts should be completely present, six being a minimally acceptable number. Specimens of inadequate lengths usually lead to understaging of fibrosis and underestimate the grade of inflammation. Cirrhotic parenchyma usually comes fragmented through biopsy, thus leading to approximately 20% sampling errors [15, 16].

As it is appreciated that a liver biopsy specimen represents 1/50 000 of the total organ mass, discussions regarding how representative it can be for diffuse lesions always existed in the literature [8, 17]. It is however appreciated that most diffuse (steatosis or inflammation etc.) or focal lesions (both malignant and benign), as well as structural lesions such as fibrosis can be visualized with a fairly high degree of accuracy, if the minimum amount of liver parenchyma and the required number of portal spaces are present. It was however demonstrated that the size of the sample is directly correlated to an underestimation of inflammatory changes [18], this paradigm being extended to fibrotic changes and has a direct effect on the subsequent grading and staging [1, 19, 20].

Another issue highly debated in literature is the inter-observer variability; even with the wide usage of quantification scores for both inflammation and fibrosis such as the Knodell [21] scoring system and the revised Ishak version [22] or the METAVIR score [23]. All interpretations are subjected to the experience and training of the pathologist, which is an independent variable in itself, separated from the inherent sampling and procedural errors. A second opinion is always recommended, and two pathologists are usually present in most large referral centers. Collaboration between the pathologist and the clinician performing the liver biopsy is also preferred, as some studies indicated [24–26].

The most important quantification parameters refer to its geometry and relationship between the principal compartments – portal tracts and the elements of the arterial vascular system; the configuration adopted by hepatocyte plates; the sinusoids and the perisinusoidal compartment; the amount of connective tissue, fat and the number of ducts present, as well as other normal cellular infiltrates of lymphoid origin [8]. Regenerative nodular hyperplasia or macronodular cirrhosis can be sometimes classified as normal parenchyma, and the inherent variations of normal inflammatory cellular infiltrate can be misleading for an inexperienced pathologist when observing low grade inflammatory lesions [8, 27].

4. Risks, complications and post-procedural complaints of liver biopsies

The main risks for a patient subjected to liver biopsy were already briefly discussed in the previous paragraphs. Their frequency and predisposition in certain patient groups are determinant factors for choosing one biopsy technique in favor of another. The risk of bleeding cannot be excluded with any instrument, and liver biopsy is not recommended in most cases of suspected primary liver cancers because of a needle track seeding of tumor cells. These however do not exclude liver biopsy as a last resort diagnostic tool, when imagistic or serum tests proved constantly inconclusive or do not converge to an outcome.

The most commonly occurring complication of percutaneous liver biopsy is pain, present in up to 84% of procedures and ranging from mild discomfort to severe pain [28]. It is usually located in the right upper quadrant and it is referred to the right shoulder, with various intensities and time of installment. Moderate to severe pain is present in fewer than 5% of all patients, and may be the sign of a more severe complication such as bleeding or the puncturing of the gallbladder [16, 29]. Mechanisms that lead to pain after the biopsy maneuver are not fully understood, however it is likely to be caused by bile or blood extravasation with subsequent capsule swelling (the only liver component with sensitive nervous terminations) [30]. Another cause of upper abdominal pain is the traction of the falciform ligament after the puncture. Cervical pain, as well as pain in the right shoulder, may also be caused by the irritation of the phrenic nerve. Subcapsular hematoma may lead to respiratory pain and irritation of the pleura or peritoneum may lead to vagal stimulation and consecutive vagal shock, manifested through bradycardia, severe hypotension, weak pulse and intense pain in the upper abdomen [1]. In some cases of extreme pain, hospitalization and further imaging tests are required to determine the correct course of action for these patients.

However, the most important complication of liver biopsy is bleeding. The most severe bleedings occur intraperitoneally, when they determine a drop in vital signs and can be visualized through imaging [16, 31]. Urgent hospitalization and blood transfusion, even followed by surgery or radiological intervention may be required. Nevertheless, these cases are scarce, with 1 in 2 500 up to 10 000 biopsies incidence, while less severe cases which do not require blood transfusions or surgical maneuvers are more frequent, approximately 1 in 500 biopsies [16]. Serious bleeding-related complications usually occur within 2 hours of the procedure, and over 90% of all bleedings become evident within 24 hours of the procedure. Clinical symptoms are revelatory, as patients experience hypotension and shock. Age and the underlying conditions also are predictive factors, as older patients and liver masses are more frequently associated with post-puncture bleeding. A correlation between the needle type and the risk for bleeding was also cited in literature, as cutting needle seem to pose an increased risk compared to their suction counterparts [15]. Other factors are related to operator experience, the diameter of the needles and their diameter [16].

A correlation between conventional coagulation tests and the risk of bleeding has not been sufficiently demonstrated until now; therefore no certain recommendations in this regard are currently in place [16]. The option to insert coagulation agents on the needle tract is considered, especially in the US, with no definite data on its ability to prevent possible bleedings. As already mentioned, the transvenous approach is preferred in certain categories of patients as it is considered safer, even though several pooled analyses showed similar risks with standard percutaneous methods [10,16].

The singular major complication of liver biopsy, caused in turn by consecutive severe bleeding is patient death. No consistent data regarding post-procedural mortality exists in the literature, the most commonly quoted rate being less or equal to 1 in 10 000 biopsies [16], and seems to be greater after biopsies of malignant liver masses compared to diffuse parenchymal disease [6].

Other complications of liver biopsies include the perforation of other viscous organs, bile peritonitis (major complication which can result in death), infections (especially in post-transplant patients due to immunosuppressive medication), hemobilia, pneumothorax (instantly recognized on radiographs, essentially to diagnose quickly due to high risk of death) or hemothorax. Correct usage of imaging methods both when choosing the biopsy site and for surveillance of the procedure minimizes many of these risks, especially those related to puncturing adjacent structures [16]. The risk of needle track seeding when puncturing liver malignancies exists in 1 to 3% of all cases [32], as will be detailed below.

5. Current recommendations regarding conditions that require liver biopsy

The indications for liver biopsy were greatly reduced since the recent introduction of accurate non-invasive tests which can evaluate liver parenchyma with minimal or no patient trauma. The concept of liver biopsy may evolve even further, if in vivo direct histological methods such as pCLE will provide important additional data. It is most likely that the recommendations for liver biopsy will suffer further changes in following years. A series of these advancements will be discussed separately within this chapter. Below, we will describe some of the main indications for liver biopsy, either for diagnostic purposes or for evaluating and staging liver disease.

5.1. Grading and staging of chronic viral hepatitis

The recent outburst of viral hepatitis cases (especially as a result of the increasing number of newly diagnosed virus C infections) represents a major health burden worldwide. With almost four million people being infected in the United States alone, and between 130 and 170 million worldwide, chronic hepatitis C virus (HCV) infections and more than double those figures for hepatitis B virus (HBV) infections, this ensemble of viral diseases currently represent the main cause of liver-related morbidity [33, 34].

Nowadays, the role of liver histology in the positive diagnosis of chronic viral hepatitis has greatly diminished. However, it still plays a central role when assessing both activity and progression of the disease [8, 35]. Sampling issues arise when evaluating liver parenchyma affected by chronic hepatitis, as the quality of the obtained specimens can greatly influence the semi-quantitative scores developed in the last four decades to quantify disease progression. There are a number of changes present within the liver and their heterogeneity makes the "10-complete portal spaces" paradigm essential when evaluating disease severity. All scoring systems are bound to yield significantly different results, primarily because of sample variability, but also as a result of the different levels of expertise from the pathologist involved in their evaluation. All modifications of the liver parenchyma – inflammation, necrosis or fibrosis – exhibit particularities and can be subjectively interpreted even in a scoring system [8].

The first approach to liver biopsy scoring for chronic hepatitis dates from the early 1980s when the histological activity index (HAI) was introduced by Knodell and Ishak [21]. This model did not clearly delimited between disease grades (that is, the importance of any inflammatory activity present) and stage, which refers to the degree of fibrosis and parenchymal remodeling. The later modification performed by Ishak resolves most of these issues and is currently used worldwide, partially replacing or at least complementing the earlier alternative Knodell classification. The preferred approach is a parallel evaluation using several scoring methods, such as the modified HAI, the Scheuer or the Ludwig systems and the Knodell classification, or the METAVIR algorithm devised in France [23].

5.2. Abnormal hepatic biochemical tests, alcoholic and non-alcoholic liver disease

Chronically elevated hepatic biochemical parameters are a common concern for many patients during routine screenings or general consults. Gastroenterologists facing abnormal aspartate aminotransferase/alanine aminotransferase, gamma-glutamyltransferase or alkaline phosphatase levels have to conduct a thorough anamnesis to determine the underlying condition. Many such patients either acknowledge high alcohol consumption or are diagnosed with non-alcoholic liver disease (NAFLD) associated with their lifestyle, while few remain undiagnosed until they begin to display signs of liver cirrhosis (cryptogenic cirrhosis or cirrhosis of unknown etiology). The latter two classes are usually diagnosed through liver biopsy, as no other condition can be found from either their background or non-invasive investigations and blood tests [8, 16].

The most common aspect revealed by liver biopsy in these patients is macrovesicularsteatosis, intracellular lipid accumulation exceeding 5% of the total cellular population. This macrosteatosis is generally coined as fatty liver disease (FLD) and can either be identified as either alcoholic liver disease (ALD), when regular alcohol consumption above established thresholds is established, or NAFLD when obesity, type 2 diabetes mellitus and/or hyperlipidemia are associated. Steatohepatitis, either of alcoholic origin (alcoholic steatohepatitis – ASH) or metabolic (non-alcoholic steatohepatitis – NASH) share histological similarities. NASH is recognized as a form of NAFLD with ballooning hepatocytes and necroinflammatory changes, as well as fibrosis and parenchymal remodeling. The NAFLD activity score (NAS) was developed in an attempt to objectively quantify the extension of this disease. This score sums the three pathologic features – steatosis, lobular inflammation and hepatocellular ballooning on a 0 to 8 scale, 5 being the cut-off point for a certain diagnose of NASH and 3–4 being labeled as borderline steatohepatitis [36, 37].

Currently, even though liver biopsy is still regarded as the "gold standard" when diagnosing these conditions, no consensus has been reached. Liver biopsy remains therefore a controversial decision which ultimately has to be performed only when a clear diagnosis cannot be extracted from serum values, imagistic findings and clinical features [38].

5.3. Metabolic liver disease

Diseases that determine intrahepatic iron accumulation are the main indications for liver biopsy when a metabolic condition is suspected, besides NAFLD or ALD. Hereditary hemochromatosis, in its various forms identified today, is routinely diagnosed and staged through liver biopsy [8, 39]. The metabolic syndrome (syndrome X) represents the increased accumulation of iron within hepatocytes, in the context of NAFLD. These deposits are not distributed equally among various regions of the liver, therefore deeper biopsies are needed in order to collect more tissue for analysis [8, 40]. For this purpose, at least two scores are currently used – the Deugnier and the Brissot scores [41, 42]. The hepatic iron index is calculated through a mathematical formula which takes into account the hepatic iron concentration (evaluated by liver biopsy), its atomic weight as well as the age of the patients. An index above 1.9 is an indicator of hemochromatosis; however its sensitivity is low as it is dependent on the timing of the liver biopsy [8].

5.4. Focal liver lesions

Discovery of a focal liver lesions (FLL) can occur after imaging tests used routinely for either screening or diagnosis. The practitioner may encounter lesions of various sizes, number and location, some of them being associated with pre-existing conditions. This is especially the case of primary liver malignant tumors, either hepatocellular carcinoma (HCC) or cholangyocarcinoma (CC). Early discovery of a FLL is possible in up to 60% of all cases, especially in developed countries where surveillance programs are well established and health services are available to the majority of the population, irrespective of their location and economic status [43, 44].

Imaging alone is currently the main diagnostic procedure for HCC, as modern contrast-enhanced techniques, either by CT or MRI, are sufficient to highlight the hallmark pattern of tumor vascularization. Diagnostic criteria in the United States of America, Europe and Asia stipulate that imaging techniques are sufficient to diagnose the majority of HCC lesions, biopsy being reserved for the few situations where imaging is unclear, discordance between two methods exists, or tumor size does not allow a precise imaging diagnosis [43–45]. A defining criteria for evaluating FLLs is the presence of an underlying hepatic condition such as hepatitis or cirrhosis.

When HCC is suspected in cirrhotic patients, criteria for liver biopsy are set by the size of the tumor. In nodules between 1 and 2 centimeters, diagnosis should ideally be based on non-invasive criteria; however, confirmation through biopsy should be sought whenever possible. The evaluation should be performed ideally by a pathologist with extensive experience in evaluating liver biopsies. In case of inconclusive findings after the initial biopsy, a second one should be performed if no other imaging criteria are present during the evaluation period. Nodules larger than 2 centimeters discovered through routine US should be ideally diagnosed through non-invasive procedures; however, when radiological findings are atypical, a liver biopsy should be obtained as confirmation [43–45]. A panel of immunohistochemical markers was proposed as diagnostic when evaluating liver biopsies for HCC. A combination of glypican 3, heat shock protein 70 and glutamine synthetase are recommended for the differential diagnosis between early HCC and high grade dysplastic nodules [46] (Di Tomaso et al, 2009). A final recommendation of the EASL-EORTC guidelines is that liver biopsy should be performed within controlled settings of scientific research, for identifying new markers for HCC and for tissue bio-banking[44].

The current tendency in diagnostic medicine is to avoid liver biopsy when evaluating HCC [44]. The main reasons against performing liver biopsy are the high rate of sampling errors which would diminish the sensitivity of the investigation; a higher rate of recurrence post-transplant in patients who underwent liver biopsy and finally the small but well-established risk of needle track seeding. In transplant referral centers, liver biopsy is performed more frequently, as there is an increased need for a correct final diagnosis; however, these procedures are subject to wide variation depending on country-specific regulations [43, 44]. Another argument for liver biopsy in HCC cases that benefit from chemotherapy would be the importance of histological grading. Response to local or systemic anti-angiogenic or anti-proliferative agents might be dictated by the microscopic configuration of the tumor and the amount of angiogenesis markers present on histological samples [16].

The second most important primary liver malignancy is CC. It can also develop in the presence of an underlying liver condition, such as chronic biliary tract diseases. Imaging diagnosis is sometimes difficult, as it may present similar contrast-enhancing patterns to those of HCC – the majority of CCs are solitary masses present in the hilum, while a minority can develop in other regions [43, 44]. Mixed forms of CC/HCC may also be present, their non-invasive diagnosis being even more difficult. All these forms of either atypical CCs or mixed presentations are usually subjected (with various degrees of variability, depending on setting and context) to liver biopsy. Surgical intervention, either by resection or liver transplant, are the approaches that yield the best survival chances for the patient. Therefore, liver biopsy may be indicated, as well as concomitant biopsy of lymph nodes in the upper abdominal area [16].

Metastases have the overall highest incidence amongst malignant liver lesions [47]. When a secondary malignant liver lesion is suspected and the physician cannot identify the primary point, liver biopsy is usually diagnostic, even when imaging fails to provide enough detail. If an underlying parenchymal disease is also suspected, biopsy should be performed outside the lesion site as well, for an extended and more precise diagnosis. A vast panel of markers may be employed in an immunohistochemistry study; however, the histologic architecture identified through normal techniques may be sufficient for an expert pathologist to determine the primary site of origin [1, 16].

Other rare primary liver parenchyma or bile duct malignant or benign neoplasms can ultimately be identified through histological analysis, after careful imaging-guided liver biopsy is performed. This diagnosis is often not possible on cross-sectional imaging studies as well as tumor serum markers, as their specificity for such lesions is inadequate. An expert hepatologist should closely collaborate with an experimented pathologist, as the diagnosis is difficult most of the times. These lesions may develop in the presence of an underlying liver condition, which would aid the clinical diagnosis or suspicion on the part of the clinician [1, 16].

The majority of lesions discovered through imaging techniques in patients without pre-existing liver conditions are benign in origin, mostly solitary or occasionally multiple. They exhibit particular vascular patterns in contrast-enhanced imaging techniques and are thus easily diagnosed without the use of invasive techniques. Such is the case of liver hemangiomas, mostly solitary benign tumors with characteristic contrast enhancement throughout all phases of an imaging investigation. Other lesions such as focal nodular hyperplasia are also usually solitary and may display distinct features such as "central scarring" or particular enhancement patterns (spiked wheel enhancement etc.). All these particularities have a morphological substrate: central hypoechoic areas which do not show vascular hyperenhancement usually correspond to areas of necrosis; intense signal enhancement zones are indicators of high microvessel density and neo-angiogenesis vessels; the US or CT peripheral rim translate in certain particularities of fibrous capsules [1, 16, 44].

Overall, lesions may present as cystic, solid or vascular; all these particularities usually being identified through non-invasive procedures prior to liver biopsy. In the USA for instance, liver biopsy is performed by imagists as they can perform the pre-biopsy or real-time assessment of the procedure, while in Europe most gastroenterologists or hepatologists perform the procedure themselves, under US surveillance [43, 44]. A core biopsy is usually preferred to fine-needle aspiration, as histology is considered superior from a diagnostic perspective compared to cytology; another reason being that experts in evaluating histology are more numerous compared to cytologists. The risk of puncturing blood vessels, either major arteries in the normal parenchyma, or intra-tumoral vessels is considerably diminished by real-time imaging guidance, for instance US with color Doppler. The risk of track seeding exists, even if extremely low (one study estimates a risk of 0.13%, while in other studies no such incidents were reported) [48, 49]. A certain dependency on the technique and size of the needle was also proven [50]. Infectious lesions may be biopsied; even if echinococcal cysts were considered an absolute contraindication as puncturing can be associated with anaphylactic shock and death, it was proven that these lesions can be aspirated with 19 or 22-gauge needles, taking all preparations for possible anaphylaxis [51].

6. Novel techniques in liver biopsy; modern non-invasive alternatives

6.1. Probe-based confocal laser endomicroscopy

The latest development in histological evaluation of gastrointestinal structures is confocal laser endomicroscopy. It allows for the in vivo evaluation of dysplasia and malignancies of the gastrointestinal tract, or in order to obtain directed biopsies that would allow rapid and more precise diagnoses [52, 53]. The first embodiments of this technique required dedicated endoscopes to be used for evaluating cavitary structures accessible from both ends of the digestive tracts.

Recent advancements however were able to miniaturize the technology so the imaging microprobe can be connected to 30,000 fiber-optic threads that enable point-to-point real-time detection at 12 frames/sec. The imaging device by itself measures less than 1.5 millimeters in diameter, thus allowing its use through 19G or tru-cut biopsy needles, or insertion by laparoscopy or NOTES [53]. This technology will allow in vivo, real-time imaging of liver histology, technically enhancing the capabilities of liver biopsy [54]. A few studies on animal models exist in the literature, detailing pCLE use for liver histological imaging [14, 55, 56]. The technique can be used for assessing the state of hepatocytes and the morphology of the liver tissue, or can be limited to the study of the exterior liver capsule, yielding interesting preliminary results in the setting of cirrhosis. Mennone et al reported interesting results regarding a fibrotic pattern and collagen deposits in animal models with cirrhosis induced by bile duct ligation [14]. The technology shows promise and may someday allow for safer histological assessment of patients with chronic liver disease irrespective of its advancement, either cirrhotic or having any extreme complications, such as HCC.

6.2. Non-invasive imaging and serum tests for the assessment of fibrosis

Transient elastography (TE, Fibroscan® developed by Echosens, Paris, France) and Acoustic radiation force impulse (ARFI) are two ultrasound-based methods for quantifying liver fibrosis without the need for histological assessment. Another approach is through serum markers of fibrosis quantification, processed in complex mathematical formulas which give a quantitative result for liver stiffness, such as the Fibrotest, Biopredictive and the aspartate transaminase to platelets ratio index (ARPI) approaches.

TE is a novel and rapid non-invasive examination which involves minimal patient discomfort over a relatively low time period (one examination may take up to 5-10 minutes depending on the skeletal and adipose conformations of the patient). The device consists of a hand-held vibrating unit with an ultrasound transducer probe mounted on its axis, which generates medium amplitude vibrations at a low frequency, thus inducing an elastic shear wave in the underlying tissue. The hand-held probe is connected to a modified tower US machine which registers the result and through the on-screen software interface presents the user with an elastogram as a function of depth in time. The patient lies on his/her side and the probe is placed against the skin on the median clavicle line, directed towards the anatomical location of the liver, at a 90 degrees angle with the skin surface. Its results are presented as kilo Pascals (kPa), units of applied force. A series of 10 measurements are mediated to present a final value of the liver stiffness, which is equivalent to an F-stage fibrosis measurement obtained through biopsy [2].

ARFI is another technology that uses short-duration, high-intensity acoustic pulses which in turn exert mechanical excitation upon the tissues, generating local displacement resulting in shear waves. Their velocity can be assessed in a selected cylindrical area of interest of 0.5 cm (length) x 0.4 cm (diameter), up to 5.5 cm below skin level. Its results are expressed as velocities, in m/s [4].

Fibrotest-Actitest (Biopredictive, France) is a serologic marker-based algorithm which represents an alternative to invasive biopsy techniques. It received clinical validation in patients with chronic hepatitis B and C, ALD and NAFLD. Fibrotest consists of a panel of markers designed for appreciating liver fibrosis: Gamma-glutamyltranspeptidase (GGT), Total bilirubin Alpha-2-macroglobulin, Haptoglobin, and Apolipoprotein A1. Necroinflammatory activity is appreciated through the Actitest component, which adds Alanine transaminase (ALT) to the above mentioned serum markers [3, 57]. All these tests are performed in validated laboratories due to their complexity and variability of their different components and their results are inserted in a complex mathematical formula through a web-based interface, the end-result being correlated with other quantitative score systems such as METAVIR, Knodell or Ishak [58].

The best results are provided by a combination of two or more non-invasive methods, one study in particular finding that Fibrotest and Fibroscan offers the best diagnosis performance compared to liber biopsy as a gold standard, at least for advanced fibrosis (F values beyond 2) or cirrhosis (F3 or F4) [2]. This conclusion was reached by another, more recent study performed by Boursier and his collaborators [59]. They diminish the number of patients who require liver biopsy, however, this procedure is not excluded in all cases. Some studies have shown a high variability between Fibroscan results, dependent of the body-mass index and population factors [60, 61]. A discordance between liver biopsy staging and the estimation provided by non-invasive methods has also been identified [34]. It was approximated that 30–40% of all patients investigated by a combination of non-invasive imagistic and marker-based methods still require liver biopsy, during either sequential or simultaneous protocols [60, 61].

7. Conclusion

Despite all its limitations and the advances in modern lesser invasive techniques, liver biopsy remains the gold standard for evaluating a wide array of liver diseases.

The main concern when turning to tissue sampling through biopsy is the risk/benefit ratio, the decision ultimately belonging to the clinician involved. The risks may at times be higher than the implied diagnostic outcome, in which case other methods are preferred for the diagnosis.

Currently, it is recommended that all interpretations should be based on proper tissue blocks, with the correct technique applied. It is preferred that more than one pathologist with extensive experience in liver pathology should formulate the final histological diagnosis. This is especially true for FLLs and liver malignancies, as benign features may at times overlap, making the diagnosis uncertain.

Modern imagistic techniques allow for precise non-invasive evaluation of liver fibrosis in the context of hepatitis; however, the correct methodology for interpreting these tests is yet to be established. Novel imagistic approaches may in time open new perspectives for liver biopsy, by providing in vivo, real time data on liver parenchymal features which would prove useful for accurate diagnosing of otherwise difficult to interpret pathologies.

Author details

Letiția Adela Maria Streba, Eugen Florin Georgescu and Costin Teodor Streba

University of Medicine and Pharmacy of Craiova, Romania

References

[1] Kuntz E, Kuntz H–D. Liver biopsy and laparoscopy. In: Hepatology: Textbook and Atlas. 3rd Edition (2008); pp 149–176. Springer, USA. 3540768386.

[2] Castéra L, Vergniol J, Foucher J et al. Prospective comparison of transient elastography, Fibrotest, APRI, and liver biopsy for the assessment of fibrosis in chronic hepatitis C.Gastroenterology. 2005;128:343-50.

[3] Halfon P, Munteanu M, Poynard T. FibroTest-ActiTest as a non-invasive marker of liver fibrosis". GastroenterolClin Biol. 2008; 32: 22–39

[4] Crespo G, Fernández-Varo G, Mariño Z, et al. ARFI, FibroScan®, ELF, and their combinations in the assessment of liver fibrosis: A prospective study. J Hepatol. 2012;57:281-7.

[5] Goetz M, Kiesslich R, Dienes HP et al. In vivo confocal laser endomicroscopy of the human liver: a novel method for assessing liver microarchitecture in real time. Endoscopy. 2008;40:554-62.

[6] Myers RP, Fong A, Shaheen AA. Utilization rates, complications and costs of percutaneous liver biopsy: a population-based study including 4275 biopsies. Liver Int 2008, 28:705-12.

[7] Bravo AA, Sheth SG, Chopra S. Liver biopsy. N Engl J Med. 2001;344:495-500.

[8] Zimmermann A. Biopsy and laparoscopy. In: Textbook of hepatology: From Basic Science to Clinical Practice, 3rd Edition. Rodes J (Ed.). (2007); pp 489–99. Wiley-Blackwell. Massachusetts, USA. 978-1-4051-2741-7.

[9] Mammen T, Keshava SN, Eapen CE, Raghuram L, Moses V, Gopi K, Babu NS, Ramachandran J, Kurien G. Transjugular liver biopsy: a retrospective analysis of 601 cases. J VascIntervRadiol 2008, 19:351-8.

[10] Kalambokis G, Manousou P, Vibhakorn S, et al. Transjugular liver biopsy - Indications, adequacy, quality of specimens, and complications - A systematic review. J Hepatol 2007;47:284-294.

[11] Cholongitas E, Senzolo M, Standish R, Marelli L, Quaglia A, Patch D, Dhillon AP, Burroughs AK. A systematic review of the quality of liver biopsy specimens. Am J ClinPathol 2006, 125:710-21.

[12] Denzer U, Arnoldy A, Kanzler S, et al. Prospective randomized comparison of minilaparoscopy and percutaneous liver biopsy: diagnosis of cirrhosis and complications. J ClinGastroenterol 2007;41:103-110.

[13] Steele K, Schweitzer MA, Lyn-Sue J, Kantsevoy SV. Flexible transgastricperitoneoscopy and liver biopsy: a feasibility study in human beings (with videos). GastrointestEndosc 2008;68:61-66.

[14] Mennone A, Nathanson MH. Needle-based confocal laser endomicroscopy to assess liver histology in vivo. GastrointestEndosc. 2011;73:338-44.

[15] Goessling W, Friedman FS (2006). Evaluation of the Liver Patient. In: The clinician's guide to liver disease, K. Rajender Reddy (Ed.),. SLACK Inc. USA: 1–31.

[16] Rockey DC, Caldwell SH, Goodman ZD et al. Liver biopsy. Hepatology. 2009;49:1017-44.

[17] Guido M, Rugge M. Liver biopsy sampling in chronic viral hepatitis. Semin Liver Dis. 2004;24: 89–97.

[18] Colloredo G, Guido M, Sonzogni A et al. Impact of liver biopsy size on histological evaluation of chronic viral hepatitis: the smaller the sample, the milder the disease. J Hepatol, 2003; 39, 239–244.

[19] Regev A, Berho M, Jeffers LJ et al. Sampling error and intra-observer variation in liver biopsy in patients with chronic HCV infection. Am J Gastroenterol. 2002; 97, 2614–2618.

[20] Siddique I, El-Naga HA, Madda JP et al. Sampling variability on percutaneous liver biopsy in patients with chronic hepatitis C virus infection. Scand J Gastroenterol. 2003; 38, 427–432.

[21] Knodell RG, Ishak KG, Black WC, et al. Formulation and application of a numerical scoring system for assessing histological activity in asymptomatic chronic active hepatitis. Hepatology 1981;1:431-435.

[22] Ishak K, Baptista A, Bianchi L, et al. Histological grading and staging of chronic hepatitis. J Hepatol 1995;22:696-699.

[23] METAVIR Cooperative Study Group. Intraobserver and interobserver variations in liver biopsy interpretation in patients with chronic hepatitis C. Hepatology. 1994; 20, 15–20.

[24] Bejarano PA, Koehler A, Sherman KE. Second opinion pathology in liver biopsy interpretation. Am J Gastroenterol 2001;96:3158-3164.

[25] Tomaszewski JE, Bear HD, Connally JA, et al. Consensus conference on second opinions in diagnostic anatomic pathology. Who, what, and when. Am J ClinPathol 2000;114:329-335.

[26] Hahm GK, Niemann TH, Lucas JG, Frankel WL. The value of second opinion in gastrointestinal and liver pathology. Arch Pathol Lab Med 2001;125:736-739.

[27] Kay EW, O'Dowd J, Thomas R et al. Mild abnormalities in liver histology associated with chronic hepatitis: distinction from normal liver histology. J ClinPathol. 1997; 50, 929–931.

[28] Eisenberg E, Konopniki M, Veitsman E, Kramskay R, Gaitini D, Baruch Y. Prevalence and characteristics of pain induced by percutaneous liver biopsy. AnesthAnalg 2003;96:1392-1396.

[29] Janes CH, Lindor KD. Outcome of patients hospitalized for complications after outpatient liver biopsy. Ann Intern Med 1993;118:96-98.

[30] Caldwell SH. Controlling pain in liver biopsy, or "we will probably need to repeat the biopsy in a year or two to assess the response". Am J Gastroenterol 2001;96:1327-1329.

[31] Huang JF, Hsieh MY, Dai CY, Hou NJ, Lee LP, Lin ZY, et al. The incidence and risks of liver biopsy in non-cirrhotic patients: An evaluation of 3806 biopsies. Gut 2007;56:736-737.

[32] Yu SC, Lo DY, Ip CB, et al. Does percutaneous liver biopsy of hepatocellular carcinoma cause hematogenous dissemination? An in vivo study with quantitative assay of circulating tumor DNA using methylation-specific real-time polymerase chain reaction.AJR Am J Roentgenol. 2004;183(2):383-5.

[33] Lavanchy D. The global burden of hepatitis C. Liver Int. 2009;29 Suppl 1:74-81

[34] Kim SU, Kim JK, Park YN, Han K-H. Discordance between Liver Biopsy and FibroScan® in Assessing Liver Fibrosis in Chronic Hepatitis B: Risk Factors and Influence of Necroinflammation. PLoS ONE. 2012; 7(2): e32233.

[35] Gebo KA, Herlong HF, Torbenson MS et al. Role of liver biopsy in management of chronic hepatitis C – a systematic review. Hepatology, 2002; 36:S161–S172.

[36] Zafrani ES. Non-alcoholic fatty liver disease: an emerging pathological spectrum. Virchows Arch, 2004;444:3–12.

[37] Mendler MH, Kanel G, Govindarajan S. Proposal for a histological scoring and grading system for non-alcoholic fatty liver disease. Liver International. 2005; 25:294–304.

[38] Streba LAM, Cârstea D, Mitruţ P, Vere CC, Dragomir N, Streba CT. Nonalcoholic fatty liver disease and metabolic syndrome: a concise review. Rom J MorpholEmbryol 2008;49:13-20.

[39] Franchini M, Veneri D. Recent advances in hereditary hemochromatosis. Ann Hematol. 2005;84:347–352.

[40] Moirand R, Mendler MH, Guillygomarc'hA et al. Nonalcoholic steatohepatitis with iron: part of insulin resistance-associated hepatic iron overload? J Hepatol. 2000;33:1024–26.

[41] Deugnier YM, Turlin B, Powell LW et al. Differentiation between heterozygotes and homozygotes in genetic hemochromatosis by means of a histological hepatic iron index: a study of 192 cases. Hepatology. 1993;17:30–34.

[42] Brissot P, Bourel M, Herry D et al. Assessment of liver iron content in 271 patients: areevaluation of direct and indirect methods. Gastroenterology. 1981; 80:557–565.

[43] Bruix J, Sherman M. Management of Hepatocellular Carcinoma: An Update. Hepatology. 2011 53(3):1020-2.

[44] EASL-EORTC Clinical Practice Guidelines: Management of hepatocellular carcinoma. Journal of Hepatology 2012;56: 908-943.

[45] Omata M, Lesmana LA, Tateishi R, et al. Asian Pacific Association for the Study of the Liver consensus recommendations on hepatocellular carcinoma. Hepatol Int. 2010; 4:439-474.

[46] Di Tommaso L, Destro A, Seok JY, et al. The application of markers (HSP70 GPC3 and GS) in liver biopsies is useful for detection of hepatocellular carcinoma. J Hepatol. 2009;50:746-54.

[47] Kasper HU, Drebber U, Dries V, Dienes HP. [Liver metastases: incidence and histogenesis].Z Gastroenterol. 2005;43(10):1149-57.

[48] Tung WC, Huang YJ, Leung SW, Kuo FY, Tung HD, Wang JH, et al. Incidence of needle tract seeding and responses of soft tissue metastasis by hepatocellular carcinoma postradiotherapy. Liver Int 2007;27:192-200.

[49] Bialecki ES, Ezenekwe AM, Brunt EM, Collins BT, Ponder TB, Bieneman BK, et al. Comparison of liver biopsy and noninvasive methods for diagnosis of hepatocellular carcinoma. ClinGastroenterolHepatol 2006; 4:361-368.

[50] Maturen KE, Nghiem HV, Marrero JA, Hussain HK, Higgins EG, Fox GA, et al. Lack of tumor seeding of hepatocellular carcinoma after percutaneous needle biopsy using coaxial cutting needle technique. AJR Am J Roentgenol 2006;187:1184-1187.

[51] Khuroo MS, Wani NA, Javid G, Khan BA, Yattoo GN, Shah AH, et al. Percutaneous drainage compared with surgery for hepatic hydatid cysts. N Engl J Med 1997;337:881-887.

[52] Hsiung PL, Hardy J, Friedland S, et al. Detection of colonic dysplasia in vivo using a targeted heptapeptide and confocal microendoscopy. Nat Med. 2008;14:454–458.

[53] Hoffman A, Goetz M, Vieth M, et al. Confocal laser endomicroscopy: technical status and current indications. Endoscopy. 2006;38:1275–1283.

[54] Ray K. Imaging: confocal endomicroscopy enables deeper in vivo imagingof human liver. Nat Rev GastroenterolHepatol 7: 417, 2010.

[55] Becker V, Wallace MB, Fockens P, et al. Needle-based confocal endomicroscopyfor in vivo histology of intra-abdominal organs: first results ina porcine model (with videos). GastrointestEndosc. 2010;71: 1260–1266.

[56] Goetz M, Deris I, Vieth M et al. Near-infrared confocal imaging during minilaparoscopy:a novel rigid endomicroscope with increased imaging planedepth. J Hepatol. 2010; 53: 84–90.

[57] Ngo Y, Munteanu M, Messous D, et al. A prospective analysis of the prognostic value of biomarkers (FibroTest) in patients with chronic hepatitis C. Clin Chem. 2006; 52: 1887–96.

[58] Imbert-Bismut F, Messous D, Thibault V, et al. Intra-laboratory analytical variability of biochemical markers of fibrosis (Fibrotest) and activity (Actitest) and references ranges in healthy blood donors. ClinChem Lab Med. 2004;42: 323–333.

[59] Boursier J, Vergniol J, Sawadogo A, et al. Thecombination of a blood test and FibroScan improves the non-invasivediagnosis of liver fibrosis. Liver Int 2009;29:1507–1515.

[60] Kim SU, Choi GH, Han WK, et al.What are 'true normal' liver stiffness values using FibroScan?: a prospectivestudy in healthy living liver and kidney donors in South Korea.Liver Int 2010;30:268-274.

[61] Das K, Sarkar R, Ahmed SM, Mridha AR et al."Normal" liver stiffness measure (LSM) values are higher in both leanand obese individuals: a population-based study from a developing country.Hepatology. 2012;55:584-593.

Chapter 6

Current Trends in Liver Biopsy Indications for Chronic Liver Diseases

Jean-François Cadranel and
Jean-Baptiste Nousbaum

Additional information is available at the end of the chapter

http://dx.doi.org/10.5772/52618

1. Introduction

At the present time, pathological examination of a liver fragment obtained by liver biopsy remains an essential diagnostic tool of numerous chronic liver diseases [1] Indications for liver biopsy (LB) have changed considerably over recent years due to the development of sensitive and specific tests for diagnosis of several chronic liver diseases (i.e., serology for hepatitis C, antimitochondrial M2 in primary biliary cirrhosis, genetic screening for hereditary hemochromatosis), but also because of intensive development during the last decade of non-invasive assessment of fibrosis using serum tests (FibroTest®, FibroMeter®, APRI score) and/or by physical methods such as pulsed elastography (FibroScan®), in particular, for chronic hepatitis C. Ultrasound-guided liver biopsy is often necessary to obtain a tumor fragment in cases of suspected primary or secondary liver malignancy and will not be discussed here [1]. In the present article, we will limit ourselves to indications of liver biopsy in diffuse parenchymal disease of the liver and its relative and absolute contraindications. Modalities for performing liver biopsy and complications will not be discussed here. Liver biopsy is an invasive procedure with possible complications; thus, individual benefits for the patient must be weighed against possible risks. Liver biopsy is indicated when the expected amount of information obtained exceeds the risks related to the procedure, when the diagnosis required for establishing a prognosis cannot be obtained without pathological examination of the liver, and finally, when the treatment decision depends on pathological results [1].

2. Indications for LB

Indications for liver biopsy in chronic liver disease have evolved (Tables 1,2). The main advantages of LB with respect to the etiology of liver disease are shown in Table 2 and will be detailed later. The indication for liver biopsy is appropriate when the treatment or prognosis will be modified by results of histopathological examination of the liver. However, liver biopsy is not appropriate when the therapeutic decision and/or establishment of a diagnosis does not depend on histological findings [1].

Indications	
For diagnostic purposes	- Combination of several parenchymal liver diseases - Abnormal liver tests of unknown origin *. - Fever of unknown origin. - Focal or diffuse abnormalities on imaging studies.
For prognostic purposes	- Assessment of known parenchymal liver diseases.
For research purposes	- Development of treatments related to results of histological analysis

* After complete check-up, according to (2)

Table 1. Indications for liver biopsy

Cause of liver disease	Diagnosis	Evaluation of fibrosis	Prognosis	Management
Hepatitis B	-	+++	+ (+)	+++
Hepatitis C	-	+++ (Non-invasive markers of fibrosis)	+ (+)	++++
Hemochromatosis	+/-	+++	+ (+)	+
Wilson's disease	++	+++	+	-
α-1 Antitrypsin deficiency	+	+++	Depends on lung status	+
Autoimmune hepatitis In particular, seronegative	+++	+++	+	++++
Primary biliary cirrhosis / overlap syndrome	++	+++	+++	++
Primary sclerosing cholangitis	++	+/0	0	+
Alcoholic liver disease	+/-	++	++	+
Severe acute alcoholic hepatitis	+++	NA	NA	+
Steatosis / steatohepatitis	+++	+++	+	+
Infiltrative lesions of the liver	++++	NA	NA	+
Medicinal cause	++	NA	NA	+
Follow-up after liver transplantation	++++	+++	+	+

NA: not applicable

Table 2. Utility of liver biopsy in clinical practice for diffuse parenchymal damage

http://dx.doi.org/10.5772/52618

Etiology	1997 Study [31] of 2,084 biopsies (%)	2009 Study [13] of 8,580 biopsies (%)
Hepatitis C	54.1	33.6
Delta hepatitis B	5.8	14.4
Hereditary hemochromatosis	4.3	1
Cholestatic disease of the liver (primary biliary cirrhosis. primary sclerosing cholangitis. chronic cholestasis)	4.3	3.7
Autoimmune hepatitis	1	3.5
Liver transplantation	3	12.
Miscellaneous	17.6	12.2
Metabolic steatopathy	unlisted	8.9

Table 3. Indications for liver biopsy. Evolutionary trend in France.

2.1. Chronic hepatitis C

Liver biopsy has long been the only reference for assessing necroinflammatory lesions and fibrosis in hepatitis C. Liver biopsy is most useful for evaluating the existence of co-morbidities: alcoholic liver disease, non alcoholic fatty liver disease and iron overload, which are especially common in patients with chronic hepatitis C. In 2002, the French consensus conference no longer recommended systematic liver biopsy in patients with consistently normal transaminases [2]. At that time, for patients recently contaminated with genotype 2 or 3 infection, without co-morbidity and/or when the indication was viral eradication independently of fibrosis data, then antiviral treatment could be undertaken without requiring LB [2]. Furthermore, liver biopsy is not useful when diagnosis of cirrhosis is obvious [2]. While abdominal ultrasonography is satisfactory for assessing the existence of steatosis, liver biopsy is needed in order to evaluate the existence of steatohepatitis, iron overload or alcoholic liver disease associated with hepatitis C. Such lesions are associated with more rapid fibrosis progression and a less favorable response to treatment. The major development over the last ten years, spurred by French teams, of non-invasive assessment of fibrosis during the course of hepatitis C has significantly reduced indications for liver biopsy in patients with chronic hepatitis C. Several serum tests (FibroTest®, FibroMeter®, Hepascore®) are currently being validated by the French High Authority of Health for establishing extent of fibrosis in patients with untreated chronic hepatitis C and no co-morbidity [3-5]. The FibroTest has been validated by numerous studies and several independent teams [6]. The FibroMeter ® virus [9] has also been the subject of independent validations by different teams. FibroScan ® is useful for confirming or ruling out the presence of cirrhosis [7, 8], and for patients with HIV-HCV co-infection. In a recent survey, the use of liver biopsy was reduced by 50 % for chronic hepatitis C patients [9]. Most hepatologists in France no longer recommend first-line liver biopsy for chronic hepatitis C (Table 4). Discrepancy between results of serum fibrosis markers and FibroScan®, when performed simultaneously, is an indication for liver biopsy.

Transparietal liver biopsy	Transjugular liver biopsy
Absolute contraindications:	Hydatid cyst
Absence of patient cooperation	Cholangitis
Clotting abnormalities (see text)	Bile duct dilatation
Need to maintain anticoagulants or antiplatelets	Uncorrected hemostasis deficits
Vascular lesion along the puncture route	
Non-percussive or non-identifiable liver	
Hydatid cyst	
Suspicion of amyloidosis	
Relative contraindications	
Morbid obesity	
Ascites	
Infection of the right pleural cavity	

Table 4. Contraindications to transjugular and transparietal liver biopsy

2.2. Hepatitis B and hepatitis B-delta

Serum markers of non-invasive necroinflammatory lesions and fibrosis in hepatitis B and B-delta have not been fully validated, nor has the FibroScan [10, 11]. Scientific institutions recommend that liver biopsy be performed prior to any treatment decision in the context of chronic hepatitis B or B-delta. Liver biopsy is the best means of assessing necroinflammatory lesions and fibrosis in chronic hepatitis B [12]. The evolutionary trend in indications for liver biopsy for hepatitis C and B has been inverted over the last twelve years: the number of liver biopsies for hepatitis C in 2009 represented 33.6%, compared to 54.1% in 1997, this trend being related to development of non-invasive measures for assessing fibrosis; however, the number of liver biopsies for hepatitis B and delta-B has tripled in France [13] (Table 4). This is probably related to the increased number of patients with hepatitis B in France and the emergence of more effective treatment, along with insufficient validation of non-invasive fibrosis assessment methods.

2.3. Alcoholic liver disease

Liver biopsy remains essential in case of severe acute alcoholic hepatitis with Maddrey function above 32. In this situation, lesions of acute alcoholic hepatitis are absent in 20% of cases [14], while the benefit of corticosteroids in the absence of alcoholic hepatitis lesions has not been demonstrated with an increased risk of bacterial infection. However, this point has been debated by some authors [15]. When there are no signs of severe acute alcoholic hepatitis and if extensive fibrosis or cirrhosis is suspected, then the Fibrotest® [16]and FibroScan® [17] give satisfactory diagnostic performances.

2.4. Non alcoholic fatty liver disease

In patients with hepatic steatosis as part of the metabolic syndrome, liver biopsy is useful for differentiating fatty lesions from steatohepatitis (NASH), the evolutionary potential of which is much more severe (risk of cirrhosis and hepatocellular carcinoma). The presence of body mass index > 30 kg/m^2, AST/ALT ratio > 1, hypertriglyceridemia > 1.7 mmol/L, age > 50 years and a syndrome of insulin resistance are predictors of steatohepatitis and fibrotic lesions. When elements of metabolic syndrome exist with or without steatosis visualized on ultrasonography, then LB performed for what is referred to as "unexplained" cytolysis leads to a diagnosis of steatosis and steatohepatitis lesions in 60% of the cases [18]. Liver biopsy enables accurate diagnosis of lesions and evaluation of the degree of fibrosis [1]. It should be noted, however, that in this setting, steatosis FibroMeter ® [19] and Fibromax® [20] can provide evidence of the existence of fibrosis and can predict the existence of NASH.

2.5. Cholestatic liver diseases, and autoimmune diseases of the liver

Diagnosis of primary biliary cirrhosis is based on identification of cholestasis associated with antimitochondrial M2 antibodies. Liver biopsy is not useful for diagnosis of primary biliary cirrhosis [21], but is very useful for assessing the activity and extent of fibrotic lesions. FibroScan® in this indication can assess the presence or absence of cirrhosis [22]. Liver biopsy is useful in case of a poor response to ursodeoxycholic acid and/or in case of a drastic increase of transaminases. Liver biopsy is able to reveal moderate to severe lymphocytic piecemeal necrosis that may fit into the context of overlap syndrome, requiring a change in therapy and the addition of corticosteroids. During the course of autoimmune hepatitis [1, 23] , liver biopsy is necessary to assess piecemeal necrotic lesions and fibrosis stage. It is especially helpful in the absence of antibodies. In autoimmune hepatitis, no method of noninvasive evaluation of fibrosis has been developed. Liver biopsy is also necessary prior to discontinuation of immunosuppressive therapy, since the presence of histological piecemeal necrotic lesions is associated with almost constant recurrence of outbreaks of cytolysis deleterious to the liver [24]. When confronted with possible chronic cholestasis, the diagnosis of primary sclerosing cholangitis is based on data from the magnetic resonance cholangiopancreatography (MRCP)[21]. Liver biopsy often confirms the diagnosis, but can appear normal in 25% of the cases. When MRCP is normal, liver biopsy enables diagnosis of cholangitis of small bile ducts and, in all cases, helps to clarify lesions due to hepatic fibrosis [1, 21].

2.6. Genetic hemochromatosis

Diagnosis of hereditary HFE-gene-related hemochromatosis is based on the association of hyperferritinemia with elevated saturation of transferrin and presence of the C282Y mutation in the homozygous state. Thus, liver biopsy is not mandatory for diagnosis. It is still indicated, however, when serum ferritin is higher than 1,000 μg/L, and/or when the AST are increased and/or if hepatomegaly is present [25]. Simple markers (platelet count and transaminases, possibly combined with the dosage of hyaluronic acid and/or use of FibroScan) can indicate the existence or absence of extensive fibrosis and help to guide indications for liver biopsy.

2.7. Unexplained abnormal liver tests

Liver biopsy is often proposed in case of unexplained abnormal liver tests, when physical examination, biochemical and serological tests, imaging investigation could not establish a diagnosis. In one study including 354 patients, non alcoholic fatty liver disease was the definite diagnosis in 64 % of the cases. Other lesions included drug induced liver injury, alcohol-related liver disease, auto-immune hepatitis, primary sclerosing cholangitis,primary and secondary biliary cirrhosis, hemochromatosis, amyloid and glycogen storage disease, and cryptogenic hepatitis [26]. In another study including 272 patients, NAFLD represented 59.5 % of the cases [18].

2.8. Other indications (Table 3)

Liver biopsy is essential for the diagnosis of rare diseases of the liver such as Wilson's disease, wherein the hepatic copper concentration has to be measured, a deficiency in alpha-1 antitrypsin with evidence of PAS-positive cells, overload diseases such as Gaucher's disease, and amyloidosis, when there exists no other alternative [2]. In case of amyloidosis, liver biopsy should be performed via the transjugular route, since there is a major risk of bleeding in case of LBP performed via the transparietal route. Liver biopsy also helps in diagnosing rare diseases (nodular regenerative hyperplasia, congenital hepatic fibrosis) in case of prolonged abnormal liver function tests [1]. In case of severe acute hepatitis, emergency liver biopsy performed via the transjugular route may be particularly useful for diagnosing seronegative autoimmune hepatitis, infiltrative lesions of the liver, hepatitis or herpes [1]. Liver biopsy is essential for diagnosis of abnormalities in liver function tests when monitoring patients after liver transplantation in order to give a positive differential diagnosis of the following anomalies: rejection, infection, drug-induced liver injury, bile duct injury and viral reinfection. In case of hepatitis C virus recurrence in the liver transplant, liver biopsy is indicated; however, the FibroScan® is currently being assessed for evaluating damage from hepatic fibrosis. In case of suspected drug-induced hepatitis, liver biopsy may be useful if biochemical abnormalities persist beyond 3 months after cessation of treatment or if there is evidence suggesting injury to the bile ducts, such as a prolonged cholestatic syndrome.

It is essential that the pathologist be provided with relevant and complete clinical and biological information. Such information should be available before performing liver biopsy in suspected cases of rare diseases of the liver, or when bacteriological seeding or special staining has to be performed [1], so that the fresh liver fragment is immediately transmitted to the pathology or microbiology laboratory.

http://dx.doi.org/10.5772/52618

3. Limitations

Liver biopsy has remained the "gold standard" for years. However, it is imperfect since a large biopsy is required to make an accurate assessment of fibrotic stage and inflammatory grade. Pathologists estimated that a 25 mm-long fragment obtained with a 16-G needle was necessary to accurately determine the grade of chronic liver disease [27]. Colloredo et al. showed that eleven to fifteen complete portal tracts was the minimal number below which disease stage was significantly underestimated [28]. In a large review of the literature including 10,027 LB, Cholongitas et al. showed that the mean ± SD length was 17.7±5.8 mm and the mean ± SD number of portal tract was 7.5±5.8 [29]. This implies that at least two passes would be necessary to obtain a 2.5 cm long specimen, thus potentially increasing the risk of complications.

4. Optimal methods for carrying out lb in 2012

Methods for performing LB will not be detailed here, but are available in practical guidelines [30]. Several issues will be addressed:

When all conditions are met, then "ambulatory" liver biopsy may be performed [30]. In the study published in 2000 (completed in 1997) [31], 27% of liver biopsies were performed on an outpatient basis, most often for chronic hepatitis C; this figure is currently at 45% [13]. Several French teams have shown that outpatient liver biopsy is a safe and effective procedure and that liver biopsy performed on an outpatient basis reduces discomfort and increases the acceptability of subsequent examination conducted under the same conditions. If all conditions are not met and/or if organizational arrangements do not permit it, then liver biopsy should be performed via traditional hospitalization.

LB is carried out by hepatogastroenterologists, radiologists and occasionally by surgeons. Currently, liver biopsy is performed in France by a hepatogastroenterologist in 63.5% of cases, by a radiologist in 34.8% of cases and by a surgeon in 1.7% of cases [13]. The increasing number of liver biopsies performed by radiologists in France is linked to an increased number of biopsies performed using ultrasound guidance or guided real-time ultrasonography [30] and by the development of the transvenous route as compared to the transparietal route. Indeed, in 1997, 9% of liver biopsies were performed via the transvenous route compared to 22.4% in 2009 [13]. In the US, 50% of biopsies are performed by radiologists. In that country, it is felt that the number of LB performed in order to gain sufficient expertise is at least 40, carried out in the presence of an experienced radiologist [1].

5. Absolute and relative contraindications for LB

Absolute and relative contraindications for LB depend on the surgical approach recommended. Contraindications for liver biopsy using the transjugular or transparietal route [1, 30] are summarized in Table 4.

5.1. Lack of patient cooperation

Absence of patient cooperation is an absolute contraindication for transparietal LB. Indeed, in case of uncontrolled respiratory movements or agitation of the patient, the biopsy needle may cause a tear in the liver capsule, bleeding or a pneumothorax. If the patient is unable to maintain breath holding, or in the absence of expected cooperation, the question of the appropriateness of the indication for liver biopsy must be raised. If this indication is maintained, then liver biopsy under general anesthesia might be necessary, eventually via the transvenous route.

5.2. Hemostasis disorders, history of unexplained bleeding, hemostatic disease

It is recommended that transparietal liver biopsy should not be performed if the prothrombin rate is less than 50%, the platelet count is below 50 Giga/L or 60 Giga/L, if activated partial thromboplastine time is greater than 1.5-fold that of the control or when bleeding time is lengthened. The need for maintaining an anticoagulant or an antiplatelet is also a contraindication to transparietal LB. Likewise, the existence along the puncture route of a hemangioma or a vascular tumor is a contraindication for liver biopsy without real-time guidance. In this case, ultrasound-guided liver biopsy may eventually be used [1]. For patients with hemophilia, transvenous liver biopsy can be performed safely after correction of anomalies. In this indication, non-invasive blood markers of fibrosis and FibroScan® are particularly useful.

5.3. Impossibility of carrying out liver detection

The incapacity to detect the liver by percussion or ultrasound is an absolute contraindication to performing transparietal liver biopsy, as is suspicion of hydatid cyst.

5.4. Dilatation of extrahepatic or cholangitic bile ducts

Dilatation of the extrahepatic bile ducts and cholangitis are contraindications to transparietal liver biopsy [1].

5.5. Relative contraindications

Morbid obesity, severe ascites persisting after evacuation and infection of the right pleural cavity are contraindications for transparietal liver biopsy [1]. The transvenous route can be used in all these settings, and especially in case of significant ascites, morbid obesity, vascular liver, anticoagulant or antiplatelet treatment that cannot be stopped, hemodialysis, chronic renal failure or suspicion of amyloidosis when liver biopsy is necessary. Contraindications for the transvenous route include bacterial cholangitis, hydatic cyst and uncorrected deficits in hemostasis [1, 30].

6. Reducing the risk of complications

Compliance with absolute and relative contraindications for liver biopsy should lead to a decrease in serious accidents due to LB, the presentation of which is beyond the scope of this paper. Liver biopsy is an invasive procedure with the possible risk of severe complications, approximately 0.5/1,000 [1, 30]. Liver biopsy is a procedure for which there exists residual mortality [32]. Although serious complications have decreased over time, mortality after performing transparietal liver biopsy remains at 0.2% and deaths related to liver biopsy for diffuse parenchymal liver amount to 1 out of 10,000 LB [32].This risk, however, has decreased dramatically over time because of improvement in indications for liver biopsy and compliance with contraindications [32].

7. Conclusion

Liver biopsy remains useful for making an etiological diagnosis and a prognostic evaluation of many non-viral liver diseases, particularly in the context of autoimmune liver diseases, as well as for monitoring liver transplant patients. Liver biopsy is of great value in cases of several associated parenchymal diseases, so as to determine the extent of each, especially in hepatitis C. However, within the setting of isolated hepatitis C without co-morbidity, we feel that first-line LB is no longer appropriate.

The authors declare that they have no conflicts of interest.

Author details

Jean-François Cadranel[1] and Jean-Baptiste Nousbaum[2]

1 Service d'Hépato-Gastroentérologie et de Nutrition,Centre Hospitalier Laënnec, France

2 Service d'Hépato-Gastroentérologie, Hôpital de la Cavale Blanche, Brest, France

References

[1] Rockey DC, Caldwell SH, Goodman ZD, Nelson RC, Smith AD. Liver biopsy. Hepatology. 2009; 49(3):1017-44..

[2] Dhumeaux D, Marcellin P, Lerebours E. Treatment of hepatitis C. The 2002 French consensus. Gut. 2003; 52(12):1784-7.

[3] Imbert-Bismut F, Ratziu V, Pieroni L, Charlotte F, Benhamou Y, Poynard T. Biochemical markers of liver fibrosis in patients with hepatitis C virus infection: a prospective study. Lancet. 2001; 357(9262):1069-75.

[4] Leroy V, Hilleret MN, Sturm N, Trocme C, Renversez JC, Faure P, et al. Prospective comparison of six non-invasive scores for the diagnosis of liver fibrosis in chronic hepatitis C. Journal of hepatology. 2007; 46(5):775-82.

[5] Cales P, Oberti F, Michalak S, Hubert-Fouchard I, Rousselet MC, Konate A, et al. A novel panel of blood markers to assess the degree of liver fibrosis. Hepatology. 2005; 42(6):1373-81.

[6] Halfon P, Bourliere M, Deydier R, Botta-Fridlund D, Renou C, Tran A, et al. Independent prospective multicenter validation of biochemical markers (fibrotest-actitest) for the prediction of liver fibrosis and activity in patients with chronic hepatitis C: the fibropaca study. The American journal of gastroenterology. 2006; 101(3): 547-55.

[7] Castera L, Vergniol J, Foucher J, Le Bail B, Chanteloup E, Haaser M, et al. Prospective comparison of transient elastography, Fibrotest, APRI, and liver biopsy for the assessment of fibrosis in chronic hepatitis C. Gastroenterology. 2005; 128(2):343-50.

[8] Ziol M, Handra-Luca A, Kettaneh A, Christidis C, Mal F, Kazemi F, et al. Noninvasive assessment of liver fibrosis by measurement of stiffness in patients with chronic hepatitis C. Hepatology. 2005; 41(1):48-54.

[9] Castera L, Denis J, Babany G, Roudot-Thoraval F. Evolving practices of non-invasive markers of liver fibrosis in patients with chronic hepatitis C in France: time for new guidelines? Journal of hepatology. 2007; 46(3):528-9; author reply 9-30.

[10] Myers RP, Tainturier MH, Ratziu V, Piton A, Thibault V, Imbert-Bismut F, et al. Prediction of liver histological lesions with biochemical markers in patients with chronic hepatitis B. Journal of hepatology. 2003; 39(2):222-30.

[11] Marcellin P, Ziol M, Bedossa P, Douvin C, Poupon R, de Ledinghen V, et al. Non-invasive assessment of liver fibrosis by stiffness measurement in patients with chronic hepatitis B. Liver International (2009); 29(2):242-7.

[12] EASL Clinical Practice Guidelines: management of chronic hepatitis B. Journal of hepatology. 2009; 50(2):227-42.

[13] Cadranel JF, Nousbaum, Hanslik B. Major trends in liver biopsy practices in France: Results of an national multicenter survey in 2009 and comparison with 1997. Journal of hepatology. 2011; 54:S137.

[14] O'Shea RS, Dasarathy S, McCullough AJ. Alcoholic liver disease. Hepatology. 2010; 51(1):307-28..

[15] Forrest EH, Gleeson D. Is a liver biopsy necessary in alcoholic hepatitis? Journal of hepatology. 2012; 56(6):1427-8.

[16] Naveau S, Gaude G, Asnacios A, Agostini H, Abella A, Barri-Ova N, et al. Diagnostic and prognostic values of noninvasive biomarkers of fibrosis in patients with alcoholic liver disease. Hepatology. 2009; 49(1):97-105.

[17] Nguyen-Khac E, Chatelain D, Tramier B, Decrombecque C, Robert B, Joly JP, et al. Assessment of asymptomatic liver fibrosis in alcoholic patients using fibroscan: pro-

spective comparison with seven non-invasive laboratory tests. Alimentary pharmacology & therapeutics. 2008; 28(10):1188-98.

[18] de Ledinghen V, Ratziu V, Causse X, Le Bail B, Capron D, Renou C, et al. Diagnostic and predictive factors of significant liver fibrosis and minimal lesions in patients with persistent unexplained elevated transaminases. A prospective multicenter study. Journal of hepatology. 2006; 45(4):592-9.

[19] Cales P, Laine F, Boursier J, Deugnier Y, Moal V, Oberti F, et al. Comparison of blood tests for liver fibrosis specific or not to NAFLD. Journal of hepatology. 2009; 50(1): 165-73.

[20] Poynard T, Ratziu V, Charlotte F, Messous D, Munteanu M, Imbert-Bismut F, et al. Diagnostic value of biochemical markers (NashTest) for the prediction of non alcoholosteato hepatitis in patients with non-alcoholic fatty liver disease. BMC gastroenterology. 2006; 6,34.

[21] EASL Clinical Practice Guidelines: management of cholestatic liver diseases. Journal of hepatology. 2009; 51(2):237-67.

[22] Corpechot C, El Naggar A, Poujol-Robert A, Ziol M, Wendum D, Chazouilleres O, et al. Assessment of biliary fibrosis by transient elastography in patients with PBC and PSC. Hepatology. 2006; 43(5):1118-24.

[23] Manns MP, Czaja AJ, Gorham JD, Krawitt EL, Mieli-Vergani G, Vergani, D., et al. Diagnosis and management of autoimmune hepatitis. Hepatology, 2010; 51(6):2193-213.

[24] Verma S, Gunuwan B, Mendler M, Govindarajan S, Redeker A. Factors predicting relapse and poor outcome in type I autoimmune hepatitis: role of cirrhosis development, patterns of transaminases during remission and plasma cell activity in the liver biopsy. The American journal of gastroenterology. 2004; 99(8):1510-6.

[25] Guyader D, Jacquelinet C, Moirand R, Turlin B, Mendler MH, Chaperon, J., et al. Noninvasive prediction of fibrosis in C282Y homozygous hemochromatosis. Gastroenterology. 1998; 115(4):929-36.

[26] Skelly MM, James PD, Ryder SD. Findings on liver biopsy to investigate abnormal liver function tests in the absence of diagnostic serology. Journal of hepatology. 2001; 35(2):195-9.

[27] Bedossa P, Dargere D, Paradis V. Sampling variability of liver fibrosis in chronic hepatitis C. Hepatology. 2003; 38(6):1449-57.

[28] Colloredo G, Guido M, Sonzogni A, Leandro G. Impact of liver biopsy size on histological evaluation of chronic viral hepatitis: the smaller the sample, the milder the disease. Journal of hepatology, 2003; 39(2):239-44.

[29] Cholongitas E, Senzolo M, Standish R, Marelli L, Quaglia A, Patch D, et al. A systematic review of the quality of liver biopsy specimens. American journal of clinical pathology. 2006; 125(5):710-21.

[30] Nousbaum JB, Cadranel JF, Bonnemaison G, Bourliere M, Chiche L, Chor H, et al. [Clinical practice guidelines on the use of liver biopsy]. Gastroenterologie clinique et biologique. 2002; 26(10):848-78.

[31] Cadranel JF, Rufat P, Degos F. Practices of liver biopsy in France: results of a prospective nationwide survey. For the Group of Epidemiology of the French Association for the Study of the Liver (AFEF). Hepatology. 2000; 32(3):477-81.

[32] West J, Card TR. Reduced mortality rates following elective percutaneous liver biopsies. Gastroenterology. 2010; 139(4):1230-7.

Chapter 7

Primary and Metastatic Tumours of the Liver: Expanding Scope of Morphological and Immunohistochemical Details in the Biopsy

Ilze Strumfa, Janis Vilmanis, Andrejs Vanags, Ervins Vasko, Dzeina Sulte, Zane Simtniece, Arnis Abolins and Janis Gardovskis

Additional information is available at the end of the chapter

http://dx.doi.org/10.5772/52838

1. Introduction

Evaluation of liver biopsy for tumour diagnostics is a highly practical task with major clinical influence. The liver is frequently affected by wide spectrum of neoplasms including benign tumours as well as primary malignancies [1-3]. In addition, due to the rich dual blood flow to liver, secondary malignant tumours also often develop here. In order to ensure the optimal management of the patient, a correct diagnosis is necessary. At present, biopsy is the gold standard in oncology [4-5].

The scope of liver neoplasms can be following. The benign tumours include hepatic adenoma, bile duct adenoma, cavernous haemangioma and angiomyolipoma, among others. The primary liver malignancies embrace hepatocellular carcinoma [6,7], cholangiocarcinoma [3] and hepatoblastoma [8]. The diagnostics of hepatocellular carcinoma (HCC) is especially urgent topic due to high incidence in Asia and rising – in Europe and USA, possibly because of high prevalence of chronic hepatitis C [4,9]. Also, prognostic data should be reported including the features of early vs. progressed HCC, presence of stem cell immunophenotype, multicentric growth or metastatic spread [7]. Among mesenchymal malignant tumours, epithelioid haemangioendothelioma and angiosarcoma [10,11] are notable. Metastatic tumours represent the bulk of malignancies in Western countries [2]. Cystic liver tumours include biliary cystadenoma and biliary cystadenocarcinoma [12-14].

Most of the above mentioned neoplastic processes can be diagnosed in core biopsy. The key aspects include the following. First, the biopsy must be representative regarding the biological process and radiologically detected changes [15]. Further, the obtained tissue must be subjected to adequate technological process. Innovations here allow shortening the turnover time significantly. Next, the evaluation of morphology must be done searching for the characteristic traits of the above noticed tumours. However, due to the limited tissue amount in the biopsy, the tumour architecture sometimes is difficult to identify embarrassing the distinction between nodular hyperplastic process, benign tumour or low-grade malignancy. In contrast, high-grade malignancies can show significant cytological atypia by few signs of differentiation embarrassing the detection of histogenesis [6] and the distinction between primary and metastatic tumour.

Immunohistochemical markers as glypican-3 [1], Hep Par 1 [3,6], CD10 [3], alpha-fetoprotein [6] and TTF-1 [16] are useful in the HCC diagnostics. Alterations of CD31 and CD34-positive endothelial cell network reflect vascular remodelling during hepatic carcinogenesis [7]. Cytokeratin (CK) 19 and 7 are characteristic for cholangiocellular carcinoma [3]. In metastases, organospecific markers including CDX2, mammaglobin, nuclear expression of TTF-1 or presence of neuroendocrine markers can confirm extra-hepatic origin [17]. As colorectal, breast, lung and neuroendocrine cancers are frequent cause of metastatic liver damage [2] high diagnostic value of immunohistochemistry (IHC) can be expected. However, the exact detection of histogenesis can be difficult with metastatic pancreatic or gastric tumours and high-grade malignancies. IHC is mandatory for the diagnostics of haematological neoplasms and epithelioid haemangioendothelioma. Assessment of tumour biological potential can be done by IHC, evaluating Ki-67, Cyclin D1, FOXJ1, stem cell markers, matrix metalloproteinases and other markers [7-8,18-22]. Novel markers appear continuously as heat-shock protein 70 [23].

Nowadays, pathology is not any more purely descriptive but it is becoming more functional and clinically relevant. The classic morphologic characteristics must be combined with integrated evaluation of neoplastic process in the liver, including histogenesis, grading, clonal changes, type and extent of vascularisation, immunophenotype, heterogeneity, prediction of treatment sensitivity and the clinical behaviour [7]. New technologies as proteomic profiling and genomic marker analysis should be applied in the evaluation of liver tumours [4]. MicroRNA studies can lead to new findings in cancer pathogenesis and prediction of treatment efficacy [24,25].

The aim of the following chapter is to describe morphological and immunohistochemical characteristics of primary and secondary liver tumours in order to develop logistic basis for differential diagnosis of these processes in biopsy materials. Short discussion about the genesis and clinical course of each tumour will be included as well.

2. Benign epithelial liver tumours

Liver cell adenoma and bile duct adenoma will be discussed here. The regenerative processes with the emphasis on focal nodular hyperplasia are described considering the differential diagnosis.

2.1. Liver cell adenoma and its differential diagnosis with focal nodular hyperplasia

Liver cell adenoma or hepatic adenoma is defined as benign tumour arising from hepatocytes. The epidemiology is characterised by female predominance (90%) and strong association with oral contraceptive use [26-27] as 85% of affected persons have such history. Liver cell adenoma was rare before the era of oral contraceptives [27]. At present, the incidence has increased but is still low: 3-4 /100 000 per year in long-term users of oral contraception [27-29]. The patients mostly are 20-39 years old. The other risk factors of hepatic adenoma include androgen burden. The tumours can also arise spontaneously or occasionally can be related toglycogen storage diseases or diabetes mellitus. Clinically, the patients mostly are symptomatic. Abdominal fullness can be attributed to the presence of mass lesion; pain can be caused by necrosis [27]. Rupture and bleeding (40%) represent dangerous complications [27,29-31]; the risk of these events is increased in pregnant ladies affected by liver cell adenoma due to prior use of hormonal contraceptives. Risk of malignant transformation also is recognised [29,32]. By literature analysis, Farges and Dokmak concluded that 5% of resected hepatic adenomas bear HCC foci [32]. The risk of malignant transformation is higher in adenomas exceeding the size of 5 cm irrespectively of the number of adenomas as well as in males. Grossly, liver cell adenomas are mostly unifocal (80%) and subcapsular. The tumours can be quite large (5-20 cm). In most cases (75%) adenomas are encapsulated [27]. However, the capsule can be thin or absent [10]. In contrast to HCC, adenomas usually are not associated with cirrhosis [31]. Otherwise, radiological similarities exist between adenoma and HCC as both can be large, have rich vascularity and can undergo necrosis [31]. Microscopically, the tumour is composed by hepatocytes lacking anaplasia and arranged in thin (1-2 cells) trabeculae [27,29]. Cellular atypia and macrotrabeculae must be absent. Single arterioles, a pair of arteriole and venule or isolated biliary ducts are scattered throughout the lesion. However, well-formed triads enveloped in connective tissue are absent within the lesion. The tumour can be distinguished from normal liver by larger size of neoplastic cells, presence of capsule and lack of triad-containing portal tracts. Steatosis, hydropic degeneration or Mallory hyaline can be observed. Fibrous tissue, haemosiderin and calcifications can develop in the consequence of haemorrhage. The immunophenotype is characterised by expression of Hep Par 1 and other antigens that confirms the hepatic origin and by lower proliferation than in HCC. Molecular typing is emerging for liver cell adenoma as well. At present, up to 4 molecular types are identified:

1. hepatic adenoma with *TCF1* gene inactivation;
2. inflammatory hepatic adenoma;
3. beta-catenin-mutated non-inflammatory hepatic adenoma;
4. hepatic adenoma not displaying any before described feature or unsuitable for analysis [29].

The hepatic adenomas with *TCF1* gene mutation comprise 35-40% of liver cell adenomas. The patients are female. The tumour loses the expression and functions of hepatocyte nuclear factor 1 (HNF1) encoded by *TCF1* gene. Inactivation of the gene can be caused by mutation in both alleles or by combination of a mutation and 12q deletion leading to loss of heterozygosity in the corresponding region [33]. Germ-line mutation of *HNF1* gene manifests as maturity-onset diabetes of the young (MODY), type 3, in association with liver adenomatosis [34]. However, the spectrum of *HNF1A* somatic mutations in liver cell adenoma differs from that in patients with MODY3 and suggests genotoxic damage [35]. By IHC, loss of liver fatty acid binding protein can be observed. Not surprisingly, the adenomas show steatosis [29].

Inflammatory hepatic adenomas constitute 50% of liver cell adenomas and can be associated with obesity, smoking and alcohol use. Pathogenetically, inflammatory hepatic adenoma is characterised by IL-6 pathway activation centred on gp130 protein in IL-6 receptor. The receptor can be subjected to ligand-independent activation due to mutation in *IL6ST* gene, or the levels of gp130 can be elevated. The IL-6 receptor activation leads to recruitment of inflammatory cells through gp130-mediated production of chemokine CCL20. The mutation was found in 60% of inflammatory adenomas [36]. However, the IL-6 pathway activation is universal in the inflammatory hepatic adenoma. Microscopically, inflammatory infiltrates are observed in addition to the architecture and cytologic details of adenoma. Occasional bile ductules, dilated sinusoids and arterioles can be present. Haemorrhage is frequent. By IHC, expression of acute phase reactants serum amyloid A and C-reactive protein is marked [29].

A group of hepatic adenomas is associated with *beta-catenin* mutation [37-38].The beta-catenin pathway is not affected in *TCF1* inactivated group [29,38]. Beta-catenin activation can be assayed by immunohistochemical over-expression of glutamine synthetase or by aberrant nuclear localisation of beta-catenin. However, the tumours can show dysplastic changes more characteristic for HCC thus possibly this group will be reclassified into well-differentiated HCC [29,36].

The last group of hepatic adenomas (5%) lacking *TCF1* inactivation, inflammatory signature and beta-catenin mutation [29] could represent distinct group with peculiar pathway of molecular pathogenesis or result of technological shortcomings.

The differential diagnosis of hepatic adenoma in biopsy includes low-grade HCC and hyperplastic lesions like focal nodular hyperplasia, nodular regenerative hyperplasia and partial nodular transformation [27].

Focal nodular hyperplasia (FNH) is a comparatively frequent differential diagnosis of hepatic adenoma. The FNH incidence is estimated as 3% [29-30,39]. FNH is characterised by presence of hypervascular stellate scar in liver parenchymal nodule. The blood vessels are located in the middle of star-like fibrous tissue while the periphery is occupied by proliferating bile ductules. The morphologically remarkable abundant vascularity is in accordance with the hypothesis of the FNH origin due to microscopic arterial malformation [40-42]. The crucial difference between FNH and adenoma is pathogenetic as the former is thought to be hyperplastic lesion, while adenoma is a neoplasm. The presence of stellate scar and lack of peripheral capsule in FNH contrasts with presence of peripheral capsule and almost complete lack of connective tissue or portal triads within adenoma. If the architecture is incompletely represented in the biopsy, molecular characteristics should be able to discriminate between the two inherently different processes, the hyperplasia and tumour. The immunohistochemical markers of biliary differentiation have been employed in the differential diag-

http://dx.doi.org/10.5772/52838

nostics between FNH and hepatic adenoma. As described by Walther and Jain, CK19 and CD56 detect rich network of proliferating biliary ducts in the fibrous septa of FNH but reveal only few isolated ducts within the parenchyma of hepatic adenoma. Expression of CK7 is remarkable for the focal presence in parenchyma of liver cell adenoma in contrast to FNH while both lesions show expression of CK7 in biliary ducts. Thus, panel of CK19, CD56 and CK7 can be advised to solve the differential diagnosis in core biopsy [29]. Immunohistochemical expression pattern of glutamine synthetase differs between normal liver tissue, FNH and liver cell tumours as well. In healthy tissue, glutamine synthetase is present in perivenular hepatocytes. These positive areas are expanded in FNH [39]. In hepatic adenomas, glutamine synthetase expression is either diffuse of negative. In the last situation, the negativity in the tumour can be incomplete, with focally preserved expression in the tumour periphery [29] and thus difficult to interpret, especially in small biopsies where the preserved positive focus seems to be dominant.

In nodular regenerative hyperplasia, the liver contains many small regenerative nodules. Partial nodular transformation affects hilar area and is characterised by group of regenerative nodules surrounded by fibrous tissue [27].

Considering the differential diagnosis with HCC, thick trabecular cords, cytologic anaplasia and invasive growth reveal the malignant biological potential. The thickening of trabeculae is defined as presence of more than 2 cell layers in the trabeculae. The anaplasia is recognised by nuclear hyperchromasia, prominent nucleoli and increase in the nucleo: cytoplasmic ratio. Presence of mitoses practically excludes the diagnosis of hepatic adenoma. Atypical mitoses are absolute evidence of malignancy. The invasive growth can manifest as invasion through the capsule, infiltration into liver parenchyma and true invasion into blood vessels [27].

2.2. Bile duct adenoma

Bile duct adenoma is defined as a benign neoplasm of portal bile ducts. The epidemiologic data suggest rare occurrence. However, as the tumours mostly are small and asymptomatic [27], the true incidence and prevalence is unknown. Grossly, bile duct adenomas are mostly solitary (83%), subcapsular (95%) and small (below 1 cm). By light microscopy, the lesion is characterised by demarcated proliferation of bile ducts lacking atypia. The immunophenotype repeats the staining characteristics of biliary ducts exhibiting expression of cytokeratins 7 and 19 [27]. The differential diagnosis can include small foci of low-grade cholangiocarcinoma or metastatic low-grade adenocarcinoma, but the benign cytological appearance is helpful. Von Meyenburg hamartoma differs from bile duct adenoma, as the hamartomas would be multiple and show traits of cholestasis. However, the exact separation might not be of crucial importance due to benign course of biliary adenoma and pathogenetic suggestion that biliary adenoma represent a reactive process rather than true neoplasm.

3. Malignant epithelial primary liver tumours

Three primary liver tumours are of utmost importance. Hepatocellular carcinoma is the most frequent primary epithelial liver tumour with grave prognosis. Cholangiocarcinoma ranks second by the incidence except for endemic regions. Hepatoblastoma is notable for the occurrence in the infancy.

3.1. Hepatocellular carcinoma

Hepatocellular carcinoma is defined as malignant tumour developing from hepatocytes and/or showing hepatocellular differentiation. It is the most common primary malignant tumour of the liver constituting 80-85% of primary epithelial liver malignancies [29,43]. Considering the epidemiology, the worldwide burden of hepatocellular carcinoma can reach 1 million of new cases per year. The incidence shows major geographic differences. HCC is the 2nd most common cancer in Asia, and the 4th – in Africa [10]. The annual age-standardised incidence is the highest in East Asia, including China and Japan. Low-risk areas comprise Europe, esp. northern and western parts; North and South America, Australia and New Zealand [10].The age-adjusted incidence rates in Mozambique are as high as 112.9 and 30.8/100 000 in males and females, respectively. In China these values reach 34.4 and 11.6. In contrast, the age-adjusted incidence rates in British males and females are 1.6 and 0.8, respectively [31]. The HCC risk factors include liver cirrhosis independently of cause, chronic hepatitis B or C, ethanol consumption and non-alcoholic liver steatosis as well as mycotoxins. The aflatoxin B1 or other mycotoxins produced by *Aspergillus* fungi could be responsible for part of HCC in areas where grains, rice and peanuts are stored in hot and humid conditions [31]. Most of HCC cases develop from dysplastic cirrhotic nodule [29], thus the differential diagnostics between dysplastic nodule and cancer represent evaluation of one point in a complex road of pathogenesis. Clinically, most of the patients approach doctor due to symptoms attributable to mass lesion in the liver (abdominal pain, sensation of fullness), tumour-related intoxication (weight loss, weakness, lack of appetite) and loss of liver functions (jaundice). Alternatively, the symptoms can be related to pre-existing cirrhosis and the tumour could be identified during routine control of cirrhotic patient or during workup for unspecific or unrelated symptoms [31]. Radiologically, the number and size of tumour masses can be evaluated. Ultrasonography can be used for screening. Typical findings regarding vascularity include hypervascularity and thrombosis of portal vein, frequently due to invasion. If it is necessary to confirm invasion into portal vein, biopsy can be obtained from it [31].

By microscopy, the typical patterns include trabecular, acinar and ductular structure. The neoplastic cells in low-grade cases resemble liver cells by possessing wide eosinophilic cytoplasm and distinct cell borders. Nuclear atypia is present and nucleo: cytoplasmic ratio is increased, although to different degree. Mitoses can be present; atypical mitoses can be observed (Figure 1). The architecture shows unequivocal deviations from normal structure such as thick trabeculae with more than 2 cell layers (in contrast to adenoma), solid areas, duct-like or gland-like structures. However, careful evaluation of the architecture under high power magnification must be carried out. There are many secondary phenomena raising the similarity between HCC and liver tissue: presence of macrovesicular or microvesicular fat, Mallory hyaline and bile. The capillaries can be dilated [27]. Among the histochemical staining methods, absent reticulin staining [44] is characteristic. PAS stain can reveal glycogen and intracytoplasmic globules; the latter structure remains positive after diastase digestion [27,44]. With some experience, morphology is helpful to distinguish finely granular glycogen or rounded globules in HCC from mucus droplets in metastatic adenocarcinoma or cholangiocarcinoma.

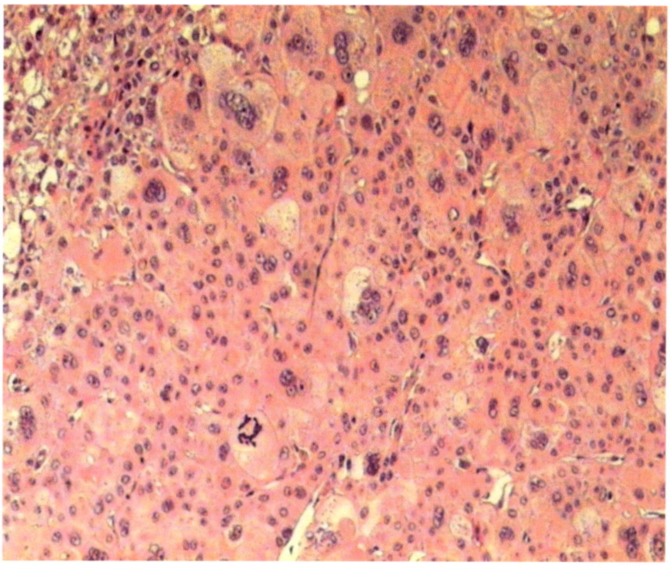

Figure 1. Hepatocellular carcinoma displaying marked cytologic atypia. Note the presence of atypical mitosis. Haematoxylin-eosin (HE), original magnification (OM) 100x.

Fibrolamellar hepatocellular carcinoma (FLHC) has distinctive aetiology, epidemiology and course. The general HCC risk factors are not associated with this subtype [31]. FLHC is rare, constituting only 1-4% of HCC [27]. It is less common in high-risk areas than in North America and Europe. The patients are young adults or even children [10]. FLHC is diagnosed at the mean age of 25 years in contrast to mean age of 52 years in typical HCC patient group [27]. Controversial data are reported about the sex predilection: some but not all authors have noted that females are mostly affected [10,31]. Clinically, symptoms attributable to liver enlargement, parenchymal damage (elevated liver enzyme level) or tumour-related intoxication (weight loss or fever) can be present. Cirrhosis is absent. The tumour can be multifocal, and metastases can affect lungs and regional lymph nodes [31]. The histological structure is remarkable for the lamellar fibrosis. The stroma is composed of thick, parallel strands of hyalinised collagen [27]. The cells are large, polygonal, with wide eosinophilic cytoplasm. The vesicular nuclei possess large nucleoli. Cytoplasmic pale bodies are more frequent (up to 50% of cases) and more abundant than in other types [10,27]. The pale bodies are rounded and very lightly eosinophilic thus staining paler than the surrounding cytoplasm. These structures represent cystically dilated endoplasmic reticulum. Pale bodies can be positive for fibrinogen by IHC. The immunophenotype is remarkable for diffuse expression of CK7. The hepatocellular differentiation can be confirmed by Hep Par 1; alpha-fetoprotein is present in approximately 20% of cases. The FLHC prognosis is better than in the general group. The mean survival is 32 months in contrast to 5.9 months in trabecular HCC [27]. However, it is found that the beneficial prognosis of FLHC is different from cancer in cirrhotic liver but not from HCC in the absence of liver cirrhosis [10].

IHC has an important role in the diagnostics of HCC. Frequently tested antigens include glypican-3, Hep Par 1, alpha-fetoprotein, CD10, carcinoembryonic antigen CEA, TTF-1, arginase-1, evaluation of cytokeratins and endothelial network as well as MOC-31 and markers of extra-hepatic tumours.

Glypican-3 is a cell surface protein [1] that is involved in the control of cell proliferation and survival. Glypican-3-knockout mice exhibit alterations in Wnt signalling [45]. Glypican-3 also interacts with Hedgehog signalling pathway [46]. In the practical surgical pathology, the value of glypican-3 is associated with the cancer diagnostics as it is expressed in 70-75% HCC but not in benign liver tissue [48-49] or cholangiocellular carcinoma [1]. Hepatoblastoma can be positive as well. However, glypican-3 can be expressed in metastatic melanoma [50], ovarian clear-cell carcinoma [51], choriocarcinoma, yolk sac tumour [52-53] as well as in blastomas including neuroblastoma and Wilms' tumour [54]. In addition, 10% of gastric cancer cases are positive for glypican-3 [55]. In melanoma, 80% of tumours contain detectable level of glypican-3 protein and mRNA [1]. Regarding ovarian cancer, the rate of glypican expression could be as high as 18% of all ovarian cancer cases and 60% of clear cell carcinoma cases [51]. However, negative reports regarding clear cell carcinoma of ovary are published as well [53]. Glypican-3 is silenced in breast cancer, lung adenocarcinoma and mesothelioma [56-58]. Another problem has been highlighted by Abdul-Al *et al.*, who have described frequent granular cytoplasmic expression of glypican-3 in chronic active hepatitis C [59]. Regenerative changes were suggested as the explanation. Authors emphasized that membranous staining was not observed in hepatitis [59]. Glypican-3 has prognostic significance in HCC as it is associated with poor prognosis [60] and shorter recurrence-free period after liver transplantation [49]. The applications of glypican-3 could extend beyond liver biopsy – and return to it. It could possible to use glypican-3 plasma levels for diagnostics and monitoring of HCC [61-63]. Immunotherapy could be guided towards glypican-3; the present research is exploring both antibody and cell-based immunological mechanisms [64-65]. Cancer vaccine could be generated against this molecule [1]. Glypican-3 is among genes that are distinctly expressed in liver cancer stem cells; it is suggested that glypican could be promising candidate for gene therapy without inducing damage to normal liver stem cells [66].

Hep Par 1 is positive in normal liver, liver adenomas and HCC. The antibody was developed in 1993 using an immunogen from failed liver allograft. The target antigen has been identified as carbamoyl phosphate synthetase. This enzyme catalyses the rate-limiting step in the urea cycle and is located in the mitochondria [67]. The specifity and sensitivity of this

http://dx.doi.org/10.5772/52838

marker in HCC diagnostics exceeds 80% and has reached 90% in several studies [6,67]. Unfortunately, sensitivity is lower in high-grade HCC. The expression in non-hepatocellular tumours including colorectal, pancreatic, breast, urothelial, prostate cancer, neuroendocrine tumours, renal cell carcinoma, melanoma and angiomyolipoma is either negative or focal. However, few gastric, colorectal and lung adenocarcinomas can be positive [6,67]. In the biopsy material, heterogeneity in the HCC can cause diagnostic problems [6].

Arginase-1 is an enzyme involved in the urea cycle as well. It is found in benign hepatocytes and hepatocellular neoplasms. The antibody has received high sensitivity estimates of 96% and favourable performance characteristics [68,69].

Alpha-fetoprotein is an oncofetal protein produced by the liver and yolk sac endoderm. The antigen is remarkable for expression in malignant hepatocellular tumours (Figure 2) in contrast to benign liver tissue, and for the high specifity. However, sensitivity is low (30-50%) and heterogeneity adds further problems in biopsy evaluation [6]. Nevertheless, positive expression is valuable.

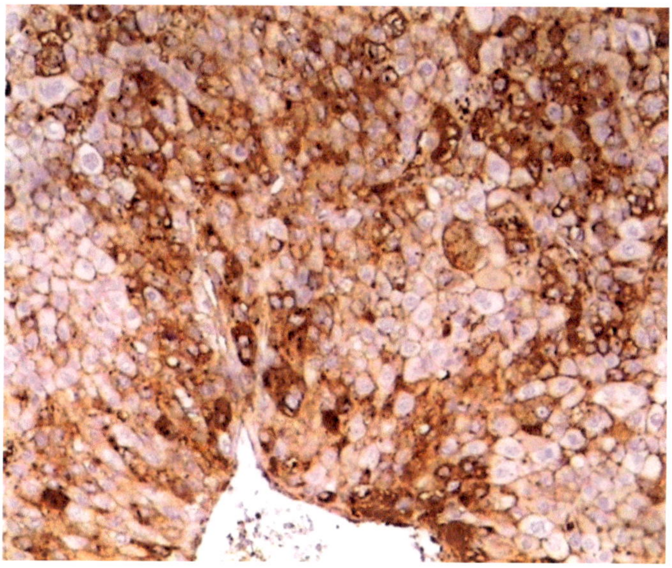

Figure 2. Heterogeneous intense cytoplasmic expression of alpha-fetoprotein in hepatocellular carcinoma. Immunoperoxidase (IP), anti-alpha-fetoprotein, OM 100x.

Polyclonal antibodies against carcinoembryonic antigen (CEA) yield positive reaction more than in 70% of HCC cases, while monoclonal anti-CEA only rarely stains HCC. Reactivity with polyclonal CEA antibodies mostly is observed in canaliculi; this pattern can be observed in benign or malignant liver tissues and is attributable to cross-reaction with biliary glycoprotein on the canalicular surface [67]. The canalicular pattern is specific for HCC and can be used to exclude cholangiocarcinoma and metastatic adenocarcinoma. It is not useful in the differential diagnosis between HCC and benign hepatocellular mass lesions. Although good general sensitivity has been reported, it is higher in well or moderately differentiated HCC that present less problems regarding the differential diagnosis with cholangiocellular carcinoma or metastasis [67]. Cytoplasmic stain is not observed in healthy liver or benign neoplasms; it is characteristic of malignancy but seen mostly in cholangiocellular carcinoma and metastatic neoplasms. The rate of cytokeratin fraction expression is 15% for CK7, 20% for CK20 and 10% for CK19. Diffuse strong expression of endothelial markers CD31 and CD34 is not characteristic for normal liver tissue in contrast to HCC [27]. The visualisation of endothelial layer is valuable also in estimating the thickness of trabeculae. However, pattern of diffuse, strong endothelial marker expression has low sensitivity of 20-40%. The patchy expression is also difficult to evaluate in liver biopsies. The visualisation of endothelium thus is not recommended for the distinction between adenoma and carcinoma [6].

The transcription factor TTF-1 is expressed as intense granular cytoplasmic staining in normal liver parenchyma [16] and hepatocellular tumours (Figure 3). The reaction is ensured by cross-reactivity with hepatocyte mitochondrial antigen and is seen with the clone 8G7G3/1 [69]. The reported sensitivity is 60-70%. However, it parallels the expression of Hep Par 1 decreasing the practical value [6]. Its expression can be retained even in metastatic HCC [16].

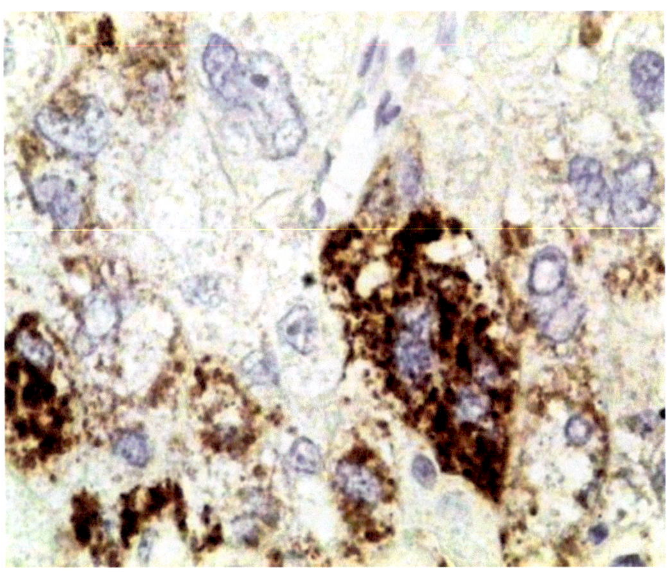

Figure 3. Granular cytoplasmic expression of TTF-1 in hepatocellular carcinoma. IP, Anti-TTF-1, OM 400x.

MOC-31 is an epithelial cell surface glycoprotein of unknown function. Evaluating liver biopsies, it is valuable as non-hepatocellular marker. MOC-31 is negative in HCC but positive in most metastatic adenocarcinomas and cholangiocellular cancer [67]. However, mesothelioma is MOC-31 negative as well; calretinin should be used in the panel to exclude this possibility [17].

http://dx.doi.org/10.5772/52838

Molecular subtyping is emerging for HCC. The subtypes are distinguished by high proliferation and chromosomal instability; by activation of Wnt signalling pathway and by interferon signalling due to tumour-infiltrating cells [70-77].

The requests for clinically relevant classification have resulted in the separation of HCC into early and progressed entities. The early HCC is recognized as small (not exceeding the diameter of 2 cm), well differentiated and lacking vascular invasion. The invasion into portal tracts can be present and is highlighted by lack of proliferating ductules. Macrovesicular steatosis is present in 40% of early HCC but appears mostly in Eastern cohorts. It can be attributable to incomplete neoarterialisation – the process of portal tract replacement by unpaired arteries outside the portal tracts. In early HCC, there is still comparatively large venous flow. The tumours in general may be radiologically hypovascular. The early HCC is more likely to become the biopsy target due to equivocal findings at imaging. Progressed HCC includes HCC of higher grade (moderate or poor differentiation degree, G2 or G3), possessing vascular invasion, larger size or stem/progenitor cell immunophenotype and mixed hepatobiliary differentiation. The stem cell immunophenotype can be detected by IHC for CK19, EpCAM, CD133, and mixed hepatobiliary immunophenotype – by expression of CK7 and CK19 [7]. The 5-year survival is 89% in the early HCC group in contrast to 48% in the progressed group. The intrahepatic metastatic spread must be distinguished from multifocal carcinoma that is prognostically better disease. The multifocal disease is characterised by "nodule in nodule" structure or by presence of at least one G1 nodule [7].

The differential diagnosis includes benign hepatic lesions, metastatic malignancies and cholangiocarcinoma. IHC is of major importance. Markers, that are expressed both in benign and malignant liver cells (CEA by polyclonal antibody, CD10, Hep Par 1, TTF-1 and (occasionally) cytokeratins [27]) identify the hepatocellular origin of tumour but cannot be used to prove the malignant biological potential of suspicious biopsied tissue. If these are found in high-grade tumour, diagnosis of HCC is preferable in contrast to metastasis. The expression of alpha-fetoprotein and glypican-3 is typical for malignant tumour of hepatocellular origin [27]. These findings are important in differential diagnosis with non-hepatocellular and/or metastatic tumour in line with other markers specific for particular histogenesis. Regarding the differential diagnosis of HCC and dysplastic cirrhotic nodule, a panel of immunohistochemical stains is recommended employing glypican-3, glutamine synthetase and heat-shock protein 70 [48,78-80]. In biopsy, the panel has lower sensitivity although good specifity: accuracy 60.8% for 3 markers and 78.4% for 2 markers with 100% specifity. The findings were acceptable even in the group of low-grade HCC: the accuracy still was 57% for 3 markers and 72.9% for 2 markers with 100% specifity [23].

HCC (except fibrolamellar type) mostly is associated either with cirrhosis or chronic active hepatitis with fibrosis that has not reached the degree of cirrhosis. To facilitate the differential diagnosis between HCC and liver adenoma or FNH it is wise to take separate biopsies-from the lesion and from distant liver tissues if possible.

The future pathways for molecular diagnostics of HCC include mRNA analysis of *GPC3*, *survivin* and *LYVE1* genes [78]. Glypican-3, encoded by *GPC3*, and survivin is up-regulated in parenchymal HCC cells while LYVE1 protein is down regulated in endothelial cells in case of malignancy. MYC pathway studies could also bring new information [29].

In addition, molecular studies can predict the HCC prognosis. Down-regulation of p57 accelerates the growth and invasion of HCC cells [18]. The reduced p57 expression correlates with larger tumour size, higher TNM stage, presence of extrahepatic metastases and decreased survival. In cell lines, the down-regulation of p57 increases the expression of cyclin D1 and CDK2, enhancing the cellular proliferation. The matrix metalloproteinase-1 (MMP-1) and protease activated receptor-1 (PAR-1) are expressed in HCC but not in normal liver. The up-regulation of MMP-1/PAR-1 axis has prognostic value [20] and potentially could be used in the identification of malignancy. Co-expression of stem cell transcription factors Oct4 and Nanog indicates aggressive tumour behaviour and predicts recurrence after HCC resection [22]. FOXJ1 is over-expressed in HCC. It is associated with histological grade, poor prognosis and with tumour cell proliferation [19]. Hedgehog signalling pathway mediates invasion and metastasis of HCC via ERK pathway. Up-regulation of cell proliferation is associated with down-regulation of p27 and p21 and up-regulation of cyclin D1 [81]. Osteopontin plays role in the proliferation of HCC through interaction with the cell surface receptor CD44 [82] and is considered the key mediator for vasculogenic mimicry [83]. Bax-interacting factor is over-expressed in HCC and correlates with shortened survival [84]. NY-ESO-1 protein is a potential marker for early recurrence after surgical treatment [85]. Hepatocyte nuclear factor 4 suppresses the HCC development [86]. Sulfatase 2 protects HCC cells against apoptosis [87]. Interleukins as IL-17 and IL-6 have tumour-promoting role [88]. Interaction with matrix metalloproteinases 2 and 9 is likely [89]. Up-regulation of sirtuins has been identified [90]. Typing of immune cells in biopsy is mostly done for research purposes [91]. If any of those parameters will show prognostic and predictive value, the relevant IHC analysis should be included in the protocol of liver biopsy evaluation. The technological future developments include virtual microscopy. Fractal analysis [92] and quantitative IHC can be applied [93].

Methylation studies have been carried out in HCC [94]. The expression of microRNAs is undergoing active analysis in HCC [95-96]. MicroRNAs are non-coding, short RNA molecules that can bind to messenger RNA and to prevent their translation into protein, providing additional regulation of gene expression. MicroRNAs act as large-scale molecular switch due to ability simultaneously down-regulate many genes. MicroRNA-181 down-regulates the differentiation and maturation of hepatocytes [96]. Suppression of microRNA-181 expression leads to reduced motility and invasion of HCC stem cells [25]. MicroRNA-182 could promote metastasis [97]. MicroRNA-183 inhibits apoptosis [98]. MicroRNA expression can be subjected to regulation with IL-6 [25]. Reduced expression of microRNA-26 in HCC is associated with poor prognosis. However, better response of interferon alpha postoperative adjuvant therapy can be expected [95]. MicroRNA-21 induces resistance to the anti-tumour effect of interferon and fluorouracil combination therapy [99]. Circulating microRNAs are valuable in tumour diagnosis and monitoring the treatment [24].

http://dx.doi.org/10.5772/52838

3.2. Hepatoblastoma

Hepatoblastoma is defined as a primary malignant blastomatous liver tumour showing complex differentiation towards fetal and embryonal hepatocytes as well as mature tissues including osteoid, connective tissue and striated muscle. Epidemiologically, hepatoblastoma is a rare malignant liver tumour of childhood with the incidence of 1 case / 1 million [8,10]. In children, hepatoblastoma is the most common primary liver tumour. Characteristically, the tumour develops within first five years of life: 4% of hepatoblastomas are present at birth, 69% have developed by 2 years of age and 90% - by 5 years of age. Only 3% of patients are older than 15 years [100]. The risk of hepatoblastoma is increased in *APC*-mutation-carrying children from familial adenomatous polyposis (FAP) kindreds. Clinically, enlarging abdomen can be the first sign. The other possible manifestations include weight loss, anorexia, nausea, vomiting and abdominal pain. Jaundice is rarely observed [100]. Paraneoplastic syndromes can occur. Among those, anaemia and thrombocytosis are frequent. Precocious puberty due to production of chorionic gonadotropin is rare. Grossly, the tumours mostly occur as single lesions [10] measuring 5-22 cm [100]. Pseudocapsule can develop due to compression of surrounding liver tissue. Microscopically, hepatoblastoma can display any of different histological patterns, or combination of these patterns. The fetal epithelial differentiation is characterised by thin trabeculae of small cuboidal cells. The nuclei are small and round with fine chromatin and small nucleolus. The cytoplasm can be either clear or finely granular resulting in "light and dark" pattern under low magnification. Foci of extramedullary haemopoesis can be present. The combined fetal and embryonal pattern is characterised by presence of small tumour cells in solid or acinar groups. The small cells have scant cytoplasm, higher nucleo: cytoplasmic ratio and coarse chromatin. Hepatoblastoma is called macrotrabecular if the cells compose 6-12 cell layers in the trabeculae in most of the tumour. Larger cells are present in the macrotrabeculae in addition to fetal and embryonal type. In teenagers, macrotrabecular hepatoblastoma must be differentiated from hepatocellular carcinoma. Small cell undifferentiated hepatoblastoma morphologically resembles small cell cancer displaying solid small blue cell pattern with focal necrosis. Mixed epithelial and mesenchymal hepatoblastomas contain mesenchymal components including fibrous tissue, osteoid, cartilage, striated muscle, bone or melanin [100]. Mixed epithelial and mesenchymal hepatoblastoma with teratoid features is recognised by the presence of endodermal, neuroectodermal and complex mesenchymal tissues. The neuroectodermal component can comprise melanin, glial and neuronal cells [10].After treatment, connective tissue, necrosis and signs of haemorrhage develop in association with residual neoplastic tissue, and squamous islands become more common. Immunohistochemically, expression of alpha-fetoprotein, beta-catenin and cell cycle markers is associated with the histological pattern. The fetal subtype is characterised by low proliferation that parallels the scant mitotic activity; alpha-fetoprotein can be present and the expression of beta-catenin is retained in the membranous localisation. The combined fetal and embryonal subtype is characterised by shift of beta-catenin expression towards the nuclei in higher grade embryonal component. An interesting circular pattern can be observed. In the rounded cell groups, the middle is occupied by progenitor-type pale, small cells displaying low proliferative activity and nuclear expression of beta-catenin. The progenitor-type cells are surrounded by intensively proliferating embryonal type cells characterised by mixed nuclear and cytoplasmic expression of beta-catenin. The outermost layer of these concentric structures is composed by fetal type cells with low proliferative activity and retained membranous expression of beta-catenin. The small cell subtype lacks alpha-fetoprotein but has high proliferative activity, usually reaching 80%; cytokeratins are expressed as well. Even in the mixed epithelial and mesenchymal hepatoblastoma, cytokeratins and alpha-fetoprotein can be expressed even in the ostecyte-like and osteoblast-like cells embedded in or associated with the osteoid, correspondingly [10]. In the study of Purcell *et al.*, cyclin D1 and Ki-67 were two markers (out of 5, including also beta-catenin, E-cadherin and alpha-fetoprotein) that were shown to have prognostic value regarding survival [8].

3.3. Cholangiocarcinoma

Cholangiocarcinoma (CC) is defined as malignant epithelial liver tumour with biliary histogenesis or biliary differentiation. Epidemiologically, CC is a rare tumour with male predilection. It composes 15% of primary liver cancer [100] but the relative incidence range of cholangiocarcinoma is wide, from 5% in males and 12% in females in Osaka, Japan, to 90% in males and 94% of primary liver cancer cases in females in Thailand. The age-standardized incidence per 100 000 males ranges from 84.6 in Thailand to 2.8 in Osaka, Japan; 1.0 in France or 0.9 in Italy. The known risk factors include association with ulcerative colitis and primary sclerosing cholangitis [27]. The rate of cholangiocarcinoma in primary sclerosing cholangitis patients is estimated as 10-20%. The presence of parasites, especially *Clonorchis sinensis* and *Opisthorchis viverrini*, also increases the risk of cholangiocarcinoma. The high-incidence area in Laos and North and Northeast Thailand corresponds to the endemic area of *Opisthorchis viverrini*. Korea has high rate of cholangiocellular cancer due to endemic spread of *Clonorchis sinensis.* Clinically, the patients can present with painless jaundice [31], general malaise, mild abdominal pain and weight loss [100]. Grossly, several types exist. Peripheral tumours arise from portal bile ducts. Hilar lesions arise in large ducts. The diffuse intraductal papillomatosis involves ducts as widespread carcinoma *in situ* lacking dominant mass but leading to severe obstruction of bile flow. Histologically, cholangiocarcinoma has adenocarcinomatous structure characterised by tubular complexes and moderate amount of desmoplastic stroma. The architectural variants include high-grade tumour lacking the characteristic architecture, signet-ring cell tumour with presence of signet-ring cells, mucinous type with extensive secretion of extracellular mucin, adenosquamous type with focal squamous differentiation and spindle cell type with pseudosarcomatoid structure, presence of malignant spindle cells and signs of epithelial differentiation. The tumour has no functional connection with bile excretory system although morphological connection in the form of invasion or cancer in situ can exist. CC arises from ductal epithelium and not from hepatocytes. Due to these two reasons, presence of bile in the lumina of malignant glands is not characteristic but eosinophilic or mucinous secretion can be present. Mucin stains as PAS or mucicarmine can be positive [44]. The immunophenotype is derived from the immunophenotype of bile duct epithelium, with expression of following cytokeratins: CK19 (100%), CK7 (80-100%), CK20 (20%). Diffuse cytoplasmic expression of CEA is found by polyclonal antibody in almost all cases and is frequent by monoclonal antibody as well [27]. However, it is

http://dx.doi.org/10.5772/52838

suggested that morphology cannot reliably distinguish cholangiocarcinoma from metastatic pancreatic or colorectal cancer [31]. In case of pancreatic adenocarcinoma, the marked cellular atypia disproportionally to better preserved architecture can be a clue. Colorectal adenocarcinoma in typical cases is characterised by columnar morphology and diffuse intense expression of CK20, CDX2 and CEA and lack of CK7. Other authors have drawn attention to the impossibility to distinguish cholangiocarcinoma from metastatic gastric cancer and cancer of gall bladder; metastatic pancreatic cancer also remains a problem [6]. The morphological differential diagnosis includes benign proliferation of bile ducts, hepatocellular carcinoma and metastatic adenocarcinoma [27]. In order to discriminate between biliary adenoma and cholangiocarcinoma, invasion (including single invasive cells and perineural invasion) and cellular atypia should be sought for. Radiologic findings are helpful as bile duct adenoma usually is smaller than 1 cm, but cholangiocarcinomas are large. The differential diagnosis with hepatocellular carcinoma can rely both on morphology and immunophenotype. Immunohistochemically, markers of biliary differentiation CK7 and CK19 are positive in cholangiocellular carcinoma. Hep Par 1 can be used to exclude hepatocellular differentiation [6,29]. Proteomic analysis of differentially expressed proteins in peripheral cholangiocarcinoma is under research [101].

4. Vascular tumours

Cavernous haemangioma, epithelioid haemangiendothelioma and angiosarcoma are endothelial tumours representing the whole spectrum of biological potential. Haemangioma is entirely benign although can cause complications due to large size; epithelioid haemangioendothelioma is notable for the peculiar structure leading to marked difficulties in the biopsy diagnostics, and angiosarcoma is a frank malignancy with grave prognosis. In addition, angiomyolipoma will be discussed as well although it should be noted that this tumour has complex structure including rich vascularity as one component.

4.1. Cavernous haemangioma

Haemangioma is defined as benign endothelial tumour [102]. Due to bleeding risk, it is only rarely seen in liver biopsy; in addition, the possibilities of radiological diagnostics are good and the prognosis only rarely necessitates active treatment. However, epidemiologically the lesion is the most common benign tumour of the liver with incidence 0.4% [27]. Clinically, haemangioma usually are asymptomatic due to small size and slow expansive growth. Occasionally, a giant haemangioma (10-30 cm) can cause pain due to mass effect. Thrombosis and bleeding can be dangerous complications. In neonates, blood shunting can lead to heart failure. Grossly, haemangiomas are mostly solitary (90%), of small or moderate size (less than 5 cm) and subcapsular. Microscopic structure is similar to cavernous haemangioma elsewhere in the body. Cavernous, lake-like blood spaces can be seen, separated by hypocellular fibrous septa (Figure 4). Thrombosis can be present. The immunophenotype reflects the endothelial origin. In the rare situation, when biopsy is obtained from cavernous haemangioma, the differential diagnosis can include hepatic tumours with rich vascularity as adenoma and cholangiocellular carcinoma. These are diagnosed by the presence and cytological properties of liver cells. Other vascular tumours could be considered, including infantile haemangioendothelioma, angiomyolipoma, epithelioid haemangioendothelioma and angiosarcoma. The infantile haemangioendothelioma can be recognized by capillary structure and occurrence in infants [27]. Angiomyolipoma shows combination of fat, smooth muscle and blood vessels with radiating immature smooth muscle cells. The higher cellularity and presence of fat are features incompatible with cavernous haemangioma. Epithelioid haemangioendothelioma is discussed separately; the occurrence of vascular lakes usually is not observed. Angiosarcoma can have cavernous architecture but the hallmark of it is the cellular atypia.

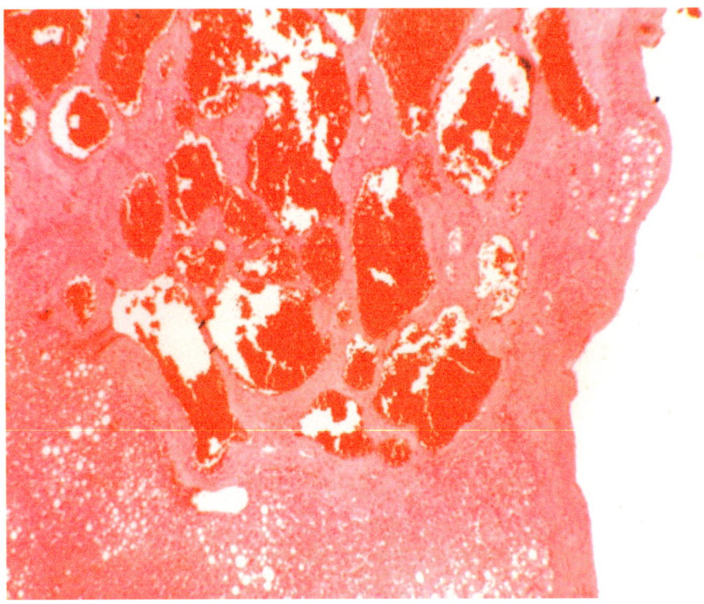

Figure 4. Cavernous haemangioma in liver tissue. Note the large, cavernous spaces filled with red blood cells. HE, OM 50x.

4.2. Angiomyolipoma

Angiomyolipoma is defined as benign mesenchymal tumour with complex structure including immature smooth muscle, blood vessels and fat. Epithelioid cells and perivascular HMB-45-positive cells can be present. Research of the tumour histogenesis has resulted in the concept of PEComa, a tumour of perivascular epithelioid cells, showing myomatous, lipomatous and melaninogenic differentiation. Epidemiologically, liver angiomyolipoma is rare. It has been diagnosed in wide age range (10-86 years). In tuberous sclerosis, the incidence of angiomyolipoma is increased. These patients may develop multiple angiomyolipomas in liver as well as kidney angiomyolipoma. Awareness of this condition is necessary to escape over-diagnosis of metastatic malignant tumour. Clinically, the tumour can be asymptomatic. However, large tumours can cause pain; rupture and bleeding is also possible. By radiologic studies, the tumour is hypervascular again. Grossly, angiomyolipoma usually is solitary (except in tuberous sclerosis), measuring 0.8-36 cm. The microscopic picture (Figure 5) is straightforward if all three components are present in liver biopsy and have typical structure. The smooth muscle cells can have epithelioid appearance leading to morphological similarity to liver parenchymal cells; the rich vascularity could lead to diagnostic confusion with hepatocellular tumour already earlier. The epithelioid cells sometimes can cause suspicion for malignancy due to large nuclei and nucleoli. However, the nucleo: cytoplasmic ratio remains low due to increased cell size.

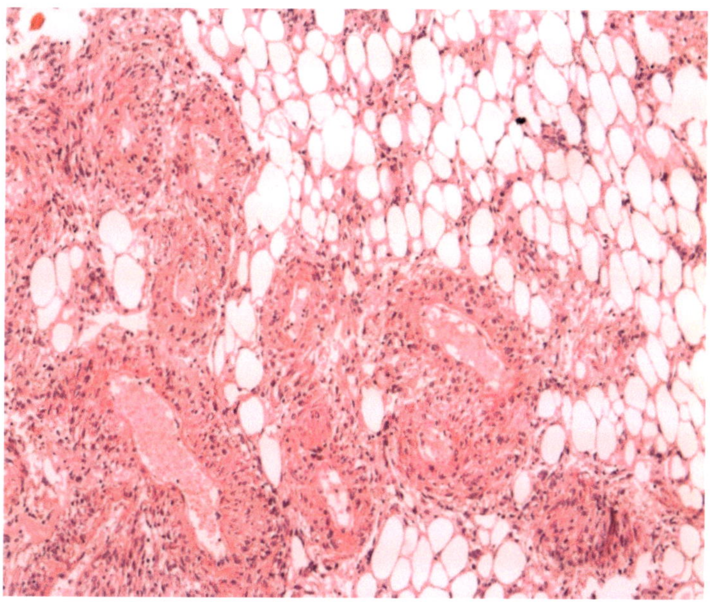

Figure 5. The microscopic structure of angiomyolipoma. Note the peculiar, thick-walled blood vessels, immature smooth muscle proliferation with high cellularity as well as the presence of fat. HE, OM 100x.

In difficult cases, IHC is helpful. The smooth muscle cells express actin (Figure 6) and fat cells – S-100 protein. HMB-45 expression can be observed in perivascular epithelioid cells (Figure 7). The differential diagnosis can include hepatocellular neoplasms or spindle cell sarcomas. Actin expression and complex histological structure helps to exclude hepatocellular origin of the tumour. Complex structure, combined immunophenotype and low proliferation help to exclude sarcoma [27].

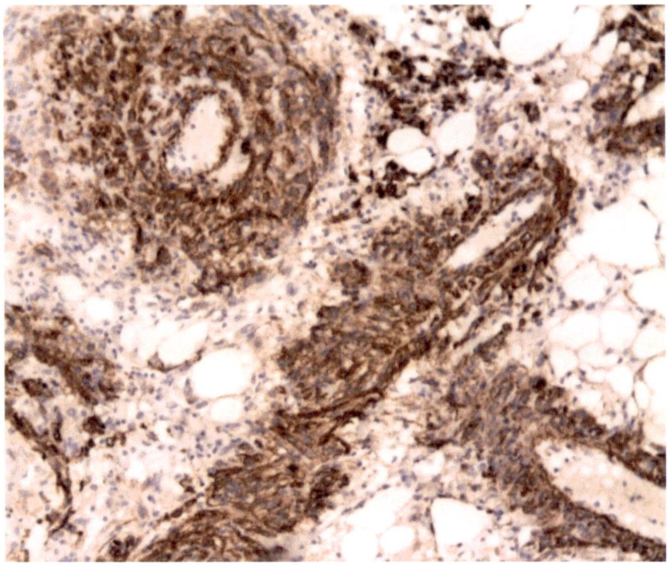

Figure 6. Actin-positive smooth muscle component in angiomyolipoma. IP, anti-actin, OM 100x.

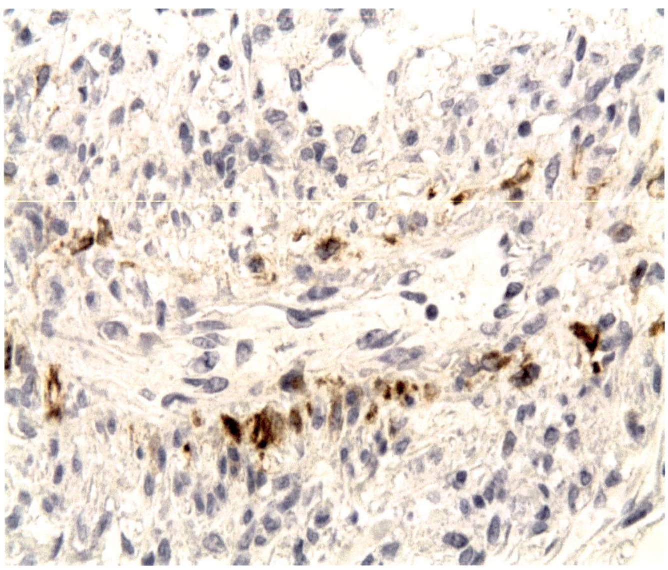

Figure 7. Expression of melanosome protein HMB-45 in angiomyolipoma. IP, anti-HMB-45, OM 400x.

4.3. Epithelioid haemangioendothelioma

Epithelioid haemangioendothelioma (EHE) is defined as intermediate-grade malignancy derived from endothelial cells. The mean age of patients is 47 years, ranging 12-86 years. The clinical picture can include symptoms related to enlarging mass in liver (abdominal pain, hepatomegaly) and tumour-related intoxication (fatigue, malaise, anorexia). Radiologically, the tumour can be found by computed tomography. EHE can be radiologically avascular [10,27,103]. This finding is probably related to fibrosis and scarcity of functioning blood vessels despite the endothelial origin of the tumour. Grossly, multiple tumours can involve liver or liver and lungs. In the lungs, epithelioid haemangioendothelioma is known also as intravascular bronchioloalveolar tumour. Despite the multifocality (Figure 8), slow progress is possible in our experience.

Biopsy material is usually sufficient to diagnose the tumour. However, in our experience, immunohistochemical investigation is crucial in order to find out the presence of tumour cells on the background of stromal fibrosis and reactive inflammation, to detect the endothelial origin and to evaluate the low biological potential as reflected by low to moderate proliferation activity by Ki-67 (Figures 9-11).

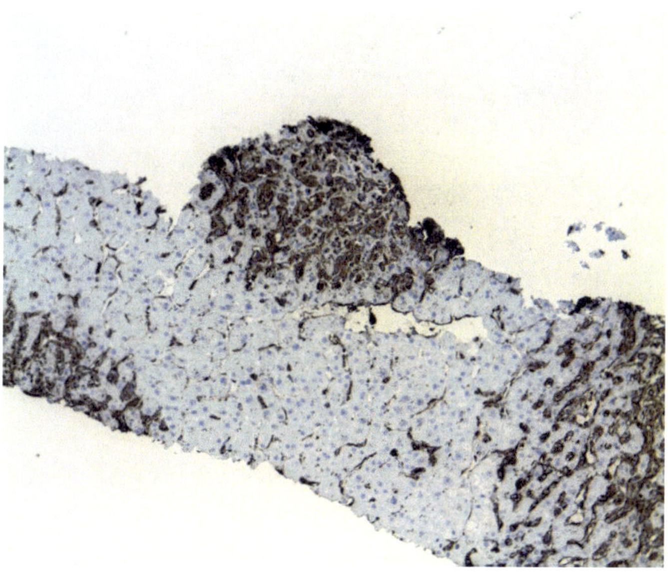

Figure 8. Multiple foci of epithelioid haemangioendothelioma in liver biopsy. The tumour is highlighted by immunohistochemical visualisation of vimentin regarding its mesenchymal nature. IP, anti-vimentin, OM 50x.

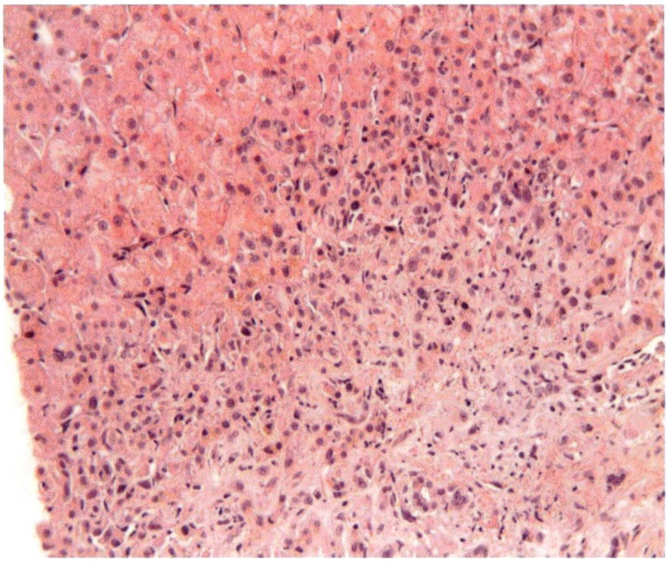

Figure 9. Epithelioid haemangioendothelioma presenting as a fibrotic focus in liver biopsy. HE, OM 100x.

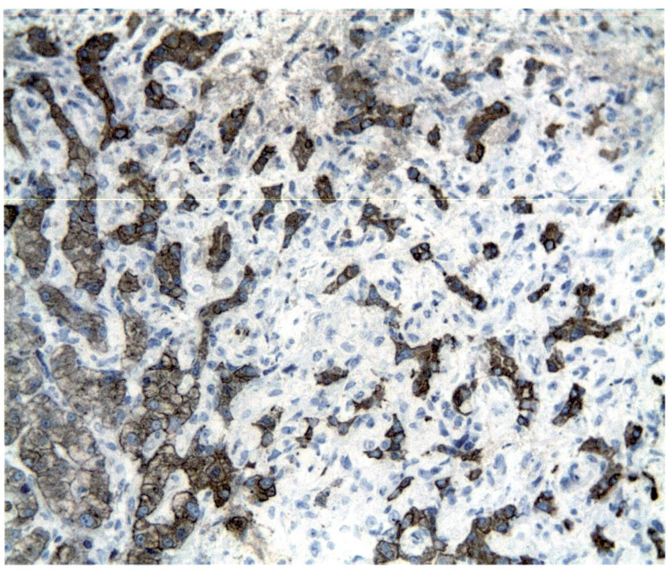

Figure 10. Loss of liver parenchyma due to infiltration of epithelioid haemangioendothelioma. IP, anti-cytokeratins AE1/AE3, OM 200x.

http://dx.doi.org/10.5772/52838

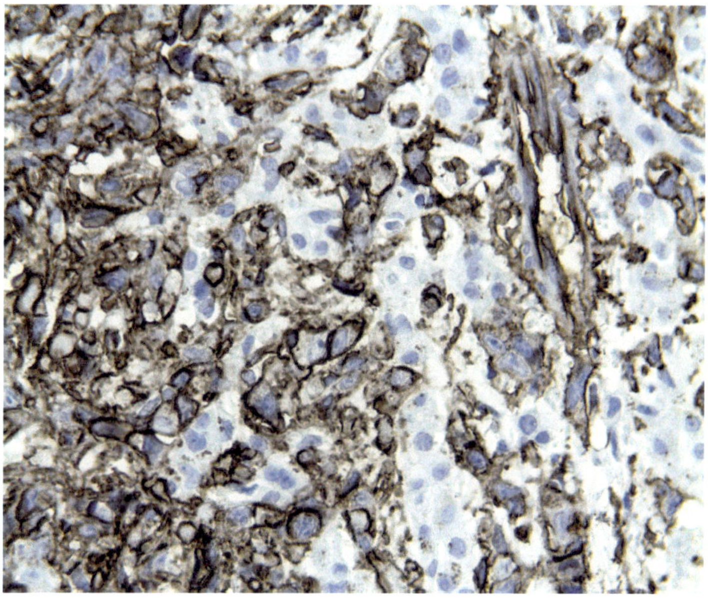

Figure 11. Expression of CD34 in epithelioid haemangioendothelioma. Note also the positive reaction in the lining of a venule. IP,anti-CD34, OM 400x.

The tumour is growing within sinusoids and venules compressing the adjacent parenchyma. As was mentioned, the expression of endothelial markers is typical. Focal expression of cytokeratin and/or actin is possible [103] and should not cause confusion if panel of immunostains is performed. Stromal fibrosis follows than and can become marked so that neoplastic cells are obscured (Figure 9). Two cell types are described: epithelioid and dendritic. The morphological differential diagnosis includes non-neoplastic fibrosis and/or inflammation and granulation tissue, angiosarcoma and metastatic cancers with marked stromal fibrosis. The non-neoplastic conditions can be ruled out by tumour architecture as revealed by immunohistochemistry. Epithelial tumours can be excluded by the predominance of endothelial markers by IHC. Among the vascular malignancies, the diagnosis of epithelioid haemangioendothelioma is preferred for lesions with low grade atypia, absence of frankly malignant spindle cells, low proliferation, limited destruction of surrounding liver tissue and absence of necrosis.

4.4. Angiosarcoma

Angiosarcoma is defined as malignant tumour of endothelial cells. Epidemiologically, it is characterised by rare occurrence in the liver constituting 2% of primary hepatic malignancies [11]. Elderly (50-60-year-old) males represent the largest group of affected patients [27]. The described risk factors include history of thorotrast use for arteriography, exposure to vinyl chloride in the plastics industry where it has been used for polymerisation, arsenic compounds (used as insecticides, possibly present in wine and used in the treatment of psoriasis), copper compounds, pesticides and other chemical carcinogens. In all cases, long latent period (6-35 years) embarrass the data collection. The clinical picture can show signs and symptoms of liver damage (hepatomegaly, local pain, jaundice), disorders of blood cell function (anaemia, thrombocytopenia, disseminated intravascular coagulation), and tumour-related intoxication manifesting as weight loss. Ascites, bleeding into abdominal cavity and liver failure is possible [27]. Grossly, multiple masses with signs of haemorrhage are present. Morphologically, the cellular atypia as well as vascular differentiation can be observed in variable extent. High-grade tumours exhibit solid growth with few vascular spaces. Immunohistochemically, endothelial markers CD31 and CD34 are expressed. However, the immunophenotype can be not straightforward. In our experience, it is important to use several endothelial markers. At first, the reactivity can be uneven [27]. Even more, CD34 is technologically beneficial antibody characterised with high affinity. However, during the evaluation it is necessary to consider CD34 expression in non-endothelial tumours including gastrointestinal stromal tumour and solitary fibrous tumour, among others.

5. Metastatic liver tumours

In Western countries, metastatic tumours represent the most common malignant liver lesion with the rate 94-98% among all malignant liver tumours [27]. Almost all malignant tumours, including carcinomas, sarcomas, melanomas and haematological malignancies, can secondary involve the liver by haematogenous, lymphogeneous or transperitoneal spread. Theoretically, metastatic tumour retains the morphological characteristics of the primary site. However, the balance between anaplasia and differentiation can shift towards anaplasia in such degree that signs of differentiation towards specific tissue or cell type are hardly recognisable. Some tumours like squamous cell cancer and melanoma lack specifity regarding the organ of origin. Even adenocarcinomas retain few specific features. Therefore the differential diagnostics between primary and secondary liver tumours represents a complicated practical task. Clinical data can be absent if metastatic liver lesion presents as cancer of unknown origin. The diagnosis can be reached by logical analysis of morphology, IHC and molecular data. If the establishment of exact histogenesis is unsuccessful, the biopsy investigation should be directed towards the analysis of treatment possibilities. Pathologist should comment in detail morphological and immunophenotype data that could either prove or disregard any particular type of treatment.

In case of liver metastasis, the primary tumour most frequently is located in colon, pancreas, stomach, breast, oesophagus, genitourinary organs [100, 103]. Lung cancer can metastasize to liver as well [6]. Neuroendocrine tumours, even small, can give rise to hepatic metastases. The clinical course in this case can be prolonged and occasionally characterised by carcinoid syndrome including flushing, diarrhoea and palpitations.

The spectrum of metastatic tumours in liver biopsies depend on the frequency of different tumours, the biological properties of different neoplasms predicting the possibility of metastatic spread to liver as well as by the medical paradigm considering the indications for liver biopsies. In the files of single university hospital, metastatic tumours constituted 45% of tumours or tumour-like liver lesions. Adenocarcinoma was the most frequent histological type of metastases (65.5%) comprising metastases of colorectal (48.2%), pancreatic (13.5%), breast (13%), gastric (6.2%), lung (4.5%) and oesophageal cancer (3.7%). Neuroendocrine carcinomas were seen frequently (16%). Lymphoma constituted 0.4% of all tumours [2]. Metastases in cirrhotic liver were rare [2]. In another study, including 130 cases of metastatic liver disease, gastrointestinal tract was found to be the most common primary location (45.3%) of cancer metastasizing to liver followed by neuroendocrine tumours (10.7%) [104]. In children, neuroblastoma, nephroblastoma and rhabdomyosarcoma are the most frequent source of metastases [103].

The spread to liver occurs in 5-10% of patients with Hodgkin's lymphoma and 15-40% of non-Hodgkin's lymphoma cases at the time of diagnosis. Leukemias can involve the liver as well. Grossly, large cell lymphoma can form masses similarly to carcinoma. In case of Hodgkin's disease, the size of nodules is variable. Leukemic infiltrate can be present without visible mass lesion. Myeloid leukemias preferentially infiltrate sinusoids, lymphoid – portal tracts, but hairy cell leukemia can involve both portal tracts and sinusoids forming small blood containing cavities, surrounded by neoplastic cells [103].

Malignant melanoma (Figures 12-14) is one of the greatest challenges in diagnostic surgical pathology [105] due to amelanotic, clear cell, sarcomatoid, small cell, haemangiopericytoid, signet-ring cell, myxoid, metaplastic and rhabdoid forms. The diagnosis largely depends on IHC. Evaluating the intermediate filaments, melanoma expresses vimentin. Despite the reported concerns of cytokeratin expression in melanoma, this is rare event (3%) in formalin-fixed tissues. Similarly, the expression of glial fibrillar acidic protein and actin is observed in 1% of melanomas [105]. Interspersed normal cells should be excluded from evaluation of cytokeratin and actin reactivity. Melanoma is characterised by nuclear and cytoplasmic expression of S-100 protein in 97.4-98%. S-100 protein can be observed in carcinomas, histiocytic neoplasms and malignant peripheral nerve sheath tumour, therefore melanoma-specific antibodies, e.g., HMB-45 and MART-1/Melan-A must be included in the panel. Melanoma can express bcl-2, CD10, CD68, CD56, CD57, CD99, CD117 antigens leading to diagnostic confusion with lymphoma, renal cell cancer, hepatocellular cancer, GIST, seminoma and other neoplasms. Expression of Melan-A is found also in metastatic adrenocortical carcinoma (50-60%) that can be recognised by inhibin expression in around 70% of cases [6]. S-100, HMB-45, Melan-A and inhibin are absent from HCC [6].

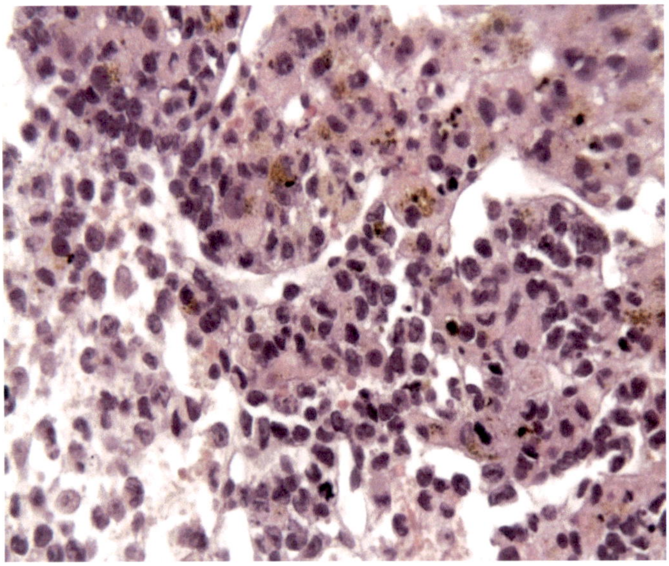

Figure 12. Diffuse sinusoidal spread of undifferentiated malignant tumour. By immunohistochemistry, metastatic melanoma was revealed (see also Figure 13). HE, OM 400 x.

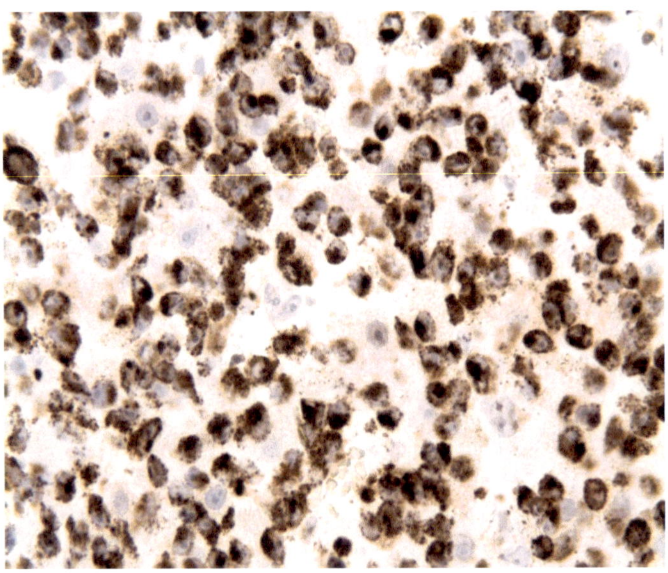

Figure 13. Intense perinuclear expression of melanosome protein HMB-45 in metastatic melanoma. IP, anti-HMB-45, OM 400x.

http://dx.doi.org/10.5772/52838

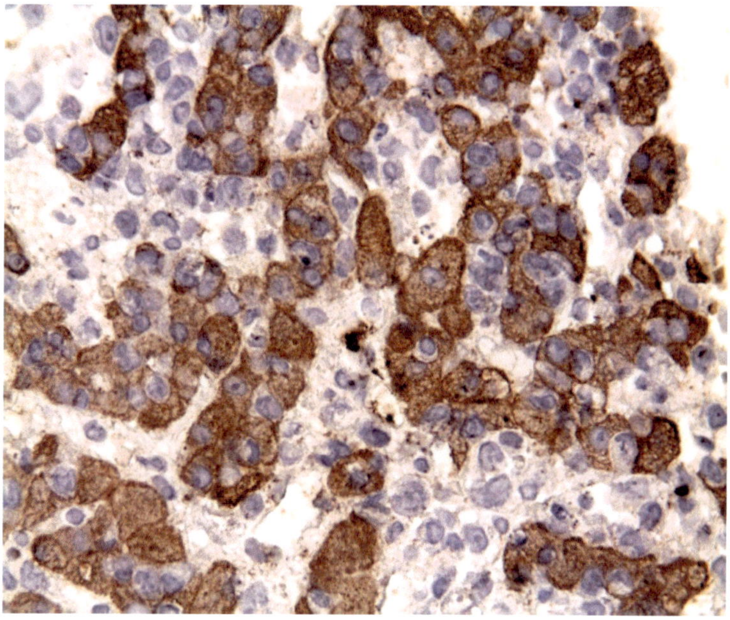

Figure 14. Lack of cytokeratins AE1/AE3 in metastatic melanoma. Note the unusual sinusoidal spread. IP, anti-AE1/AE3, OM 400x.

Metastatic breast cancer expresses CK7 but not CK20. However, this immunophenotype is shared by many adenocarcinomas. To identify the tumour as metastasis from breast primary tumour, gross cystic disease fluid protein fraction-15 (GCDFP-15) and/or mammaglobin can be detected. The specifity of GCDFP-15 is estimated as 99%, and the sensitivity ranges from 50 to 74%. Breast cancers of luminal molecular type express oestrogen (ER) and progesterone receptors (PR). Naturally, the expression of female steroid hormone receptors is shared by ovarian and endometrial cancer. Nowadays the detection of ER and PR is routine in breast cancer diagnostics but less experience is obtained with expression of hormone receptors in extra-genital carcinomas. The scientific studies report expression of ER in carcinoma of lung, stomach and thyroid [105]. The cross-reactivity can be associated by certain antibody clones. Also, HER-2 positive and triple negative molecular types of breast cancer are more prone to develop visceral metastases. Thus, negative ER/PR expression cannot exclude metastatic breast cancer, and positive findings should be interpreted with caution recognising the possibility of metastatic ovarian or endometrial cancer and cross-reactivity or true expression of hormone receptors in extra-genital tumour. ER/PR expression in lung or thyroid tumour can be controlled by TTF-1 protein expression and/or evaluation for neuroendocrine markers and calcitonin.

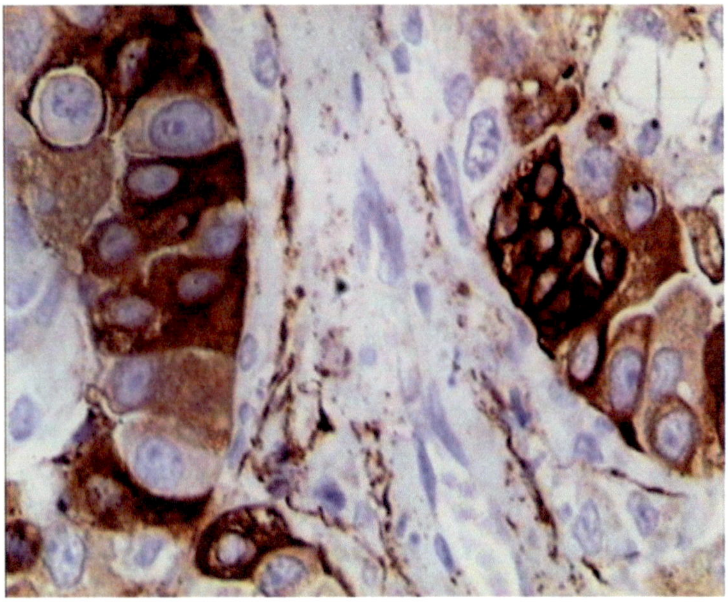

Figure 15. Surfactant A in pulmonary adenocarcinoma. IP, anti-surfactant apoprotein A, OM 400x.

Adenocarcinoma, squamous cell cancer, small cell cancer and carcinoid are the most frequent lung neoplasms. Lung adenocarcinoma is characterised by expression of CK7 (100%) and TTF-1 (60-75%). Expression of CK20 is rare. Cytokeratins 5/6 and 34betaE12 can be present but are not dominant in comparison with CK7. Vimentin can be found in lung adenocarcinomas. Nuclear expression of TTF-1 and/or cytoplasmic expression of surfactant apoprotein A (Figure 15) is an evidence of pulmonary origin. Small cell cancer expresses neuroendocrine markers and pan-cytokeratin. The expression of chromogranin A and CK AE1/AE3 can be limited to perinuclear dot reactivity. Simultaneous detection of leukocyte common antigen can be suggested to perform differential diagnosis with haematological neoplasm. Nuclear expression of TTF-1 protein is frequently present (Figures 16-18). The high proliferation fraction by Ki-67 is characteristic albeit unspecific. The immunophenotype of squamous cell cancer is unspecific and characterised by cytoplasmic expression of CK5/6 and CK 34betaE12 in association with strong nuclear reactivity with p63 protein. CK7 can be present but is not dominant. TTF-1 protein is absent. Carcinoid is characterised by neuroendocrine differentiation and low proliferative activity. The TTF-1 expression is not frequent [17,105-107].

http://dx.doi.org/10.5772/52838

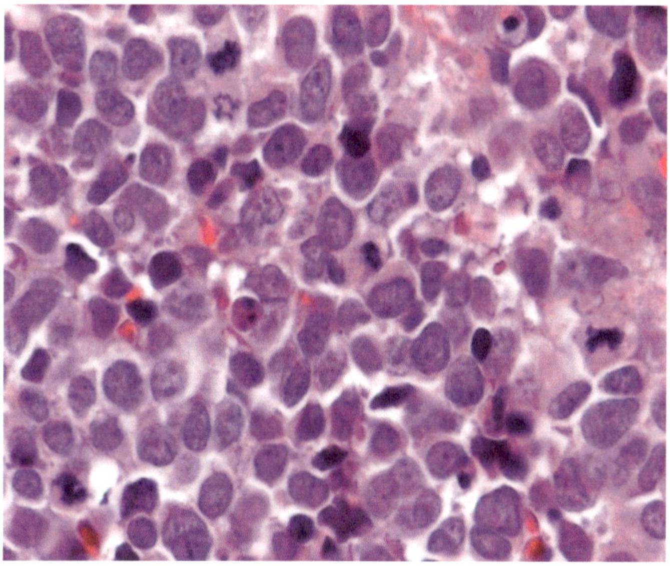

Figure 16. Small cell cancer. Note the "salt-and-pepper" chromatin and high mitotic activity. HE, OM 400x.

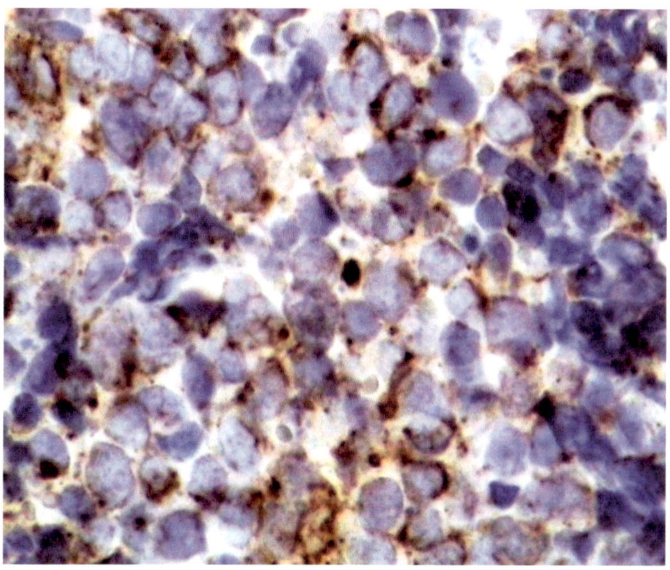

Figure 17. Granular cytoplasmic and perinuclear expression of chromogranin A in small cell cancer. IP, anti-chromogranin A, OM 400x.

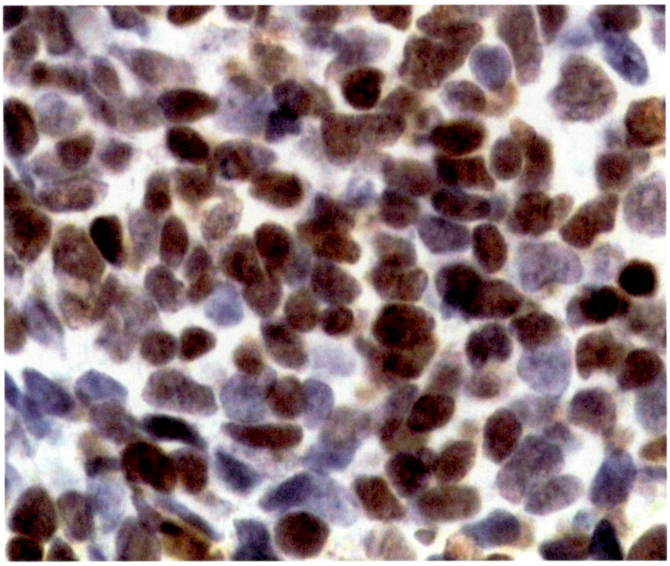

Figure 18. Nuclear TTF-1 expression in small cell cancer. IP, anti-chromogranin A, OM 400x.

Mesothelioma is characterised by expression of CK7, CK5/6, vimentin and calretinin (Figure 19). HBME-1 can be expressed as well but lacks specifity.

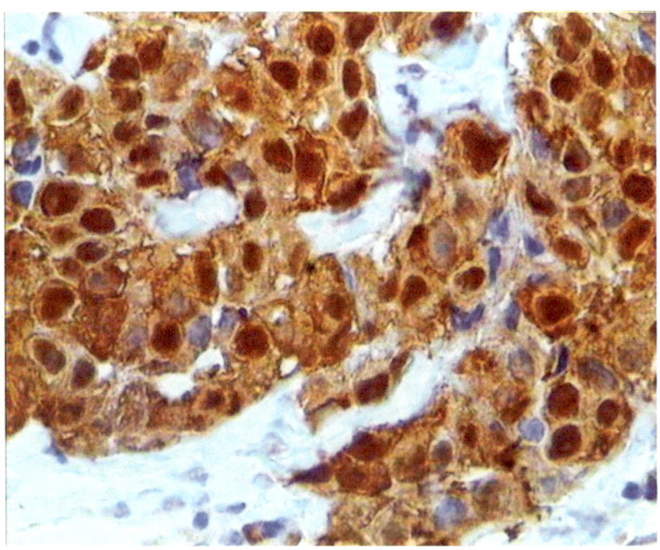

Figure 19. Nuclear and cytoplasmic expression of calretinin in epithelioid mesothelioma.IP, anti-calretinin, OM 400x.

http://dx.doi.org/10.5772/52838

Metastatic colorectal carcinoma can be recognised by diffuse intensive cytoplasmic expression of CK20 and nuclear expression of CDX2 [108]. Carcinoid of the midgut and hindgut also are positive for CDX2 [109].

Neuroendocrine tumours are characterised by strong cytoplasmic expression of chromogranin A and synaptophysin and negativity for Hep Par 1 [6]. CD56 is considered to be the most sensitive neuroendocrine marker. In our experience, it shows reliable performance in small or compressed biopsies making it especially valuable tool for the evaluation of scant tissue material. Occasional CD56 expression in HCC is described [6].

Renal cell carcinoma is characterised by negativity for Hep Par 1 and CEA expression (by polyclonal anti-CEA antibody). Unfortunately, the rate of RCC expression decreases from 50-80% in primary clear cell renal carcinoma and 60-90% in papillary renal cell cancer to 20% in metastatic renal cell carcinoma. CD10 can be present both in HCC and renal cell carcinoma. Although the pattern of expression is different this can be difficult to evaluate, especially in core biopsy. PAX-2 is advised as marker of metastatic renal cell carcinoma with the expression rate 70-80%. Expression of vimentin is more characteristic in clear cell renal carcinoma (60-70%) than in hepatocellular carcinoma; chromophobe renal cell carcinoma also is negative [6].

As tumour heterogeneity remains a source of problems [69] and the immunophenotype can be inherently complex and subjected to cross reactivity, we recommend wide IHC panels including several markers for HCC and cholangiocarcinoma as well as markers for metastatic tumour, including the organospecific antigens (see Tables 1-2).

Tumour	Immunophenotype
Malignant melanoma	Vim + CK AE1 / AE3 – S-100 + HMB-45 + MART-1 / Melan A +
Lung adenocarcinoma	CK7+ CK20- CK34betaE12-/+ TTF-1+ Surfactant apoprotein A +
Small cell cancer	CK AE1/AE3 + ChrA+ CD56 +TTF-1 +
Squamous cancer	CK34betaE12+ CK7-/+ CK20 – p63+
NET	CK AE1/AE3 + ChrA+ TTF-1 +/ - (lung) or CDX2 + (midgut, hindgut)
Breast cancer	CK 7 + CK20 – MG +/– ER +/– PR +/–
Colorectal cancer	CK20+ CK7- CDX2+ TTF-1-

Table 1. The immunophenotype of selected malignant tumours. Abbreviations in the Table: Vim, vimentin; CK, cytokeratin; TTF-1, thyroid transcription factor 1; ChrA, chromogranin A; NET, neuroendocrine tumour; MG, mammaglobin; ER, oestrogen receptor; PR, progesterone receptor

Antigen	Valuable positive expression	Notes
Glypican-3	Hepatocellular carcinoma	Occasional positivity in non-hepatocellular tumour
Arginase-1	Hepatocellular carcinoma	Sensitivity for hepatocellular carcinoma 96% Normal liver tissue positive Metastatic tumours rarely positive [69]

Hep Par 1	Hepatocellular carcinoma	Sensitivity for hepatocellular carcinoma around 50% [69] Gastric carcinoma can be positive
AFP	Hepatocellular carcinoma	Sensitivity for hepatocellular carcinoma around 15% [69]
CD10	Renal cell carcinoma Hepatocellular carcinoma	Negative in adrenal carcinoma
CK7	Cholangiocellular carcinoma Metastatic cancers	Positivity does not exclude hepatocellular carcinoma Valuable for primary evaluation of malignant tumour within liver
CK17	Cholangiocellular carcinoma Metastatic cancers	Positive tumours as pancreatic cancer (58%), squamous carcinoma (75%), urothelial carcinoma (75%) and cholangiocellular carcinoma (35%) can be distinguished from negative ones (gastric, colorectal, prostate, breast cancer, hepatocellular carcinoma)
CK19	Cholangiocellular carcinoma Metastatic cancers	Positivity does not exclude hepatocellular carcinoma
CK20	Metastatic colorectal cancer	Useful in conjuction with CK7 for initial grouping of cancers showing adenocarcinomatous structure
CDX2	Metastatic colorectal cancer and NETs	Heterogeneous focal expression in gastric and pancreatic carcinomas Mucinous ovarian cancers can be positive Morules in endometrioid carcinoma are positive
Calretinin	Mesothelioma Adrenal cortical carcinoma Sex cord-stromal tumours of the genital tract	Squamous carcinoma frequently positive
Surfactant apoprotein A	Lung adenocarcinoma. In our experience possess high affinity and is useful, if positive	Reactivity in thyroid cancer (43% in small group) has been reported Heterogeneous expression has been observed [69]
TTF-1, nuclear expression	Metastatic pulmonary adenocarcinoma (75% of non-mucinous type and 10% of mucinous type), small cell cancer (pulmonary, 50-90%; non-pulmonary, 44-80%) or thyroid cancer including papillary, follicular and medullary but not anaplastic carcinoma [69]	Regarding pulmonary adenocarcinoma, less subjected to heterogeneity-related evaluation problems than surfactant apoprotein A Endometrial (17%) or breast (2.4%) cancer occasionally positive [69]
TTF-1, cytoplasmic expression:	Hepatocellular carcinoma	Expression in benign liver parenchyma is present Gastric or prostatic cancer can show cytoplasmic positivity
Chromogranin and synaptophysin	ANET	

CD56	NET, cholangiocarcinoma	Other tumours can be positive
Oestrogen and progesterone receptors	Breast, ovarian or endometrial cancer, endometrial stromal sarcoma	Non-gynaecologic cancers can be occasionally positive, including lung cancer (4-15-67%)
CD117	GIST Seminoma	CD34 is co-expressed in GISTs PLAP is co-expressed in germ cell tumours
Mammaglobin	Breast cancer	High heterogeneity Sensitivity for breast cancer 40-85% Ovarian (17%), endometrial (40-70%) and endocervical (30%) carcinoma can also be positive [69]
GCDFP-15	Breast cancer	Sensitivity for breast cancer 50-60% High heterogeneity Not associated with mammaglobin thus simultaneous evaluation can be recommended [69]
PSA	Prostatic cancer	Negative in 5% high-grade prostate cancers. Reactivity in few breast carcinomas and rectal NETs have been observed [69]
Pax8	Thyroid cancer Female genital tract carcinomas Renal cell cancer	Sensitivity for thyroid cancer 79-100% and for renal cancer 71-98% Breast cancer is negative. Positivity is useful to discriminate breast cancer from ovarian or endometrial cancer NETs can be positive
P63	Squamous cell cancer Urothelial carcinoma	

Table 2. Panel of antibodies for liver biopsy evaluation. Abbreviations in the Table: AFP, alpha-fetoprotein; CK, cytokeratin; NET, neuroendocrine tumour; TTF-1, thyroid transcription factor 1; GIST, gastrointestinal stromal tumour; PLAP, placental alkaline phosphatase; GCDFP-15, gross cystic disease fluid protein-15; PSA, prostate specific antigen

6. Cystic biliary tumours

The cystic biliary tumours are defined by cystic structure and development of / differentiation towards intrahepatic bile duct epithelium. The group includes malignant biliary cystadenocarcinoma and benign biliary cystadenoma. Epidemiologically, cystic biliary tumours represent rare entities, with incidence of biliary cystadenocarcinoma approximately 1/10 million (corresponding to 0.01/100 000) and of biliary cystadenoma 1/100 000 - 5/100 000 [110]. Biliary cystadenocarcinoma is diagnosed mostly at the age 50-60 years [100]. Biliary cystadenoma is diagnosed in younger patients: mean age 40.6 (range 30-51) vs. 51.3 (range 41-63) years in biliary cystadenocarcinoma group [14]. In other studies even larger age difference (17 years) is found between patients affected by benign and malignant cystic biliary tumours, respectively [111-112]. Cystic biliary tumours are more common in women: 80-100% of biliary adenoma and 63-71.4% of biliary cystadenocarcinoma are described in female [14]. The clinical picture reflects the presence of mass lesion and is dominated by abdominal pain [113]. The other manifestations and complications include jaundice, cholangitis, tumour rupture [114], haemorrhage [115], compression of the portal or caval veins with possible subsequent ascites [113], hemobilia [12] and mucobilia [116]. Notably, the tumour can progress slowly [117] with the clinical history of biliary cystadenocarcinoma as long as 10-15 years [112,118]. The long course is is in accordance with the low grade of malignancy and gradual development of tumour through stages of increased epithelial proliferation, dysplasia, *in situ* cancer and, finally, invasive cancer. Thus, long anamnesis of cystic hepatic mass does not exclude the possibility of malignant tumour and the need for careful follow-up if the cyst is not removed by operation. Although biopsy can be considered in cases with unclear differential diagnosis, it is not the first choice because of the following considerations. First, simple liver cyst is the main differential diagnosis of cystic biliary tumours. Although biliary cystadenocarcinoma is rare, liver cysts have high prevalence being present in 2.5% of the population [119] and cannot be distinguished from cystic biliary tumours on the basis of CA19-9 and CEA levels [14,114]. However, core biopsy is unlikely to yield sufficient tissue in case of simple cyst or cystadenoma; it also is not suitable for the diagnostics of focal malignancy and rarely can lead to peritoneal carcinomatosis [13]. Therefore radiological diagnostics, especially computed tomography, is essential [117]. Grossly, biliary cystadenocarcinoma is multicystic. Internal mural nodules are irregularly distributed in the walls. The tumour most frequently is located within the liver (83%). Extrahepatic bile ducts (13%) or the gall bladder (0.02%) has been affected by this tumour as well [14]. The size of cystic biliary tumours (1.5-30 cm) is not helpful in the differential diagnostics between simple hepatic cyst and cystic biliary tumours; it also has no correlation with malignant biological potential [120]. The metastatic spread of biliary cystadenocarcinoma can affect the liver, regional lymph nodes in the hepatoduodenal ligament, lungs, pleura or peritoneum [100]. Histologically, biliary cystadenocarcinoma is characterised by clear-cut signs of malignancy: cellular atypia, particularly nuclear polymorphism, mitotic activity and invasion into surrounding stroma. The tumour architecture is cystic and papillary. The benign counterpart of biliary cystadenocarcinoma, the biliary cystadenoma lacks the malignant features [100] and is composed by either mucinous or serous benign epithelium. Most of cystic biliary tumours possess characteristic mesenchymal, ovarian–type stroma. Hypothetically, these tumours arise from bile ducts proximal to the hilum of the liver and share the cystic structure and presence of peculiar ovarian-type mesenchymal stroma with mucinous cystic tumours of the pancreas and retroperitoneum, leading to the hypothesis that ectopic ovarian stroma during embryogenesis can become incorporated along the biliary tree, in the pancreas and retroperitoneal space and cause the proliferation of the adjacent epithelium by production of the hormones and growth factors [121]. Origin from intrahepatic peribiliary glands [122] or from ectopic rests of primitive foregut sequestered in the liver [114] has been hypothesised. Development from pluripotential stem cells is suggested on the basis of the presence of albumin messenger RNA and biliary type cytokeratins in the tumour cells [123]. Biliary cystadenocarcinoma without mesenchymal stroma more frequently arises in males and carries poorer prognosis in comparison with the tumour possessing mesenchymal stroma [122]. By immunohistochemistry, increasing proliferative activity by Ki-67 expression as well as increasing p53 protein expression from adenoma to carcinoma was shown in biliary cystadenocarcinoma without ovarian-type stroma [124]. Expression of cytokeratin (CK) 7 and absence of CK20, CEA, alpha-fetoprotein, calretinin, CD31 and chromogranin is described [125]. However, presence of CK20, although typical for colorectal cancer, is described in cholangiocarcinoma, especially non-peripheral [126]. It might be expected in biliary cystadenocarcinoma with growing awareness about this entity.

There is evidence showing that at least some cases of biliary cystadenocarcinoma originate from pre-existing biliary cystadenoma. These data include the age difference between biliary cystadenocarcinoma and biliary adenoma patients [14] as well as morphologic findings of malignant transformation in a lesion with focally innocuous structure [127].

Radiologically, presence of internal septations allows excluding a simple cyst. Vascularity of septa is characteristic for cystic biliary tumours [14] and is considered by some specialists to be more reliable in distinguishing biliary cystadenoma from cyst than the simple presence of septations [117]. Biliary cystadenoma is characterised by smooth and thin internal septa, but presence of enhanced mural nodules in the outer wall or septa is the most important sign of malignancy. Calcification is not frequent but has been found specific for malignancy by some [14] but not all [119] authors as far as cystic biliary tumours are concerned. Size, number of septations or location of the neoplasm does not help to differentiate between benign or malignant cystic biliary tumours [14]. Some authors have postulated that preoperative differentiation between biliary adenoma and cystadenocarcinoma by radiologic imaging is not possible therefore liver resection should be performed for all cystic biliary tumours [120]. This assumption is based on the experience that internal papillae with arterial enhancement may be present in both tumours so that computed tomography and magnetic resonance imaging yield overlapping data.

The clinical differential diagnosis of cystic liver lesions, entering the differential diagnosis of biliary cystadenocarcinoma, include developmental, neoplastic, inflammatory and traumatic lesions as simple bile duct cyst, polycystic liver disease, biliary hamartoma, cystically degenerated cases of other primary or metastatic liver tumours, abscesses, hydatid cyst, extrapancreatic pseudocyst, hematoma and biloma [119,128].

7. Conclusions

In conclusion, wide variety of neoplastic processes can affect the liver. Most of non-cystic tumours can be reliably diagnosed in liver biopsy. Several demographic and clinical data should be submitted along with the liver biopsy. Patient's age and presence or absence of clinical symptoms must be known. If there is history of contraceptive use it should be reported. Radiological data have high relevance: the size, localisation in respect to liver capsule and number of focal liver lesions should be known to the pathologist. The vascularity should be described. Knowing these data, pathologist should evaluate the haematoxylin-eosin stained specimen. Wide panel of immunohistochemical stains can be recommended than.

Author details

Ilze Strumfa[1*], Janis Vilmanis[2], Andrejs Vanags[2*], Ervins Vasko[3], Dzeina Sulte[3], Zane Simtniece[1], Arnis Abolins[1] and Janis Gardovskis[2]

*Address all correspondence to: ilze.strumfa@rsu.lv

1 Department of Pathology, Riga Stradins University, Riga, Latvia

2 Department of Surgery, Riga Stradins University, Riga, Latvia

3 Faculty of Medicine, Riga Stradins University, Riga, Latvia

References

[1] Ho, M., & Kim, H. (2011). Glypican-3: a new target for cancer immunotherapy. *Eur J Cancer*, 47(3), 333-338.

[2] Kasper, H. U., Drebber, U., Dries, V., & Dienes, H. P. (2005). Liver metastases: incidence and histogenesis. *Z Gastroenterol*, 43(10), 1149-1157.

[3] Al-Muhannadi, N., Ansari, N., Brahmi, U., & Satir, A. A. (2011). Differential diagnosis of malignant epithelial tumours in the liver: an immunohistochemical study on liver biopsy material. *Ann Hepatol*, 10(4), 508-515.

[4] Marrero, J. A. (2009). Modern diagnosis of hepatocellular carcinoma: utilization of liver biopsy and genomic markers. *J Hepatol*, 50(4), 659-661.

[5] Kayser, K. (2012). Introduction of virtual microscopy in routine surgical pathology – a hypothesis and personal view from Europe. *Diagn Pathol*, 7(1), 48, http://www.diagnosticpathology.org/content/pdf/1746-1596-7-48.pdf , (accessed 04 August 2012).

[6] Kakar, S., Gown, A. M., Goodman, Z. D., & Ferrell, L. D. (2007). Best practices in diagnostic immunohistochemistry: hepatocellular carcinoma versus metastatic neoplasms. *Arch Pathol Lab Med*, 131(11), 1648-1654.

[7] Roncalli, M., Park, Y. N., & Di Tommaso, L. (2010). Histopathological classification of hepatocellular carcinoma. *Dig Liver Dis*, 42(3), S228-S234.

[8] Purcell, R., Childs, M., Maibach, R., Miles, C., Turner, C., Zimmermann, A., Czauderna, P., & Sullivan, M. (2011). Potential biomarkers for hepatoblastoma: Results from the SIOPEL-3 study. *Eur J Cancer*, 48(12), 1853-1859.

[9] Bosch, F. X., Ribes, J., Cleries, R., & Diaz, M. (2005). Epidemiology of hepatocellular carcinoma. *Clin Liver Dis*, 9(2), 191-211.

[10] Bosman, F. T., Carneiro, F., Hruban, R. H., & Theise, N. D. (2010). WHO classification of tumours of the digestive system, 4th edition. *Lyon: International Agency for Research on Cancer (IARC).*

[11] Bhati, C. S., Bhatt, A. N., Starkey, G., Hubscher, S. G., & Bramhall, S. R. (2008). Acute liver failure due to primary angiosarcoma: a case report and review of literature. *World J Surg Oncol*, 6, 104, doi:10.1186/1477-7819-6-104, http://www.wjso.com/content/6/1/104, (accessed 08 August 2012).

[12] Madariaga, J. R., Iwatsuki, S., Starzl, T. E., Todo, S., Selby, R., & Zetti, G. (1993). Hepatic resection for cystic lesions of the liver. *Ann Surg*, 218(5), 610-614.

[13] Manouras, A., Markogiannakis, H., Lagoudianakis, E., & Katergiannakis, V. (2006). Biliary cystadenoma with mesenchymal stroma: report of a case and review of the literature. *World J Gastroenterol*, 12(37), 6062-6069.

[14] Pojchamarnwiputh, S., Na, Chiangmai. W., Chotirosniramit, A., & Lertprasertsuke, N. (2008). Computed tomography of biliary cystadenoma and biliary cystadenocarcinoma. *Singapore Med J*, 49(5), 392-396.

[15] Schullian, P., Widmann, G., Lang, T. B., Knoflach, M., & Bale, R. (2011). Accuracy and diagnostic yield of CT-guided stereotactic liver biopsy of primary and secondary liver tumours. *Comput Aided Surg*, 16(4), 181-187, doi: 10.3109/10929088.2011.578367.

[16] Mishra, M., Morgan, V., Hamati, A. K., & Al-Abbadi, M. (2012). Carcinoma of unknown primary: check the liver... thanks to TTF-1. *Tenn Med*, 105(1), 35-36.

[17] Bahrami, A., Truong, L. D., & Ro, J. Y. (2008). Undifferentiated tumour: true identity by immunohistochemistry. *Arch Pathol Lab Med*, 132(3), 326-348.

[18] Guo, H., Lv, Y., Tian, T., Hu, T. H., Wang, W. J., Sui, X., Jiang, L., Ruan, Z. P., & Nan, K. J. (2011). Downregulation of p57 accelerates the growth and invasion of hepatocellular carcinoma. *Carcinogenesis*, 32(12), 1897-1904.

[19] Chen, H. W., Huang, X. D., Li, H. C., He, S., Ni, R. Z., Chen, C. H., Peng, C., Wu, G., Wang, Y. Y., Zhao, Y. H., Zhang, Y. X., Shen, A. G., & Wang, H. M. (2012). Expression of FOXJ1 in hepatocellular carcinoma: correlation with patients' prognosis and tumor cell proliferation. *Mol Carcinog*, Epub ahead of print,, doi: 10.1002/mc.21904, http://onlinelibrary.wiley.com/doi/10.1002/mc.21904/pdf, (accessed 4 July).

[20] Liao, M., Tong, P., Zhao, J., Zhang, Y., Li, Z., Wang, J., Feng, X., Hu, M., & Pan, Y. (2012). Prognostic value of matrix metalloproteinase-1/proteinase-activated receptor-1 signaling axis in hepatocellular carcinoma. *Pathol Oncol Res*, 18(2), 397-403.

[21] Lu, J. T., Zhao, W. D., He, W., & Wei, W. (2012). Hedgehog signaling pathway mediates invasion and metastasis of hepatocellular carcinoma via ERK pathway. *Acta Pharmacol Sin*, 33(5), 691-700.

[22] Yin, X., Li, Y. W., Zhang, B. H., Ren, Z. G., Qiu, S. J., Yi, Y., & Fan, J. (2012). Coexpression of stemness factors Oct4 and Nanog predict liver resection. *Ann Surg Oncol*,

Epub Mar 30 ahead of print., doi: 10.1245/s10434-012-2314-6, http://www.springerlink.com/content/h31v0112827836r2/fulltext.pdf, (accessed 04 August).

[23] Di Tommaso, L., Destro, A., Seok, J. Y., Balladore, E., Terracciano, L., Sangiovanni, A., Iavarone, M., Colombo, M., Jang, J. J., Yu, E., Jin, S. Y., Morenghi, E., Park, Y. N., & Roncalli, M. (2009). The application of markers (HSP70 GPC3 and GS) in liver biopsies is useful for detection of hepatocellular carcinoma. *J Hepatol*, 50(4), 746-754.

[24] Albulescu, R., Neagu, M., Albulescu, L., & Tanase, C. (2011). Tissular and soluble miRNAs for diagnostic and therapy improvement in digestive tract cancers. *Expert Rev Mol Diagn*, 11(1), 101-120.

[25] Meng, F., Glaser, S. S., Francis, H., De Morrow, S., Han, Y., Passarini, Stokes. A., Cleary, J. P., Liu, X., Venter, J., Kumar, P., Priester, S., Hubble, L., Staloch, D., Sharma, J., Liu, C. G., & Alpini, G. (2012). Functional analysis of microRNAs in human hepatocellular cancer stem cells. *J Cell Mol Med*, 16(1), 160-173.

[26] Barthelmes, L., & Tait, I. S. (2005). Liver cell adenoma and liver cell adenomatosis. *HPB (Oxford)*, 7(3), 186-196.

[27] Kanel, G. C., & Korula, J. (2011). Atlas of liver pathology. *3rd edition. Philadelphia: Elsevier Saunders.*

[28] Bioulac-Sage, P., Balabaud, C., & Zucman-Rossi, J. (2010). Subtype classification of hepatocellular adenoma. *Dig Surg*, 27(1), 39-45.

[29] Walther, Z., & Jain, D. (2011). Molecular pathology of hepatic neoplasms: classification and clinical significance. *Pathology Research Int*, 2011, 403929, 10.4061/2011/403929, http://www.hindawi.com/journals/pri/2011/403929/, (accessed 08 July 2012).

[30] Buell, J. F., Tranchart, H., Cannon, R., & Dagher, I. (2010). Management of benign hepatic tumours. *Surg Clin North Am*, 90(4), 719-735.

[31] Longo, D. L., Fauci, A., Kasper, D., Hauser, S., Jameson, J. L., & Loscalzo, J. (2012). Harrison's principles of internal medicine. *McGraw-Hill.*

[32] Farges, O., & Dokmak, S. (2010). Malignant transformation of liver adenoma: an analysis of the literature. *Dig Surg*, 27(1), 32-38.

[33] Bluteau, O., Jeannot, E., Bioulac-Sage, P., Marques, J. M., Blanc, J. F., Bui, H., Beaudoin, J. C., Franco, D., Balabaud, C., Laurent-Puig, P., & Zucman-Rossi, J. (2002). Biallelic inactivation of TCF1 in hepatic adenomas. *Nat Genet*, 32(2), 312-315.

[34] Reznik, V., Dao, T., Coutant, R., Chiche, L., Jeannot, E., Clauin, S., Rousselot, P., Fabre, M., Oberti, F., Fatome, A., Zucman-Rossi, J., & Bellanne-Chantelot, C. (2004). Hepatocyte nuclear factor-1 alpha gene inactivation: cosegregation between liver adenomatosis and diabetes phenotypes in two maturity-onset diabetes of the young (MODY) 3 families. *J Clin Endocrinol Metab*, 89(3), 1476-1480.

[35] Jeannot, E., Mellottee, L., Bioulac-Sage, P., Balabaud, C., Scoazec, J. Y., Tran Van, Nhieu. J., Bacq, Y., Michalak, S., Buob, D., Groupe d'etude Genetique des Tumeurs Hepatiques (INSERM Network), Laurent-Puig, P., Rusyn, I., & Zucman-Rossi, J. (2010). Spectrum of HNF1A somatic mutations in hepatocellular adenoma differs from that in patients with MODY3 and suggests genotoxic damage. *Diabetes*, 59(7), 1836-1844.

[36] Rebouissou, S., Amessou, M., Couchy, G., Poussin, K., Imbeaud, S., Pilati, C., Izard, T. B., Alabaud, C., Bioulac-Sage, P., & Zucman-Rossi, J. (2009). Frequent in-frame somatic deletions activate gp130 in inflammatory hepatocellular tumours. *Nature*, 457(7226), 200-204.

[37] Chen, Y. W., Jeng, Y. M., Yeh, S. H., & Chen, P. J. (2002). P53 gene and Wnt signaling in benign neoplasms: beta-catenin mutations in hepatic adenoma but not in focal nodular hyperplasia. *Hepatology*, 36(4 Pt 1), 927-935.

[38] Zucman-Rossi, J., Jeannot, E., Nhieu, J. T., Scoazec, J. Y., Guettier, C., Rebouissou, S., Bacq, Y., Leteurtre, E., Paradis, V., Michalak, S., Wendum, D., Chiche, L., Fabre, M., Mellottee, L., Laurent, C., Partensky, C., Castaing, D., Zafrani, E. S., Laurent-Puig, P., Balabaud, C., & Bioulac-Sage, P. (2006). Genotype-phenotype correlation in hepatocellular adenoma: new classification and relationship with HCC. *Hepatology*, 43(3), 515-524.

[39] Bioulac-Sage, P., Laumonier, H., Rullier, A., Cubel, G., Laurent, C., Zucman-Rossi, J., & Balabaud, C. (2009). Over-expression of glutamine synthetase in focal nodular hyperplasia: a novel easy diagnostic tool in surgical pathology. *Liver Int*, 29(3), 459-465.

[40] Wanless, I. R., Mawdsley, C., & Adams, R. (1985). On the pathogenesis of focal nodular hyperplasia of the liver. *Hepatology*, 5(6), 1194-1200.

[41] Bioulac-Sage, P., Laumonier, H., Cubel, G., Saric, J., & Balabaud, C. (2008). Over-expression of glytamine synthase in focal nodular hyperplasia (part 1): early stages in the formation support the hypothesis of a focal hyper-arterialisation with venous (portal and hepatic) and biliary damage. *Comp Hepatol*, 7, 2.

[42] Rebouissou, S., Bioulac-Sage, P., & Zucman-Rossi, J. (2008). Molecular pathogenesis of focal nodular hyperplasia and hepatocellular adenoma. *J Hepatol*, 48(1), 163-170.

[43] Altekruse, S. F., Mc Glynn, K. A., & Reichman, M. E. (2009). Hepatocellular carcinoma incidence, mortality, and survival trends in the United States from 1975 to 2005. *J Clin Oncol*, 27(9), 1485-1491.

[44] Bancroft, J. D., & Gamble, M. (2002). Theory and practice of histological techniques, 5th ed. *Edinburgh: Churchill Livingstone*.

[45] Capurro, M. I., Xiang, Y. Y., Lobe, C., & Filmus, J. (2005). Glypican-3 promotes the growth of hepatocellular carcinoma by stimulating canonical Wnt signaling. *Cancer Res*, 65(14), 6245-6254.

[46] Capurro, M. I., Xu, P., Shi, W., Li, F., Jia, A., & Filmus, J. (2008). Glypican-3 inhibits Hedgehog signaling during development by competing with patched for Hedgehog binding. *Dev Cell*, 14(5), 700-711.

[47] Nakatsura, T., Yoshitake, Y., Senju, S., Monji, M., Komori, H., Motomura, Y., Hosaka, S., Beppu, T., Ishiko, T., Kamohara, H., Ashikara, H., Katagiri, T., Furukawa, Y., Fujiyama, S., Ogawa, M., Nakamura, Y., & Nishimura, Y. (2003). Glypican-3, overexpressed specifically in human hepatocellular carcinoma, is a novel tumor marker. *Biochem Biophys Res Commun*, 306(1), 16-25.

[48] Yamauchi, N., Watanabe, A., Hishinuma, M., Ohashi, K., Midorikawa, Y., Morishita, Y., Niki, T., Shibahara, J., Mori, M., Makuuchi, M., Hippo, Y., Kodama, T., Iwanari, H., Aburatani, H., & Fukayama, M. (2005). The glypican 3 oncofetal protein is a promising diagnostic marker for hepatocellular carcinoma. *Mod Pathol*, 18(12), 1591-1598.

[49] Wang, Y. L., Zhu, Z. J., Teng, D. H., Yao, Z., Gao, W., & Shen, Z. Y. (2012). Glypican-3 expression and its relationship with recurrence of HCC after liver transplantation. *World J Gastroenterol*, 18(19), 2408-2414.

[50] Nakatsura, T., Kageshita, T., Ito, S., Wakamatsu, K., Monji, M., Ikuta, Y., Senju, S., Ono, T., & Nishimura, Y. (2004). Identification of glypican-3 as a novel tumor marker for melanoma. *Clin Cancer Res*, 10(19), 6612-6621.

[51] Stadlmann, S., Gueth, U., Baumhoer, D., Moch, H., Terracciano, L., & Singer, G. (2007). Glypican-3 expression in primary and recurrent ovarian carcinomas. *Int J Gynecol Pathol*, 26(3), 341-344.

[52] Zynger, D. L., Dimov, N. D., Luan, C., Teh, B. T., & Yang, X. J. (2006). Glypican 3: a novel marker in testicular germ cell tumors. *Am J Surg Pathol*, 30(12), 1570-1575.

[53] Esheba, G. E., Pate, L. L., & Longacre, T. A. (2008). Oncofetal protein glypican-3 distinguishes yolk sac tumor from clear cell carcinoma of the ovary. *Am J Surg Pathol*, 32(4), 600-607.

[54] Baumhoer, D., Tornillo, L., Stadlmann, S., Roncalli, M., Diamantis, E. K., & Terracciano, L. M. (2008). Glypican 3 expression in human nonneoplastic, preneoplastic, and neoplastic tissues: a tissue microarray analysis of 4,387 tissue samples. *Am J Clin Pathol*, 129(6), 899-906.

[55] Ushiku, T., Uozaki, H., Shinozaki, A., Ota, S., Matsuzaka, K., Nomura, S., Kaminishi, M., Aburatani, H., Kodama, T., & Fukuyama, M. (2009). Glypican 3-expressing gastric carcinoma: distinct subgroup unifying hepatoid, clear-cell and alpha-fetoprotein-producing gastric carcinomas. *Cancer Sci*, 100(4), 626-632.

[56] Murthy, S. S., Shen, T., De Rienzo, A., Lee, W. C., Ferriola, P. C., Jhanwar, S. C., Mossman, B. T., Filmus, J., & Testa, J. R. (2000). Expression of GPC3, an X-linked recessive overgrowth gene, is silenced in malignant mesothelioma. *Oncogene*, 19(3), 410-416.

[57] Xiang, Y. Y., Ladeda, V., & Filmus, J. (2001). Glypican-3 expression is silenced in human breast cancer. *Oncogene*, 20(50), 7408-7412.

[58] Kim, H., Xu, G. L., Borczuk, A. C., Busch, S., Filmus, J., Capurro, M., Brody, J. S., Lange, J., D'Armiento, J. M., Rothman, P. B., & Powell, CA. (2003). The heparan sulphate proteoglycan GPC3 is a potential lung tumor suppressor. *Am J Respir Cell Mol Biol*, 29(6), 694-701.

[59] Abdul-Al, H. M., Makhlouf, H. R., Wang, G., & Goodman, Z. D. (2008). Glypican-3 expression in benign liver tissue with active hepatitis C: implications for the diagnosis of hepatocellular carcinoma. *Hum Pathol*, 39(2), 209-212.

[60] Shirakawa, H., Suzuki, H., Shimomura, M., Kojima, M., Gotohda, N., Takahashi, S., Nakagohri, T., Konishi, M., Kobayashi, N., Kinoshita, T., & Nakatsura, T. (2009). Glypican-3 expression is correlated with poor prognosis in hepatocellular carcinoma. *Cancer Sci*, 100(8), 1403-1407.

[61] Hippo, Y., Watanabe, K., Watanabe, A., Midorikawa, Y., Yamamoto, S., Ihara, S., Tokita, S., Iwanari, H., Ito, Y., Nakano, K., Nezu, J., Tsunoda, H., Yoshino, T., Ohizumi, I., Tsuchiya, M., Ohnishi, S., Makuuchi, M., Hamakubo, T., Kodama, T., & Aburatani, H. (2004). Identification of soluble NH2-terminal fragment of glypican-3 as a serological marker for early-stage hepatocellular carcinoma. *Cancer Res*, 64(7), 418-423.

[62] Yan, B. C., Gong, C., Song, J., Krausz, T., Tretiakova, M., Hyjek, E., Al-Ahmadie, H., Alves, V., Xiao, S. Y., Anders, R. A., & Hart, J. A. (2010). Arginase-1: a new immunohistochemical marker of hepatocytes and hepatocellular neoplasms. *Am J Surg Pathol*, 34(8), 1147-1154.

[63] Yao, M., Yao, D. F., Bian, Y. Z., Zhang, C. G., Qiu, L. W., Wu, W., Sai, W. L., Yang, J. L., & Zhang, H. J. (2011). Oncofetal antigen glypican-3 as a promising early diagnostic marker for hepatocellular carcinoma. *Hepatobiliary Pancreat Dis Int*, 10(3), 289-294.

[64] Ishiguro, T., Sugimoto, M., Kinoshita, Y., Miyazaki, Y., Nakano, K., Tsunoda, H., Sugo, I., Ohizumi, I., Aburatani, H., Hamakubo, T., Kodama, T., Tsuchiya, M., & Yamada-Okabe, H. (2008). Anti-glypican 3 antibody as a potential antitumor agent for human liver cancer. *Cancer Res*, 68(23), 9832-9838.

[65] Nakatsura, T., Komori, H., Kubo, T., Yoshitake, Y., Senju, S., Katagiri, T., Furukawa, Y., Ogawa, M., Nakamura, Y., & Nishimura, Yl. (2004). Mouse homologue of a novel human oncofetal antigen, glypican-3, evokes T-cell mediated tumor rejection without autoimmune reactions in mice. *Clin Cancer Res*, 10(24), 8630-8640.

[66] Ho, D. W., Yang, Z. F., Yi, K., Lam, C. T., Ng, M. N., Yu, W. C., Lau, J., Wan, T., Wang, X., Yan, Z., Liu, H., Zhang, Y., & Fan, S. T. (2012). Gene expression profiling of liver cancer stem cells by RNA-sequencing. *PLoS One*, 7(5), e37159, 10.1371/journal.pone.0037159.

[67] Chan, E. S., & Yeh, M. M. (2010). The use of immunohistochemistry in liver tumours. *Clin Liver Dis*, 14(4), 687-703.

[68] Yan, B. C., Gong, C., Song, J., Krausz, T., Tretiakova, M., Hyjek, E., Al-Ahmadie, H., Alves, V., Xiao, S. Y., Anders, R. A., & Hart, J. A. (2010). Arginase-1: a new immunohistochemical marker of hepatocytes and hepatocellular neoplasms. *Am J Surg Pathol*, 34(8), 1147-1154.

[69] Miller, R. T. (2012, 30.04.2011). Immunohistochemistry in the diagnosis of metastatic carcinoma of unknown primary origin. Paper presented at Proceedings of the American Academy of Oral and Maxillofacial Pathology Annual Meeting, San Juan, Puerto Rico. *Proceedings of the American Academy of Oral and Maxillofacial Pathology Annual Meeting, 30.04.2011, San Juan, Puerto Rico.*, http://www.aaomp.org/annual-meeting/docs/2011_CE5_Miller--Met%20ca%20Final%20Handout.pdf, (accessed 04 August).

[70] Chiang, D. Y., Villanueva, A., Hoshida, Y., Peix, J., Newell, P., Minguez, B., Le Blanc, A. C., Donovan, D. J., Thung, S. N., Sole, M., Tovar, V., Alsinet, C., Ramos, A. H., Barretina, J., Roayaie, S., Schwartz, M., Waxman, S., Bruix, J., Mazzaferro, V., Ligon, A. H., Najfeld, V., Friedman, S. L., Sellers, W. R., Meyerson, M., & Llovet, J. M. (2008). Focal gains of VEGFA and molecular classification of hepatocellular carcinoma. *Cancer Res*, 68(16), 6779-6788.

[71] Hoshida, Y., Nijman, S. M., Kobayashi, M., Chan, J. A., Brunet, J. P., Chiang, D. Y., Villanueva, A., Newell, P., Ikeda, K., Hashimoto, M., Watanabe, G., Gabriel, S., Friedman, S. L., Kumada, H., Llovet, J. M., & Golub, T. R. (2009). Integrative transcriptome analysis reveals common molecular subclasses of human hepatocellular carcinoma. *Cancer Res*, 69(18), 7385-7392.

[72] Lee, J. S., Chu, I. S., Heo, J., Calvisi, D. F., Sun, Z., Roskams, T., Durnez, A., Demetris, A. J., & Thorgeirsson, S. S. (2004). Classification and prediction of survival in hepatocellular carcinoma by gene expression profiling. *Hepatology*, 40(3), 667-676.

[73] Lee, J. S., Heo, J., Libbrecht, L., Chu, I. S., Kaposi-Novak, P., Calvisi, D. F., Mikaelyan, A., Roberts, L. R., Demetris, A. J., Sun, Z., Nevens, F., Roskams, T., & Thorgeirsson, S. S. (2006). A novel prognostic subtype of human hepatocellular carcinoma derived from hepatic progenitor cells. *Nat Med*, 12(4), 410-416.

[74] Boyault, S., Rickman, D. S., de Reynies, A., Balabaud, C., Rebouissou, S., Jeannot, E., Herault, A., Saric, J., Belghiti, J., Franco, D., Bioulac-Sage, P., Laurent-Puig, P., & Zucman-Rossi, J. (2007). Transcriptome classification of HCC is related to gene alterations and to new therapeutic targets. *Hepatology*, 45(1), 42-52.

[75] Breuhahn, K., Vreden, S., Haddad, R., Beckebaum, S., Stippel, D., Flemming, P., Nussbaum, T., Caselmann, W. H., Haab, B. B., & Schirmacher, P. (2004). Molecular profiling of human hepatocellular carcinoma defines mutually exclusive interferon regulation and insulin-like growth factor II overexpression. *Cancer Res*, 64(17), 6058-6064.

[76] Yamashita, T., Forgues, M., Wang, W., Kim, J. W., Ye, Q., Jia, H., Budhu, A., Zanetti, K. A., Chen, Y., Qin, L. X., Tang, Z. Y., & Wang, X. W. (2008). EpCAM and alpha-

fetoprotein expression defines novel prognostic subtypes of hepatocellular carcinoma. *Cancer Res*, 68(5), 1451-1461.

[77] Villanueva, A., Hoshida, Y., Toffanin, S., Lachenmayer, A., Alsinet, C., Savic, R., Cornella, H., & Llovet, J. M. (2010). New strategies in hepatocellular carcinoma: genomic prognostic markers. *Clin Cancer Res*, 16(19), 4688-4694.

[78] Llovet, J. M., Chen, Y., Wurmbach, E., Roayaie, S., Fiel, M. I., Schwartz, M., Thung, S. N., Khitrov, G., Zhang, W., Villanueva, A., Battiston, C., Mazzaferro, V., Bruix, J., Waxman, S., & Friedman, S. L. (2006). A molecular signature to discriminate dysplastic nodules from early hepatocellular carcinoma in HCV cirrhosis. *Gastroenterology*, 131(6), 1758-1767.

[79] Di Tommaso, L., Franchi, G., Park, Y. N., Fiamengo, B., Destro, A., Morenghi, E., Montorsi, M., Torzilli, G., Tommasini, M., Terracciano, L., Tornillo, L., Vecchione, R., & Roncalli, M. (2007). Diagnostic value of HSP70, glypican 3, and glutamine synthetase in hepatocellular nodules in cirrhosis. *Hepatology*, 45(3), 725-734.

[80] Roskams, T., & Kojiro, M. (2010). Pathology of early hepatocellular carcinoma: conventional and molecular diagnosis. *Semin Liver Dis*, 30(1), 17-25.

[81] Xie, C., Song, L. B., Wu, J. H., Li, J., Yun, J. P., Lai, J. M., Xie, D. Y., Lin, B. L., Yuan, Y. F., Li, M., & Gao, Z. L. (2012). Upregulator of cell proliferation predicts poor prognosis in hepatocellular carcinoma and contributes to hepatocarcinogenesis by downregulating FOXO3a. *PLoS One*, 7(7), e40607, 10.1371/journal.pone.0040607, http://www.plosone.org/article/info%3Adoi%2F10.1371%2Fjournal.pone.0040607, (accessed 09 August 2012).

[82] Phillips, R. J., Helbig, K. J., van der Hoek, K. H., Seth, D., & Beard, M. R. (2012). Osteopontin increases hepatocellular carcinoma cell growth in a CD44 dependant manner. *World J Gastroenterol*, 18(26), 3389-3399.

[83] Liu, W., Xu, G., Jia, J., Ma, W., Li, J., Chen, K., Wang, W., Hao, C., Wang, Y., & Wang, X. (2011). Osteopontin as a key mediator for vasculogenic mimicry in hepatocellular carcinoma. *Tohoku J Exp Med*, 224(1), 29-39.

[84] Fan, R., Miao, Y., Shan, X., Qian, H., Song, C., Wu, G., Chen, Y., & Zha, W. (2012). Bif-1 is overexpressed in hepatocellular carcinoma and correlates with shortened patient survival. *Oncol Lett*, 3(4), 851-854.

[85] Xu, H., Gu, N., Liu, Z. B., Zheng, M., Xiong, F., Wang, S. Y., Li, N., & Lu, J. (2012). NY-ESO-1 expression in hepatocellular carcinoma: a potential new marker for early recurrence after surgery. *Oncol Lett*, 3(1), 39-44.

[86] Ning, B. F., Ding, J., Yin, C., Zhong, W., Wu, K., Zeng, X., Yang, W., Chen, Y. X., Zhang, J. P., Zhang, X., Wang, H. Y., & Xie, W. F. (2010). Hepatocyte nuclear factor 4 alpha suppresses the development of hepatocellular carcinoma. *Cancer Res*, 70(19), 7640-7651.

[87] Lai, J. P., Sandhu, D. S., Yu, C., Moser, C. D., Hu, C., Shire, A. M., Aderca, I., Murphy, L. M., Adjei, A. A., Sanderson, S., & Roberts, L. R. (2010). Sulfatase 2 protects hepatocellular carcinoma cells against apoptosis induced by the PI3K inhibitor LY294002 and ERK and JNK kinase inhibitors. *Liver Int*, 30(10), 1522-1528.

[88] Gu, F. M., Li, Q. L., Gao, Q., Jiang, J. H., Zhu, K., Huang, X. Y., Pan, J. F., Yan, J., Hu, J. H., Wang, Z., Dai, Z., Fan, J., & Zhaou, J. (2011). IL-17 induces AKT-dependent IL-6/JAK2/STAT3 activation and tumor progression in hepatocellular carcinoma. *Mol Cancer*, 10, 150, http://www.molecular-cancer.com/content/pdf/1476-4598-10-150.pdf, (accessed 09 August 2012).

[89] Li, J., Lau, G. K., Chen, L., Dong, S. S., Lan, H. Y., Huang, X. R., Li, Y., Luk, J. M., Yuan, Y. F., & Guan, X. Y. (2011). Interleukin 17A promotes hepatocellular carcinoma metastasis via NF-kB induced matrix metalloproteinases 2 and 9 expression. *PLoS One*, 6(7), e21816, http://www.plosone.org/article/info%3Adoi%2F10.1371%2Fjournal.pone.0021816, (accessed 04 August 2012).

[90] Chen, J., Zhang, B., Wong, N., Lo, A. W., To, K. F., Chan, A. W., Ng, M. H., Ho, C. Y., Cheng, S. H., Lai, P. B., Yu, J., Ng, H. K., Ling, M. T., Huang, A. L., Cai, X. F., & Ko, B. C. (2011). Sirtuin 1 is upregulated in a subset of hepatocellular carcinomas where it is essential for telomere maintenance and tumor cell growth. *Cancer Res*, 71(12), 4138-4149.

[91] Cariani, E., Pilli, M., Zerbini, A., Rota, C., Olivani, A., Pelosi, G., Schianchi, C., Soliani, P., Campanini, N., Silini, E. M., Trenti, T., Ferrari, C., & Missale, G. (2012). Immunological and molecular correlates of disease recurrence after liver resection for hepatocellular carcinoma. *PLoS One*, 7(3), e32493, 10.1371/journal.pone.0032493.

[92] Streba, C. T., Pirici, D., Vere, C. C., Mogoanta, L., Comanescu, V., & Rogoveanu, I. (2011). Fractal analysis differentiation of nuclear and vascular patterns in hepatocellular carcinomas and hepatic metastasis. *Rom J Morphol Embryol*, 52(3), 845-854.

[93] Szutowicz, E., & Dziadziuszko, R. (2010). Quantitative immunohistochemistry in lung cancer: clinical perspective. *Folia Histochem Cytobiol*, 48(1), 7-11.

[94] Zhang, Y., Yang, B., Du, Z., Bai, T., Gao, Y. T., Wang, Y. J., Lou, C., Wang, F. M., & Bai, Y. (2012). Aberrant methylation of SPARC in human hepatocellular carcinoma and its clinical implication. *World J Gastroenterol*, 18(17), 2043-2052.

[95] Ji, J., Shi, J., Budhu, A., Yu, Z., Forgues, M., Roessler, S., Ambs, S., Chen, Y., Meltzer, P. S., Croce, C. M., Qin, L. X., Man, K., Lo, C. M., Lee, J., Ng, I. O., Fan, J., Tang, Z. Y., Sun, H. C., & Wang, X. W. (2009). MicroRNA expression, survival, and response to interferon in liver cancer. *N Engl J Med*, 361(15), 1437-1447.

[96] Ji, J., Yamashita, T., Budhu, A., Forgues, M., Jia, H. L., Li, C., Deng, C., Wauthier, E., Reid, L. M., Ye, Q. H., Qin, L. X., Yang, W., Wang, H. Y., Tang, Z. Y., Croce, C. M., & Wang, X. W. (2009). Identification of microRNA-181 by genome-wide screening as a critical player in EpCAM-positive hepatic cancer stem cells. *Hepatology*, 50(2), 472-480.

[97] Wang, J., Li, J., Shen, J., Wang, C., Yang, L., & Zhang, X. (2012). MicroRNA-182 downregulates metastasis suppressor 1 and contributes to metastasis of hepatocellular carcinoma. *BMC Cancer*, 12(1), 227, 10.1186/1471-2407-12-227, http://www.biomedcentral.com/1471-2407/12/227/abstract, (accessed 01 August 2012).

[98] Li, J., Fu, H., Xu, C., Tie, Y., Xing, R., Zhu, J., Qin, Y., Sun, Z., & Zheng, X. (2010). miR-183 inhibits TGF-beta1-induced apoptosis by downregulation of PDCD4 expression in human hepatocellular carcinoma cells. *BMC Cancer*, 10, 354, 10.1186/1471-2407-10-354, http://www.biomedcentral.com/1471-2407/10/354accessed, (04 August 2012).

[99] Tomimaru, Y., Eguchi, H., Nagano, H., Wada, H., Tomokuni, A., Kobayashi, S., Marubashi, S., Takeda, Y., Tanemura, M., Umeshita, K., Doki, Y., & Mori, M. (2010). MicroRNA-21 induces resistance to the anti-tumour effect of interferon-alpha/5-fluoruracil in hepatocellular carcinoma cells. *Br J Cancer*, 103(10), 1617-1626.

[100] Hamilton, S. R., & Aaltonen, L. A. (2000). Pathology and genetics. *Tumours of the digestive system. Lyon: IARC Press.*

[101] Darby, I. A., Vuillier-Devillers, K., Pinault, E., Sarrazy, V., Lepreux, S., Balabaud, C., Bioulac-Sage, P., & Desmouliere, A. (2010). Proteomic analysis of differentially expressed proteins in peripheral cholangiocarcinoma. *Cancer Microenviron*, 4(1), 73-91.

[102] Bioulac-Sage, P., Laumonier, H., Laurent, C., Blanc, J. F., & Balabaud, C. (2008). Benign and malignant vascular tumors of the liver in adults. *Semin Liver Dis*, 28(3), 302-314.

[103] Mills, S. E., Carter, D., Greenson, J. K., Reuter, V. E., & Stoler, M. H. (2009). Sternberg's diagnostic surgical pathology, 5th ed. *Wolter Kluver Health / Lippincott Williams and Wilkins.*

[104] Khadim, M. T., Jamal, S., Ali, Z., Akhtar, F., Atique, M., Sarfraz, T., & Ayaz, B. (2011). Diagnostic challenges and role of immunohistochemistry in metastatic liver disease. *Asian Pac J Cancer Prev*, 12(2), 373-376.

[105] Dabbs, D. J. (2002). Diagnostic immunohistochemistry. *New York: Churchill Livingstone.*

[106] Boggaram, V. (2009). Thyroid transcription factor-I(TTF-I/Nkx2.1/TITFI) gene regulation in the lung. *Clin Sci (Lond)*, 116(1), 27-35.

[107] Capelozzi, VL. (2009). Role of immunohistochemistry in the diagnosis of lung cancer. *J Bras Pneumol*, 35(4), 375-382.

[108] Kaimaktchiev, V., Terracciano, L., Tornillo, L., Spichtin, H., Stoios, D., Bundi, M., Korcheva, V., Mirlacher, M., Loda, M., Sauter, G., & Corless, C. L. (2004). The homeobox intestinal differentiation factor CDX2 is selectively expressed in gastrointestinal adenocarcinomas. *Mod Pathol*, 17(11), 1392-1399.

[109] Moskaluk, C. A., Zhang, H., Powell, S. M., Cerilli, L. A., Hampton, G. M., & Frierson, H. F. Jr. (2003). Cdx2 protein expression in normal and malignant human tissues: an immunohistochemical survey using tissue microarrays. *Mod Pathol*, 16(9), 913-919.

[110] Koffron, A., Rao, S., Ferrario, M., & Abecassis, M. (2004). Intrahepatic biliary cystadenoma: role of cyst fluid analysis and surgical management in the laparoscopic era. *Surgery*, 136(4), 926-936.

[111] Wheeler, D. A., & Edmondson, H. A. (1985). Cystadenoma with mesenchymal stroma (CMS) in the liver and bile ducts. A clinicopathologic study of 17 cases, 4 with malignant change. *Cancer*, 56(6), 1434-1435.

[112] Davies, W., Chow, M., & Nagorney, D. (1995). Extrahepatic biliary cystadenomas and cystadenocarcinoma. Report of seven cases and review of the literature. *Ann Surg*, 222(5), 619-625.

[113] Zhang, M., Yu, J., Yan, S., & Zheng, S. S. (2005). Cystadenocarcinoma of the liver: a case report. *Hepatobiliary Pancreat Dis Int*, 4(3), 464-467.

[114] Zhou, J. P., Dong, M., Zhang, Y., Kong, F. M., Guo, K. J., & Tian, Y. L. (2007). Giant mucinous biliary cystadenoma: a case report. *Hepatobiliary Pancreat Dis Int*, 6(1), 101-103.

[115] Kitajima, Y., Okayama, Y., Hirai, M., Hayashi, K., Imai, H., Okamoto, T., Aoki, S., Akita, S., Gotoh, K., Ohara, H., Nomura, T., Joh, T., Yokoyama, Y., & Itoh, M. (2003). Intracystic hemorhage of a simple liver cyst mimicking a biliary cystadenocarcinoma. *J Gastroenterol*, 38(2), 190-193.

[116] Jan, Y. Y., Chen, M. F., & Chen, T. J. (1994). Cholangiocarcinoma with mucobilia. *J Formos Med Assoc*, 93(3), S149-155.

[117] Thomas, K. T., Welch, D., Trueblood, A., Sulur, P., Wise, P., Gorden, D. L., Chari, R. S., Wright, J. K., Jr Washington, K., & Pinson, C. W. (2005). Effective treatment of biliary cystadenoma. *Ann Surg*, 241(5), 769-775.

[118] Kubota, E., Katsumi, K., Iida, M., Kishimoto, A., Ban, Y., Nakata, K., Takahashi, N., Kobayashi, K., Andoh, K., Takamatsu, S., & Joh, T. (2003). Biliary cystadenocarcinoma, followed up as benign cystadenoma for 10 years. *J Gastroenterol*, 38(3), 278-282.

[119] Mortele, K. J., & Ros, P. R. (2001). Cystic focal liver lesions in the adult: differential CT and MR imaging features. *Radiographics*, 21(4), 895-910.

[120] Poggio, P., & Buonocore, M. (2008). Cystic tumours of the liver: a practical approach. *World J Gastroenterol*, 14(23), 3616-3620.

[121] Zamboni, G., Scarpa, A., Bogina, G., Iacono, C., Bassi, C., Talamini, Sessa. F., Capella, C., Solcia, E., Rickaert, F., Mariuzzi, G. M., & Klopel, G. (1999). Mucinous cystic tumors of the pancreas: clinicopathologic features, prognosis, and relationship to other mucinous cystic tumors. *Am J Surg Pathol*, 23(4), 410-422.

[122] Sudo, Y., Harada, K., Tsuneyama, K., Katayanagi, K., Zen, Y., & Nakanuma, Y. (2001). Oncocytic biliary cystadenocarcinoma is a form of intraductal oncocytic papillary neoplasm of the liver. *Mod Pathol*, 14(12), 1304-1309.

[123] D'Errico, A., Deleonardi, G., Fiorentino, M., Scoazec, J. Y., & Grigioni, W. F. (1998). Diagnostic implications of albumin messenger RNA detection and cytokeratin pattern in benign hepatic lesions and biliary cystadenocarcinoma. *Diagn Mol Pathol*, 7(6), 289-294.

[124] Ishibashi, Y., Ojima, H., Hiraoka, N., Sano, T., Kosuge, T., & Kanai, Y. (2007). Invasive biliary cystic tumour without ovarian-like stroma. *Pathol Int*, 57(12), 794-798.

[125] Bardin, R. L., Trupiano, J. K., Howerton, R. M., & Geisinger, K. R. (2004). Oncocytic biliary cystadenocarcinoma: a case report and review of the literature. *Arch Pathol Lab Med*, 128(2), e25-28.

[126] Rullier, A., Le Bail, B., Fawaz, R., Blanc, J. F., Saric, J., & Bioulac-Sage, P. (2000). Cytokeratin 7 and 20 expression in cholangiocarcinomas varies along the biliary tree but still differs from that in colorectal carcinoma metastasis. *Am J Surg Pathol*, 24(6), 870-876.

[127] Ishak, K. G., Willis, G. W., Cummins, S. D., & Bullock, A. A. (1977). Biliary cystadenoma and cystadenocarcinoma: report of 14 cases and review of the literature. *Cancer*, 39(1), 322-338.

[128] Karahan, O. I., Kahriman, G., Soyuer, I., & Ok, E. (2007). Hepatic von Meyenburg complex simulating biliary cystadenocarcinoma. *Clin Imaging*, 31(1), 50-53.

Chapter 8

Nonalcoholic Fatty Liver Disease: A Pathological View

Joaquín Cabezas, Marta Mayorga and Javier Crespo

Additional information is available at the end of the chapter

http://dx.doi.org/10.5772/52622

1. Introduction

Nonalcoholic fatty liver disease (NAFLD) is the most common liver disorder of our times. The spectrum of this disease goes from steatosis to non-alcoholic steatohepatitis (NASH), cirrhosis and hepatocellular carcinoma. NAFLD can appear in the context of many conditions. Probably, NAFLD could be a component of metabolic syndrome, with its complete phenotypic expression: insulin resistance, obesity, type 2 diabetes, hypertension, hypercholesterolemia, and hypertriglyceridemia.

The pathogenesis involves insulin resistance, hepatic fat deposition, increased oxidant stress, apoptosis, inflammation and fibrosis. At present day, a new hormone has been discovered. Muscle cells products this new hormone, called irisin. Irisin can induce changes in adipose tissue.

Diagnosis of NAFLD cannot be performed with a single test and it should be one of exclusion, as well.

Nowadays, there is not a single therapeutic intervention. The focus of management should be treatment of the risk factors for NASH (insulin resistance, obesity…). Principal methods used for weight management are dietary modifications and life style changes. Then, pharmacotherapy may include insulin sensitizers, cholesterol-lowering agents, anti-obesity and anti-oxidant agents. Morbid obese patients may benefit from surgical weight loss, reducing the progression of NASH.

2. Definition

NAFLD definition [1] requires that there is evidence of hepatic steatosis, either by imaging or by histology and there are no causes for secondary hepatic fat accumulation (Table 1).

NAFLD is usually associated with metabolic risk factors such as metabolic syndrome, obesity, diabetes mellitus, and dyslipidaemia.

COMMON CAUSES OF SECONDARY HEPATIC STEATOSIS
Macrovesicularsteatosis
Excessive alcohol consumption. Hepatitis C (genotype 3) Wilson's disease. Lipodistrophy Starvation Parenteral nutrition. Abetalipoproteinemia. Medication (amiodarone, methotrexate, tamoxifen, corticosteroids)
Microvesicularstatosis
Reye's syndrome. Medications (valproate, anti-retroviral medicines) Acutte fatty liver of pregnancy HELLP syndrome Inborn errors of metabolism (LCAT deficiency, cholesterol ester storage disease, Wolman disease)

Table 1. Causes of secondary fat accumulation.

NAFLD includes a constellation of histological findings that goes from steatosis, to necroinflammation, called NASH and progression to advanced fibrosis and cirrhosis.

3. Epidemiology

NAFLD is becoming the leading cause of liver disease. One of the causes is the increasing of obesity[2].

The incidence of NAFLD has been evaluated in a few number of studies, it ranges from 31-86 cases/1000 person-year in Japan to 29 cases per 100000 person-year in England [3, 4].

The prevalence of NAFLD is increasing. Recent studies presented in the Digestive Diseases Week 2012 summarizes this increased prevalence over the last 20 years [5, 6]. Investigators report an increasing in obesity. This increase is followed by a rising in steatosis and NASH, the presence of steatosis among obese people has increased from 23% in the 80s, 43% in the

90s and finally to 60% nowadays [4]. Even in non-obese patients, the prevalence of steatosis increased from 12%, to 27% and 36%, respectively [5].

In children/adolescents, over the last 20 years, obesity has increased from 11% to 21%, suspected NAFLD from 4% to 10, and the prevalence of altered aminotransferases among obese adolescents has increased from 17% to 37% [6].

4. NAFLD and liver biopsy

Liver biopsy remains the gold standard for characterizing liver histology in patients with NAFLD. However, it is expensive and carries some morbidity and very rare mortality risk. Thus, it should be performed in those who would benefit the most from diagnostic, therapeutic guidance, and prognostic perspectives.

The last guideline for NAFLD management recommends liver biopsy [1]: in patients who are at risk to have steatohepatitis and advance fibrosis; theses patients could be identified by the presence of metabolic syndrome and NAFLD fibrosis score; and a liver biopsy should be considered in patients in whom other etiologies are suspected and cannot be excluded without a liver biopsy.

Liver biopsy allows confirming the diagnosis, evaluation and semiquantitation of necroinflammatory lesions and fibrosis.

On the other hand, liver biopsy suffers from challenges. An adequate biopsy represents only 1/50000-1/65000 of the organ. Sampled area should be carefully chosen and sample length must be enough, a least 15mm. This size can reduce sample error. Finally, experienced pathologist is important to haver a greater yield of findings.

5. Histology of NAFLD

NAFLD represents a histopathologic spectrum ranging from steatosis alone, to necroinflammation, summarized as NASH; and progression to advanced fibrosis and cirrhosis.

The histologic characterization of NAFLD and NASH may include description of steatosis and cell injury in addition to inflammation and fibrosis. Kleiner and Brunt [7] propose categorizing the histologic changes when studying NAFLD as follows in table 2.

The main histological characteristic of NAFLD is the accumulation of fat in the form of triglyicerides within hepatocytes, lesion termed steatosis (Figure 1 and 2); this term is defined by the guideline [1] as NAFL – non-alcoholic fatty liver, where the risk of progression to cirrhosis and liver failure is minimal. The presence of >5% steatoic hepatocytes in a liver biopsy is accepted as the minimum criterion for thehistological diagnosis of NAFLD [8].

CATEGORY	DEFINITION
No significant evidence of fatty liver disease.	Insufficientsteatosis for diagnosis of steatosis, without other changes (ballooning, fibrosis) that would suggest steatohepatitis.
Steatosis: Steatosis with inflammation. Steatosis with nonspecific fibrosis	Steatosis without specific changes to suggest a form of steatohepatitis. This category may include spotty lobular inflammation and/or mild degrees of fibrosis of uncertain significance.
Steatohepatitis: - zone 3 borderline steatohepatitis	Form of steatoshepatitis most common in adults; defined as a zone 3 centered injury pattern that includes steatosis, inflammation, ballooning injury, (often with Mallory-Denk bodies) with or without fibrosis. Borderline steatohepatitsis has some, but not all ofthe features that would allow a diagnosis of steatohepatitis.
Zone 1, borderline pattern	Form of steatohepatitis that occurs mainly in young children, characterized by zone 1-centered (portal inflammation, portal-based fibrosis, zone 1 steatosis, ballooning injury in zone 1 if present).
Cryptogenetic fibrosis/ cirrhosis	Presence of fibrosis (usually advanced) or cirrhosis, with little ton o steatosis and no changes (ballooning, Mallory-Denk bodies) that would suggest borderline or definite steatohepatitis. Other explanations for fibrosis (besides steatohepatitis) should be considered.

Table 2. Histologic Categorization of NAFLD [7].

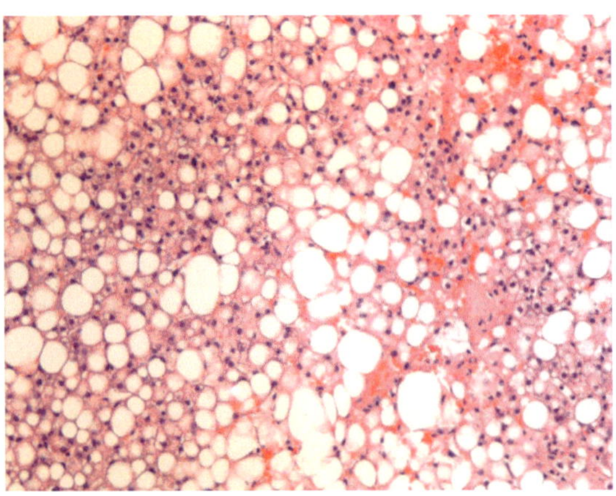

Figure 1. Steatosis. Hematoxylin-eosin stain.

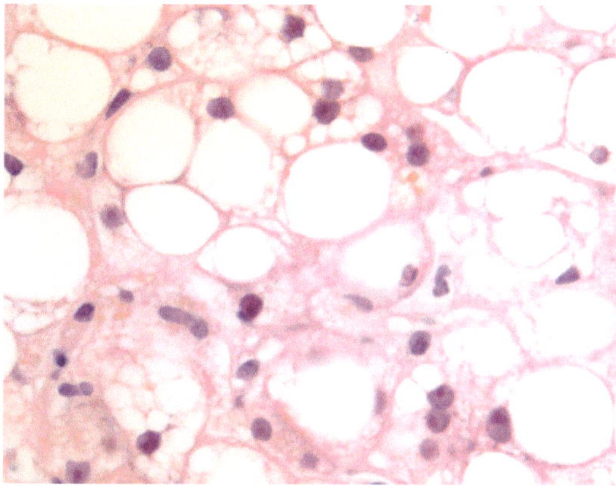

Figure 2. Steatosis. Hematoxylin-eosin stain.

Steatosis in NAFLD is usually macrovesicular, which refers to hepatocytes with single large intracytoplasmatic fat droplet or smaller well defined droplets displacing the nucleus to the cell periphery. This macrovesicularsteatosis is usually present in a zone 3 or panacinar distribution; it differs from zone 1 steatosis that is a common distribution in chronic hepatitis C. Azonal steatosis is most often seen in biopsies with advanced fibrosis [9].

The extent of steatosis can be evaluated and classified semi-quantitative. The most reproducible method follows the acinararchiqueture dividing the liver parenchyma in thirds and assessing percentage involvement bay steatoic hepatocytes [8] – table 3.

STEATOSIS SEMI-QUANTIFICATION	
Mild	0 – 33%
Moderate	33 – 66%
Severe	> 66%.

Table 3. Steatosis semi-quantification according to acinar architecture [8].

NASH, under this concept is the histology pattern of NAFLD, which is at risk of developing advance fibrosis. The minimal criteria for the histopathological diagnosis of adult NASH include steatosis, hepatocyte injury, usually in form of ballooning, and lobular inflammation, typically localized in acinar zone 3 [10, 11].

The key feature for the diagnosis of NASH is the ballooning injury (Figures 3 and 4), and it is considered a marker of apoptosis [12]. This type of cell injury is characterized by a cell that becomes enlarged and the cytoplasm becomes irregularly clumped with optically clear, nonvesiculated areas. Ballooned cells are seen most frequently in zone 3 near the hepatic veins, and lose this localization, becoming portal inflammation more prominent when the disease progresses and in severe cases. Immunostaining of hepatocyte keratins 8 and 18 might help to identify ballooned hepatocytes [13]. Ballooned degeneration is difficult to diagnose even by trained pathologist, for that reason it can show significant inter-observer variation [14].

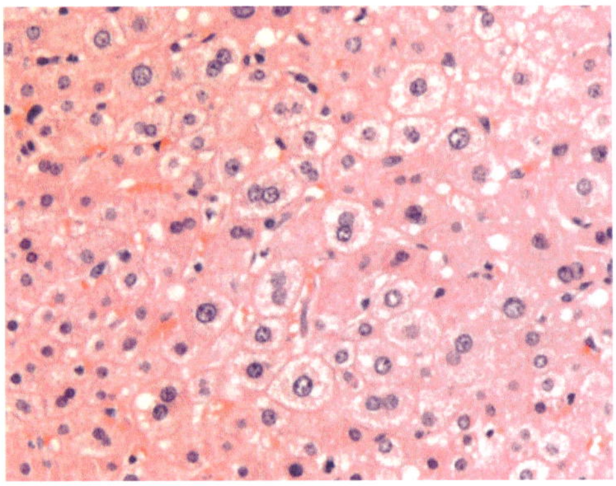

Figure 3. Hepatocyte ballooned. Hematoxylin-eosin stain.

Ballooning degeneration is associated with an increased liver-related mortality [15].

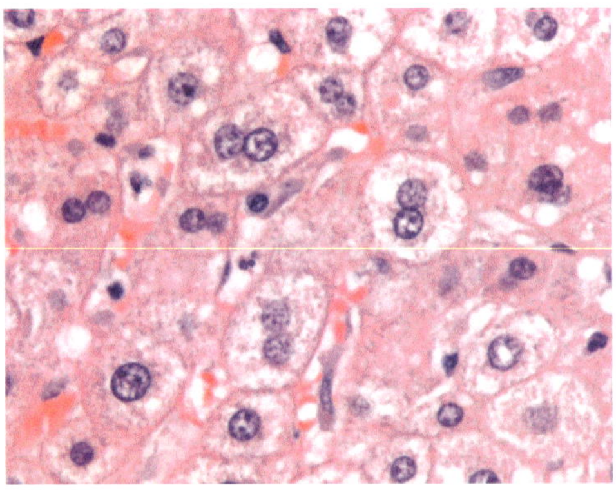

Figure 4. Ballooning hepatocyte. Hematoxylin-eosin stain.

Mallory-Denk Bodies (MDB), also known as Mallory bodies, are eosinophilic, ropey cytoplasmatic inclusion bodies in the hepatocyte of patients with chronic liver disease. This type of lesion contains abnormal cytokeratin 8 and 18 filaments that have been ubiquinated.

Mallory bodies have an importance in disease progression and it is suggested a possible prognostic role in steatohepatitis [16]. In a recent study, the presence of MBD was significantly associated with liver-related mortality [15].

Both ballooning degeneration and MDB can trigger the development of apoptosis. Apoptotic (acidophil) bodies are common in NASH. They can be identified as rounded, eosinophilic cytoplasmic fragments, which appear to be free within the sinusoids or surrounded by

Kupffer or other inflammatory cells. Apoptosis has been validated as an accurate marker for diagnosis of NASH based on immunochemistry in liver tissue [17].

Inflammatory infiltrates (Figure 5) can be seen in the hepatic acini/lobules or the portal tract. Lobular inflammation is usually mild, consists of a mixed inflammatory cell infiltrate, composed of lymphocytes, some eosinophils, and a few neutrophils. Polymorphs can be observed around ballooned hepatocytes that are called "satellitosis" (Figure 6). Kuppfer cells aggregates as lobular microgranulomas and lipogranulomas may appear [10]

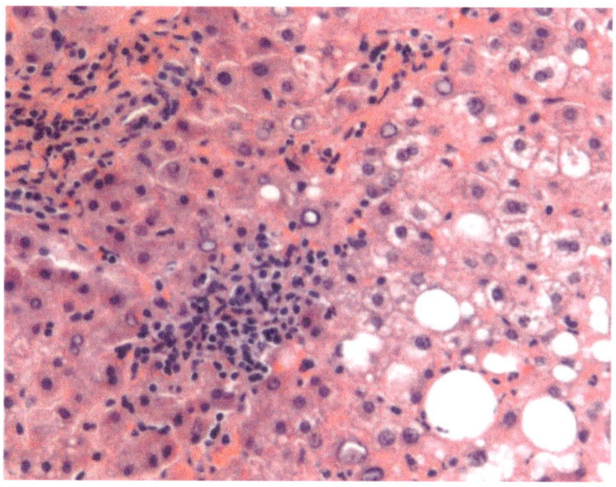

Figure 5. Mononuclear inflammatory infiltration. Hematoxylin-eosin stain.

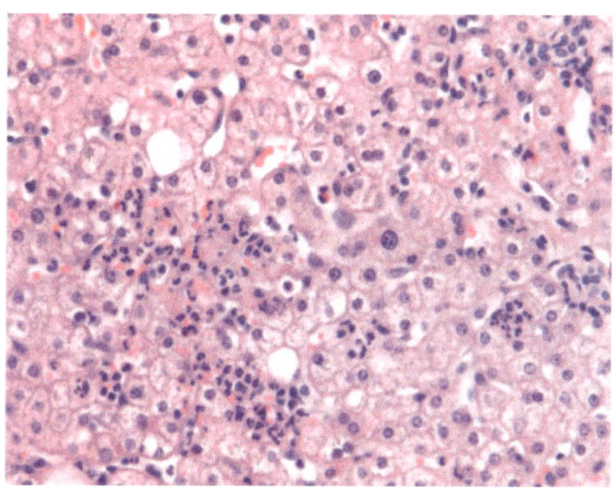

Figure 6. Polymorph around ballooned hepatocytes, "satelitosis".

Hematoxylin-eosin stain.Portal chronic mononuclear cell inflammation in adult NASH is common and mild. When portal inflammation is greater than lobular other aetiologies should be ruled out, such as chronic hepatitis C [18]. On the other side, a greater portal inflammation than lobular inflammation can be seen in successfully treated patients [19]. In a large database of liver biopsies from the NASH Clinical Research Network, including adults and children, portal chronic inflammation was associated with clinical and histologic features of severity and advance disease [20].

Vascular alterations in NAFLD. Recent paper has focused the study of NASH in microvessels of the liver [21]. This work has found an intraacinar branch of the hepatic artery in the perivenular region in active steatohepatitis. This finding is important because it can lead to confusion for a portal tract resulting in an equivocal diagnosis. Likewise, the presence of this vessel correlates with higher stage of fibrosis.

Fibrosis in adult NASH usually starts in acinar zone 3 and has characteristic "chicken wire" pattern due to deposition of collagen an other extracellular matrix fibres along the sinusoids of zone 3 and around the hepatocytes (Figure 7 and 8). Portal fibrosis has been reported in cases of morbid obesity-related NASH and in pediatric NASH. Fibrosis predicts clinical outcomes in NASH [22]. there was noter from this study that the progression of the fibrosis is accompanied of steatosis reduction. Approximately 37% to 41% of patients with NAFLD have fibrosis progression over 3 to 10 years [22, 23]. The higher rates of fibrosis progression were related to: body mass index, diabetes and low initial fibrosis [22]. When periportal fibrosis was not present, there was a 100% of negative predictive value in predicting liver-related outcomes [23]. Steatosis, inflammation, ballooning and Mallory hyaline were not associated with liver-related mortality after adjusting for the presence of fibrosis [15]. The inclusion of fibrosis explains why the recent classifications for NASH used by Younossi [15] and Matteoni [16], independently correlated with liver-related mortality. This observation shows the importance of fibrosis in NAFLD, patients with NASH and fibrosis portends a higher risk of death [24].

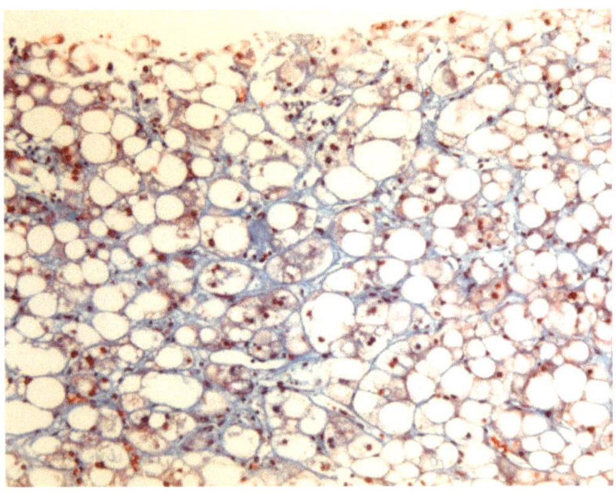

Figure 7. Fibrosis pattern: around hepatocytes. Masson trichrome stain.

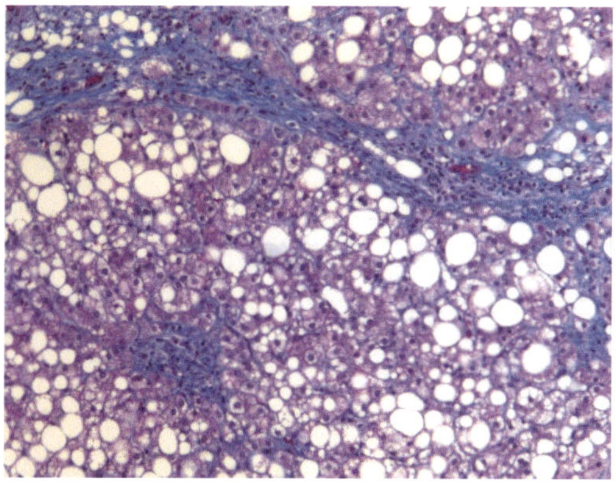

Figure 8. Zone 3 fibrosis perivenular/pericellular. Masson trichrome stain.

Other histological lesions that may be seen in NASH include megamitochondria, glycogenated nuclei and iron deposition.

Megamitochondria (giant mitochondria) are round or needle-shaped, eosinophilic, intracytoplasmatic inclusions more commonly observed in hepatocytes with microvesicularsteatosis. This abnormal mitochondria is a result of injury from lipid peroxidation or represent an adaptive change [25]. Glycogenated nuclei are vacuolated nuclei usually observed in periportal hepatocytes. Their presence is more frequent in non-alcoholic etiology and it is rare in alcoholic injury [26].

Finally, hepatic siderosis might be seen in NAFLD. One study of 293 liver biopsies (34,5% of patients with NAFLD) investigates the relationship between iron deposition and NAFLD [27]. Stainable hepatic iron described three histological patterns: hepatocellular pattern, reticuloendothelial system cell – RES - (mainly Kupffer cell) pattern and mixed. RES pattern was associated with advanced fibrosis and higher histological features of portal inflammation, ballooning and definite NASH [27].

6. Histologic scoring systems

NAFLD histologic criteria requires an accumulation of more than 5% of fat deposition, mainly in form of triglycerides. NAFLD was first described by Ludwig and colleagues [28], and since then several systems for grading and staging NAFLD have been proposed.

In 1999, Matteoni and colleagues characterized histologic subtypes that correlate with clinical outcomes [16] – table 4. In 2005, NASH Clinical Research Network developed NAFLD activity score (NAS) [8]. This score comprises four features evaluated semi-quantitatively: steatosis, lobular inflammation, hepatocellular ballooning and fibrosis. Fibrosis was classified separately – table 5. When NAS is >5 sensitivity and specificity for definite NASH were 0,75 and 0,83, respectively. Finally, a recent classification for NAFLD has been proposed by

Younossi and colleagues [15]. This classification includes the evaluation of these histologic features: steatosis with centrilobular ballooning, and/or Mallory-Denk bodies of fibrosis – see table 6.

CLASSIFICATION OF NONALCOHOLIC LIVER FATTY LIVER DISESASE (NAFLD) BY SUBTYPE		
NAFLD subtype	**Pathology**	**Clinicopathologic correlation**
Type 1	Simple steatosis alone	No NASH
Type 2	Statosis + lobular inflammation only	No NASH
Type 3	Steatosis + hepatocellular ballooning	NASH without fibrosis
Type 4	Steatosis, ballooning, Mallory bodies or fibrosis	NASH with fibrosis

Table 4. Classification of NAFLD by subtype [16].

CLASSIFICATION OF NONALCOHLIC FATTY LIVER DISEASE BY NAFLD CLINICAL RESEASCH NETWORK	
Histologic finding	Score
Steatosis	0-3
Lobular inflammation	0-3
Hepatocellular ballooning	0-2
NASH requires a score of ≥ 4 with at least 1 point o ballooning injury.	
Fibrosis type	Score
None	0
Perisinusoidal zone 3	
Mild	1A
Moderate	1B
Portal/periportal	1C
Persinusoidal and portal/periportal	2
Bridging	3
Cirrhosis	4

Table 5. Classification of NAFLD by NAFLD CRN [8].

http://dx.doi.org/10.5772/52622

CLASSIFICATION OF NAFLD BY SUBTYPE	
Pathology	**Clinicopathologic correlation**
Simple steatosis alone	No NASH
Steatosis + lobular inflammation only	No NASH
Steatosis with centrilobular ballooning and/or Mallory-Denk bodies	NASH
Any steatosis with centrilobularpericellular/perisinusoidal or briding fibrosis	NASH

Table 6. Classification of NAFLD proposed by Younossi and colleagues [15].

The most important difference between NAS and subtype classifications is that the latters include fibrosis and this provides a better prediction of liver-related mortality in patients with NAFLD [15].

7. NAFLD in special populations

Patients with insulin resistance. Insulin resistance can be estimated using the homeostasis model for assessing of insulin resistance (HOMA-IR), calculated as the product of fasting insulin level (mUI/ml) and plasma glucose level (mmol/ml), divides by 22,5 [29]. Portal fibrosis has been linked to the ductular reaction (ductularproliferation at the portal tract interface arising from progenitor cells in the periportal area and accompanied by neutrophils and stromal changes). These findings correlate the insulin resistance with advanced stages of fibrosis and provide a pathway for fibrosis progression [30].

In some cases in a study with a few number of patients treated with an insulin sensitizer, histologic evaluation of post-treatment liver biopsy showed that increased portal inflammation is a feature related to resolution of NASH, and it is associated to a change in the quality of zone 3 perisinusoidal fibrosis from dense to delicate [19].

NAFLD in bariatric surgery patients. Patients undergoing bariatric surgery for weight loss are at a risk of NAFLD. They often have comorbidities such as: severe obesity, diabetes, hypertension, sleep apnea or coronary artery disease. And high percentage will have metabolic syndrome [31] (see table 7). The prevalence of steatosis and steatohepatitis in these patients undergoing liver biopsy when surgery is performed, is 91% and 37%, respectively [32]. At least a third of morbidity obese patients have portal inflammation, and this is related to the presence of fibrosis [20, 33]. In early stage, localization of fibrosis differs from those nonbariatric populations, in bariatric is portal and in nonbariatric is perisinusoidal [19].

The Adult Treatment Panel III clinical definition of the metabolic syndrome: - Requires the presence of three or more of the following features:
Waist circumference greater than 102 cm in men or greater than 88 cm in women.
Triglyceride level 150mg/dl or greater.
High-density lipoprotein (HDL) cholesterol level less than 40 mg/dl in men and less than 50 mg/dl in women.
Systolic blood pressure 130 mmHg or greater or diastolic pressure 85 mmHg or greater.
Fasting plasma glucose level 110 mg/dl or greater.

Table 7. Definition of the metabolic syndrome [31].

NAFLD after bariatric surgery. Improvements of major histological features of disease activity, grade of steatohepatitis and rarely fibrosis following therapy (dietary, medicines or surgery) have been reported [34]. After surgical intervention liver histology improve in these features: lobular steatosis, necroinflammatory changes and fibrosis, against no improve in portal abnormalities [35]. Recent meta-analysis [36] shows that patients after bariatric surgery have improvement or resolution in steatosis (91,6%), in steatohepatitis (81,3%), in fibrosis (65,5%) and for complete resolution of NASH was 69,5%.

In the near future, we will have to get used to new types of treatment, for example, "metabolic surgery", which might be performed to non-morbid obese patients with diabetes, and to the new changes in hepatic parenchyma following endoscopic procedures performed to treat obesity.

NAFLD in children. Pediatric NAFLD can have a different histologic presentation than adult NAFLD. In the first large biopsy series of pediatric NAFLD [37], two different histologic patterns were described with differences in race and gender. Type 1 NASH: similar to adults, more common in Caucasian children. Histologic characteristics are: steatosis, ballooning degeneration and perisinusoidal fibrosis. On the other hand, Type 2 NASH was more common in Asian, Native American and Hispanics. Typical features in the liver biopsy are: steatosis with lymphocytic portal inflammation and portal fibrosis. Children with type 2 were younger and had a greater severity of obesity, and advanced fibrosis. This kind of pattern was described in adult morbid obese patients undergoing bariatric surgery, these patients mean age were slightly lower [33]. Overlap cases with characteristic of both histological types may also be observed in pediatric NASH. A multicentre retrospective cohort study reviewed 130 liver biopsies of children according to these criteria of pediatric NAFLD [38]. The majority of the biopsies presented an overlapping pattern (82%). Advanced fibrosis was associated with the presence of lobular and portal inflammation.

Portal fibrosis is common in pediatric NAFLD and may evolve to periportal fibrosis and bridging fibrosis in some patients, whereas progression to cirrhosis is observed in rare cases [39].

It is not clear, that Type 2 NASH, described as pediatric NASH, is an entity by itself or it is another stage of the spectrum of NASH which could be a predictor of those who have a severe disease [40].

http://dx.doi.org/10.5772/52622

8. Imaging tecnology in NAFLD

Ultrasonography (US), computed tomography (CT), and magnetic resonance (MR) can identify liver steatosis but not steatohepatitis, nevertheless they provide anatomical and morphological information. The sensitivity of these imaging methods is optimal for steatosis over 33%. When advance liver disease, radiology techniques can provide indirect signs of cirrhosis, such as portal hypertension, or may be useful for the screening and diagnosis of hepatocellular carcinoma (HCC)[41]. Imaging technique may help to differentiate diffuse from focal form of steatosis. Hepatic fatty infiltration can present as focal steatosis (a focal area of steatosis in an otherwise normal liver) or as focal fatty sparing (fatty change with sparing of certain areas) [42].

Abdominal US is the most commonly used imaging technique to clinically evaluate the presence of liver steatosis. Advantages include low cost, lack of radiation exposure and wide availability. The brightness of the liver echo is compared with the kidney, the attenuation of the sound beam by the fat results in relatively hypoechoic kidney. For detailed description of sonographic features for staging fatty liver see table 8. This US feature is not characteristic of NAFLD because it can be present in other diffuse parenchymal liver disease. The US can be accurate detecting hepatic steatosis when there is a moderate to severe infiltration [43]. Overall sensitivity and specificity are 60-94% and 66-95%, respectively, however the sensitivity is lower when BMI (body mass index) is over 35 Kg/m^2. Although this acceptable level of sensitivity it does not provide reproducible quantitative information. US scoring system for fatty liver is based on hyperechogenic liver tissue, the increased discrepancy of echo amplitude between liver and kidney and the loss of echoes from the walls of the portal system [44]. US cannot differentiate between steatosis and fibrosis, but with advance degrees of fibrosis an increase in coarse echoes without posterior beam attenuation can be seen.

Features	NORMAL	MILD	MODERATE	SEVERE
Liver echotexture	Liver parenchyma is homogeneous and no difference in contrast between liver and kidney	Slight increase in echo pattern	Intermediate	Gross discrepancy of the increased hepatic to renal cortical echogenicity
Echo penetration an visibility of diaphragm	Liver structure is clearly defined from the surface to diaphragm. The outline of the diaphragm is clearly visualized.	Mild attenuation of sound beam through the liver	Intermediate	Marked attenuation of sound beam through the liver, the diaphragm is not visualized.
Clarity of liver blood vessel structure	Vessel wall and lumen of vessel can clearly visualized	Slight decrease definition of portal venule walls	Intermediate	Only the main portal walls can be visualized with absence of all smaller portal venule walls

Table 8. Ultrasonographic grading system for diagnosis of fatty liver, adapted from [41].

Computer Tomography provides an accurate and a reliable visualization of whole liver, so that not only diffuse but also focal fatty infiltration of the liver parenchyma can be accurately diagnosed. CT enables the evaluation of absolute measurement of attenuation values which are given in Hounsfield units, the difference of attenuation between liver and spleen as well as the calculation of the liver-to-spleen attenuation ratio, those correlate with steatosis degree. Liver density as measured by CT attenuation units has been shown to have an inverse correlation to the degree of fatty infiltration. Non-enhanced CT provides a high performance in qualitative diagnosis of hepatic steatosis when fatty infiltration is over 30%, obtaining 82% of sensitivity and 100% specificity using histologic analysis of biopsies of liver donors as the reference standard [45], however is not sensitive in detecting mild-to-moderate amounts of steatosis between 5% and 30% [43]. New CT scanning techniques are developing, such as dual-source/dual energy scanners, but their evaluation needs further studies. A drawback of this technique is the liver iron overload because it increases the attenuation. This method is associated with radiation exposure which limits its use in children.

Magnetic Resonance can detect steatosis by exploiting the difference of resonance frequencies between water and fat proton signals. The sensitivity and specificity of MRI in detecting as low as 5% of liver fat infiltration are 85% and 100%, respectively [46]. The detection of the fatty liver can be seen in "white/bright" when applying in-phase T1 images and "black" when applying out-of-phase images, compared to the signal intensity of the spleen and paraespinal muscles. Another technic of MR imaging with fat saturation may quantify more accurately liver fat infiltration, especially in patients who have fibrosis.

MR spectroscopy can reliably quantify even minimal steatosis, as low as 0,5% [47]. In has been based on the ubiquitous protons hydrogen and phosphorus [48], and more than 5% of fat content on MR spectroscopy indicates presence of steatosis [49]. Its routine application is limited by cost and lack of availability, and it remains a research tool.

Methods (S/s)	Advantages	Disadvantage
Ultrasonography. (60-95% / 84-100%)	Noninvasive, widely aviable, low cost, repetition, Useful for screening	Operator dependent. Qualitative assessment of steatosis. Only accurate when moderate-to-severe fat infiltration.
Computer tomography, Contrast images. (50-86% / 75-87%)	Noninvasive, semiquantitative assessment of fat content. Detects focal or diffuse infiltration.	Radiation exposure. Iron overload, copper and fibrous tissue could be confounding factors. Not sensitive for mild-to-moderate amounts of steatosis.
Magnetic resonance imaging (85% / 100%)	Noninvasive, semiquantitative, and no radiation exposure. Detects focal or diffuse infiltration.	Limitation in patients with iron overload. Not suitable for patients with claustrophobia or implantable devices.
MR spectroscopy	Noninvasive, reproducible, accurate quantification.	High cost not widely available. Long time taking images.

Table 9. Pro's and con's of radiologic modalities for the study of NAFLD. S: sensitivity; s: specificity. Adapted from [41].

US, CT and MR are insensitive in differentiating hepatic steatosis from NASH, and they cannot be used to stage fibrosis [43, 48]. But in the near future, a novel method based on MRI imaging and a new software will be able to stage fibrosis and to distinguish NASH from no-NASH. Professor Romero-Gomez conducts this study and it will be soon published.

Table 9 summarizes advantages and disadvantages of these radiologic methods.

9. Non-invasive assesment in NAFLD

Liver biopsy remains a useful tool to confirm the diagnosis and exclude other disease or helps to discover concomitant chronic liver disease. It provides prognostic information by staging and grading this disease. At present non-invasive diagnostic markers could provide a new tool for differentiating fatty liver from NASH as well as for grading /staging NAFLD.

The investigation of these new diagnostic methods comes from the well known drawbacks of liver biopsy. These include sampling error, inadequate biopsy size, variability in pathologist interpretation, cost and associated morbidity (complications 0,3%, mortality rate 0,01%).

An ideal non-invasive test should be simple, reproducible, readily available, less expensive than liver biopsy, able to predict the full spectrum of liver fibrosis stages, and reflect changes occurring with therapy [48].

Some reviews provide an overview of the role of non-invasive test in NAFLD [48, 50, 51]. We will try to present many of these scores through a table (number 10) to summarize their characteristics. AUROC is a numerical data that assess the performance of a scoring system. AUROC value greater than 0,8 indicate good diagnostic performance. The closer the value to 1, the better performing the scoring system.

SCORE [Reference]	Variables	Cutoff	AUROC	Sens. (%)	Spec. (%)	PPV (%)	NPV (%)
NONINVASIVE DIAGNOSIS OF STEATOSIS							
SteatoTest [52]	6 components of FibroTest-ActiTest, BMI, cholesterol, triglycerides, glucose	0,3 0,7	0,79-0,86	85	88	46 63	93 79
Fatty liver Index (FLI) [53]	BMI, waist circumference, triglycerides, GGT	<30 >70	0,85	87	86		
NONINVASIVE ASSESSMENT IN NASH							
Palekar [54]	HA >55 mcg/l, age >50 years, female gender, AST >45 UI/ml, AAR >80.	≥3	0,763	73,7	65,7	68,2	71,4
CK-18 [17]	CK-18 plasma (apoptosis marker)	250 U/l	0,83	75	81		

SCORE [Reference]	Variables	Cutoff	AUROC	Sens. (%)	Spec. (%)	PPV (%)	NPV (%)
oxNASH [55]	Detection of lipid peroxidation products by chromatography-mass spectrometric		0,74-0,83	63-81	84-97		
SHIMADA [56]	Serum adiponectin, type 4 collagen 7s level, HOMA-IR			94	74	94	74
NASH Diagnostics [57]*	CK-18, cleaved CK-18, adiponectin, resistin	0,3825	0,73	71,4	72,7	83,3	57,1
NashTest [58]	Age, gender, BMI, triglycerides, cholesterol, alfa-2macroglobulin, GGT, haptoglobin, apolipoprotein-A1, total bilirubin		0,79	29	98	91	71
NONINVASIVE MANAGEMENT OF FIBROSIS IN NAFLD							
NAFLD fibrosis score [59]	Age, BMI, IFG/diabetes, AAR, platelet, albumin	≤1,455 ≥0,676	0,88			56 90	93 85
Pediatric NAFLD fibrosis index [60]	Age, waist circumference and triglycerides.	≥9: rule in liver fibrosis.	0,85			98,5	44,5
		<3:rule out fibrosis				75,4**	75**
						**Pre-test probability: 69%	
BARD score [61]	BMI ≥28 =1, AAR ≥0,8 =2, diabetes=1,	≥2: advanced fibrosis	0,81				96
FIB-4 [62]	Age, AST, platelet, ALT	<1,3 >2,67	0,80			43 80	90 83
APRI [63]	AST, platelet	0,98	Advanced fibrosis: 0,85	75	86	54	93
ELF [64]	HA, TIMP1, P3NP.	0,3576	For severe fibrosis 0,90.	80	90	71	94
		-0,1068	For moderate fibrosis 0,82	70	80	70	80
		ELF: -0,2070.	No fibrosis 0,76	61	80	81	79
BAAT [65]	Age ≥50years, BMI ≥28kg/m2 =1, triglycerides ≥7mmol/L=1, ALT ≥2N	0-1, for septal fibrosis	0,84	100	47		100
Fibrotest [66]		0,30	F0-1 VS F2-4: 075-085.	70			90

SCORE [Reference]	Variables	Cutoff	AUROC	Sens. (%)	Spec. (%)	PPV (%)	NPV (%)
			F0-2 VS F3-4: 0,81-0,92				
		0,70			98	73	
Fibrometer [67]	Glucose, AST, platelets, ferritin, ALT, weight, age.	<0,611	F0-1 vs F2-4: 0,936-0,952				
ULTRASOUND BASED TECHNIQUES IN FIBROSIS DETECTION IN NAFLD							
Fibroscan [68]	Transient elastography	9,9 kPa	F ≥3: 0,99	100	93	77	100
		16 kPa	F4: 0,998	100	93	86	100
ARFI [69]		4,24 kPa	F0-2 vsF3-4: 0,90	90	90		
ARFI [68]		1,77 m/sec	F ≥3: 0,973	100	91	71	100
		1,90 m/sec	F4: 0,976	100	96	75	100
MAGNETIC RESONANCE IMAGING BASED TECHNIQUES							
MR elastography[70]	Discriminating NASH from simple steatosis (SS)	2,74 kPa	SS vs NASH: 0,93	94	73	85	89
		Means: - 2,51kPa. - 3,24kPa. - 4,16kPa.	Simple steatosis. NASH no fibrosis. With fibrosis				

Abbreviations: AUROC: area under receiver operator curve. Sens.: Sensitivity; Spec.: Specificity; PPV: positive predictive value; NPV: negative predictive value; BMI: body mass index; GGT: Gamma-glutamyl-transpeptidase; HA: hyaluronic acid; AST: aspartate transaminase; AAR: AST/alanine aminotransferase, TIMP-1: tissue inhibitor of matrix metalloproteinase 1; P3NP: aminoterminal peptide of pro-collagen III; ARFI: acoustic radiation force impulse; * Sample: bariatric surgery patients. COMMENTS: BARD score can reliably exclude advance fibrosis, particularly among non-diabetics. FIB-4, as happened with BARD score, is useful in excluding advance fibrosis due its high NPV. Transient elastography and ARFI are based on the variation of the speed wave through liver tissue (generated by vibrator/short-duration acoustic pulses, respectively), this can be measured and converted to a numerical value (in kPa and m/sec, respectively, but ARFI could also be expressed as kPa) which is the liver stiffness and it is proportional to liver fibrosis. An important difference between both systems is that ARFI consists in a probe which can be plugged to a common US machine so both techniques can be performed at the same time.

Table 10. Non-invasive assessment of NAFLD.

APRI and FIB-4 have been evaluated in obese children and they might be useful in this special population [71]. Pediatric NAFLD scores is a noninvasive model evaluated in obese children, and it may help clinicians to predict liver fibrosis but external validation is needed [60].

In the future, new serologic markers, such as CD36, will help to differentiate more accurately between NAFLD stages, we would be able to distinguish simple steatosis from NASH.

Although clinical and laboratory models may be useful in identifying a group of patients at a low risk of advance fibrosis and liver biopsy might be avoided, they are not enough for staging and prognostic purposes if patients are at risk of advance fibrosis [48]. NAFLD Practice Guideline of 2012 recommends NAFLD fibrosis score to identify patients with higher likelihood of having bridging fibrosis and/or cirrhosis [1].

10. New diagnostic platforms in nafld

NAFLD is a disease with wide spectrum: from steatosis through inflammation to fibrosis and finally cirrhosis and hepatocellular carcinoma, even in absence of cirrhosis [72]. The strongest predictor of fibrosis progression in NAFLD is steatohepatitis. The most important features are hepatocellular degeneration (ballooning) and inflammatory cell infiltration.

These new techniquesinclude genomics, metabolomics and proteomics.

Genomics. Gene expression studies provide an insight into possible mechanism of pathogenesis as well as potential biomarkers of disease. One method for studying gene expression is micro-arrays of DNA. A study using this test found 34 gens with different expression in NASH vs controls, these genes where implicated in lipid metabolism and extracellular matrix remodelling [73]. Another study compared gene expression in NASH-related cirrhosis with other causes of cirrhosis. In NASH cirrhosis group genes involved in anti-oxidant stress were underexpressed, along with genes involved in fatty and glucose metabolism [74]. In our centre we used micro-arrays to study gene expression in obese patients with NAFLD [75]. Obese patients with NASH without fibrosis show an overexpression of proinflammatory and proapoptotic genes; and those with fibrosis show an overexpression of fibrogenic genes, including the leptin receptor Ob-Rb.

Most recent genomic tests, such GWAS (Genome-wide association studies) provide a method for evaluating a large number of single nucleotide polymorphisms (SNP) with the same experiment. A study performed with a GWAS study found a SNP in farnesyldiphosfatasefarnesyltransferase 1 (FDFT1) which was associated with different histological parameters (a SNP with portal inflammation and another different SNP with fibrosis stage) and the total NAFLD activity score [76]. In an earlier GWAS study [77], an SNP in PNPA3 (adiponutrin/patatin-like phospholipase-3) was strongly associated with both hepatic fat content and hepatic inflammation. The prevalence of this mutation may explain the difference in susceptibility to NAFLD seen in different ethnicities [77]. A subsequent study [78], confirmed the relationship between this SNP and histological score, the no association with metabolic syndrome.

These studies are incredibly interesting and they could help the development of new noninvasive markers, nevertheless all of them share limitations, mainly concerning to sample size. It is easily understandable given the fact that they use expensive and complex tools [51].

Proteomics. Proteomic tools look specifically at protein expression patterns and profiles. There are several approaches to proteomic studies depending on the used tool. These tools are complex; they are based on diverse types of mass-spectrometry. For more detailed information refer to [79, 80]. The different proteomic platforms support the use of either liver tissue or blood. This platform allows identifying, quantifying and comparing proteins in the study groups of interest. That novel approach has been applied for the study of NAFLD [81-84]. These studies have found several proteins related to disease progression: alfa and beta-hemoglobin [84], lumican and FABP1 (fatty acid binding protein-1) [82]; and finally fibrinogen beta-chain, retinol binding protein-4, serum amiloyd p-component, lumican, transgrelin-2 and CD5-like antigen, in 6-panel model and complement component 7, transgrelin-2 and insulin grow factor acid labile subunit, in a 3-panel model. These panels performed in the diagnosis of the diverse NAFLD stages get an area under the receiver operator curve (AUROC) ranging from 0,83 to 0,91 [83].

Metabolomics. In the natural history of NAFLD the progression to hepatic fibrosis occurs only in 10 to 25% of cases, leading to cirrhosis, end-stage liver disease or hepatocellular carcinoma. The strongest predictor of fibrotic progression, apart from pre-existing fibrosis, is steatohepatisis. A two-hit model has been proposed as an explanation for why some patients progress to NASH. In a first step, because of insulin resistance, adipose tissue has enhanced triglyceride lipolysis, which leads to increased serum free fatty acids, and impaired hepatic triglyceride export. In this model, hepaticsteatosis (hit 1) exposes the liver parenchyma to environmental and extracellular hepatic insults (hit 2), leading to inflammation, steatonecrosis and fibrosis. Impaired mitochondrial oxidation and lipid export may also contribute to hepatic fat deposition.

Leptin system is also implicated, and its receptor expression is related to fibrosis degree [85].

As it was explained in the introduction, irisin is a newly identified hormone. Irisin is produced in muscle cells induced in exercise [86-88]. Irisin activates changes in adipose tissue, and make its change from white adipose tissue to brown adipose tissue, and this causes a significant increase in total body energy expenditure and resistance to obesity-linked insulin resistance. So this advance opens new pathogenic pathways in NAFLD.

Inflammation is considered to be the central clue for the progression of NAFLD, the origins and components are considered in this review [89]. Hepatocytes injured by toxic lipid molecules play a central role in the recruitment of innate immunity involving Toll-like receptors (TLR), Kuppfer cells, lymphocytes and neutrophils and possibly inflammasome. On this way, a study was carried to determine the lipidomic signature in NAFLD [90]. Using proteomic tools (mass spectrometry) the investigators found metabolites from nonenzymatic oxidation product of arachidonic acid and from impaired peroxisomal polyunsaturated fatty acid (PUFA). This study links to another, where investigators characterize metabolic profile to distinguish steatosis and NASH [91], they also found arachidonic acid, among other substances, relation to NASH and fibrosis. Metabolomics analysis was performed to NAFLD patients showing a lower concentrations of glutathione, an antioxidant substance, in this group [92].

The key pro-inflammatory signalling pathways in NASH are nuclear factor-kappa B (NF-kB) and c-Jun N-terminal kinase (JNK). It could be possible that inflammation in NASH could originate outside the liver. Gut microbiota, the related Kupffer/TLR response, inflamed adipose tissue and circulating inflammatory cell can contribute or act as co-factors that triggers or maintain hepatic injury. In a study conducted in our centre to study the relationship between endotoxemia and NAFLD, we found higher levels of LBP (Lipopolysaccharide-binding protein) in patients with NASH when compared to patients with simple steatosis [93]. The LBP increase correlates with the level of tumor necrosis factor alfa (TNF-alfa) which is overexpressed in patient with NASH and significant fibrosis. [94] Detailed information in pathophysiology of NAFLD and NASH is not the aim of this paper, if you are interested refer to this review [89].

11. Conclusion

NAFLD is an emerging problem. The study of pathology is ever evolving which is allowing the development of new therapeutic targets, and the emergence of new diagnostic techniques allow better identification of patients who will benefit from new treatments.

Author details

Joaquín Cabezas[1], Marta Mayorga[2] and Javier Crespo[1]

1 Gastroenterology and Hepatology Unit, University Hospital "Marqués de Valdecilla", Santander, Spain

2 Pathology Department, University Hospital "Marqués de Valdecilla", Santander, Spain

References

[1] Chalasani N, Younossi Z, Lavine JE, Diehl AM, Brunt EM, Cusi K, et al. The diagnosis and management of non-alcoholic fatty liver disease: practice Guideline by the American Association for the Study of Liver Diseases, American College of Gastroenterology, and the American Gastroenterological Association. Hepatology. 2012;55(6): 2005-23. Epub 2012/04/11.

[2] Younossi ZM, Stepanova M, Afendy M, Fang Y, Younossi Y, Mir H, et al. Changes in the prevalence of the most common causes of chronic liver diseases in the United States from 1988 to 2008. Clin Gastroenterol Hepatol. 2011;9(6):524-30 e1; quiz e60. Epub 2011/03/29.

[3] Whalley S, Puvanachandra P, Desai A, Kennedy H. Hepatology outpatient service provision in secondary care: a study of liver disease incidence and resource costs. Clin Med. 2007;7(2):119-24. Epub 2007/05/12.

[4] Suzuki A, Angulo P, Lymp J, St Sauver J, Muto A, Okada T, et al. Chronological development of elevated aminotransferases in a nonalcoholic population. Hepatology. 2005;41(1):64-71. Epub 2005/02/04.

[5] Lee FY, Evans A, Kim D. Prevalence of fatty liver disease: a community-based autopsy study. Program and abstracts of Digestive Disease Week 2012; May 19-22, 2012; San Diego, California; Abstract 1054.

[6] Vos MB, Welsh J. Prevalence of suspected NAFLD is increasing among U.S. adolescents. Digestive Disease Week 2012; May 19-22, 2012; San Diego, California. Abstract 705.

[7] Kleiner DE, Brunt EM. Nonalcoholic fatty liver disease: pathologic patterns and biopsy evaluation in clinical research. Semin Liver Dis. 2012;32(1):3-13. Epub 2012/03/16.

[8] Kleiner DE, Brunt EM, Van Natta M, Behling C, Contos MJ, Cummings OW, et al. Design and validation of a histological scoring system for nonalcoholic fatty liver disease. Hepatology. 2005;41(6):1313-21. Epub 2005/05/26.

[9] Chalasani N, Wilson L, Kleiner DE, Cummings OW, Brunt EM, Unalp A. Relationship of steatosis grade and zonal location to histological features of steatohepatitis in adult patients with non-alcoholic fatty liver disease. J Hepatol. 2008;48(5):829-34. Epub 2008/03/07.

[10] Brunt EM, Tiniakos DG. Histopathology of nonalcoholic fatty liver disease. World J Gastroenterol. 2010;16(42):5286-96. Epub 2010/11/13.

[11] Tiniakos DG. Nonalcoholic fatty liver disease/nonalcoholic steatohepatitis: histological diagnostic criteria and scoring systems. Eur J Gastroenterol Hepatol. 2010;22(6): 643-50. Epub 2009/05/30.

[12] Malhi H, Gores GJ, Lemasters JJ. Apoptosis and necrosis in the liver: a tale of two deaths? Hepatology. 2006;43(2 Suppl 1):S31-44. Epub 2006/02/01.

[13] Lackner C, Gogg-Kamerer M, Zatloukal K, Stumptner C, Brunt EM, Denk H. Ballooned hepatocytes in steatohepatitis: the value of keratin immunohistochemistry for diagnosis. J Hepatol. 2008;48(5):821-8. Epub 2008/03/11.

[14] Ratziu V, Charlotte F, Heurtier A, Gombert S, Giral P, Bruckert E, et al. Sampling variability of liver biopsy in nonalcoholic fatty liver disease. Gastroenterology. 2005;128(7):1898-906. Epub 2005/06/09.

[15] Younossi ZM, Stepanova M, Rafiq N, Makhlouf H, Younoszai Z, Agrawal R, et al. Pathologic criteria for nonalcoholic steatohepatitis: interprotocol agreement and ability to predict liver-related mortality. Hepatology. 2011;53(6):1874-82. Epub 2011/03/02.

[16] Matteoni CA, Younossi ZM, Gramlich T, Boparai N, Liu YC, McCullough AJ. Nonalcoholic fatty liver disease: a spectrum of clinical and pathological severity. Gastroenterology. 1999;116(6):1413-9. Epub 1999/05/29.

[17] Feldstein AE, Wieckowska A, Lopez AR, Liu YC, Zein NN, McCullough AJ. Cytokeratin-18 fragment levels as noninvasive biomarkers for nonalcoholic steatohepatitis: a multicenter validation study. Hepatology. 2009;50(4):1072-8. Epub 2009/07/09.

[18] Brunt EM. Nonalcoholic steatohepatitis: pathologic features and differential diagnosis. Semin Diagn Pathol. 2005;22(4):330-8. Epub 2006/08/31.

[19] Neuschwander-Tetri BA, Brunt EM, Wehmeier KR, Oliver D, Bacon BR. Improved nonalcoholic steatohepatitis after 48 weeks of treatment with the PPAR-gamma ligand rosiglitazone. Hepatology. 2003;38(4):1008-17. Epub 2003/09/27.

[20] Brunt EM, Kleiner DE, Wilson LA, Unalp A, Behling CE, Lavine JE, et al. Portal chronic inflammation in nonalcoholic fatty liver disease (NAFLD): a histologic marker of advanced NAFLD-Clinicopathologic correlations from the nonalcoholic steatohepatitis clinical research network. Hepatology. 2009;49(3):809-20. Epub 2009/01/15.

[21] Gill RM, Belt P, Wilson L, Bass NM, Ferrell LD. Centrizonal arteries and microvessels in nonalcoholic steatohepatitis. Am J Surg Pathol. 2011;35(9):1400-4. Epub 2011/08/13.

[22] Adams LA, Sanderson S, Lindor KD, Angulo P. The histological course of nonalcoholic fatty liver disease: a longitudinal study of 103 patients with sequential liver biopsies. J Hepatol. 2005;42(1):132-8. Epub 2005/01/05.

[23] Ekstedt M, Franzen LE, Mathiesen UL, Thorelius L, Holmqvist M, Bodemar G, et al. Long-term follow-up of patients with NAFLD and elevated liver enzymes. Hepatology. 2006;44(4):865-73. Epub 2006/09/29.

[24] Pagadala MR, McCullough AJ. The relevance of liver histology to predicting clinically meaningful outcomes in nonalcoholic steatohepatitis. Clin Liver Dis. 2012;16(3): 487-504. Epub 2012/07/25.

[25] Caldwell SH, Chang CY, Nakamoto RK, Krugner-Higby L. Mitochondria in nonalcoholic fatty liver disease. Clin Liver Dis. 2004;8(3):595-617, x. Epub 2004/08/28.

[26] Pinto HC, Baptista A, Camilo ME, Valente A, Saragoca A, de Moura MC. Nonalcoholic steatohepatitis. Clinicopathological comparison with alcoholic hepatitis in ambulatory and hospitalized patients. Dig Dis Sci. 1996;41(1):172-9. Epub 1996/01/01.

[27] Nelson JE, Wilson L, Brunt EM, Yeh MM, Kleiner DE, Unalp-Arida A, et al. Relationship between the pattern of hepatic iron deposition and histological severity in nonalcoholic fatty liver disease. Hepatology. 2011;53(2):448-57. Epub 2011/01/29.

[28] Ludwig J, Viggiano TR, McGill DB, Oh BJ. Nonalcoholic steatohepatitis: Mayo Clinic experiences with a hitherto unnamed disease. Mayo Clin Proc. 1980;55(7):434-8. Epub 1980/07/01.

[29] Levy JC, Matthews DR, Hermans MP. Correct homeostasis model assessment (HOMA) evaluation uses the computer program. Diabetes Care. 1998;21(12):2191-2. Epub 1998/12/05.

[30] Richardson MM, Jonsson JR, Powell EE, Brunt EM, Neuschwander-Tetri BA, Bhathal PS, et al. Progressive fibrosis in nonalcoholic steatohepatitis: association with altered regeneration and a ductular reaction. Gastroenterology. 2007;133(1):80-90. Epub 2007/07/17.

[31] Grundy SM, Cleeman JI, Daniels SR, Donato KA, Eckel RH, Franklin BA, et al. Diagnosis and management of the metabolic syndrome: an American Heart Association/

National Heart, Lung, and Blood Institute Scientific Statement. Circulation. 2005;112(17):2735-52. Epub 2005/09/15.

[32] Machado M, Marques-Vidal P, Cortez-Pinto H. Hepatic histology in obese patients undergoing bariatric surgery. J Hepatol. 2006;45(4):600-6. Epub 2006/08/11.

[33] Abrams GA, Kunde SS, Lazenby AJ, Clements RH. Portal fibrosis and hepatic steatosis in morbidly obese subjects: A spectrum of nonalcoholic fatty liver disease. Hepatology. 2004;40(2):475-83. Epub 2004/09/16.

[34] Vuppalanchi R, Chalasani N. Nonalcoholic fatty liver disease and nonalcoholic steatohepatitis: Selected practical issues in their evaluation and management. Hepatology. 2009;49(1):306-17. Epub 2008/12/10.

[35] Dixon JB, Bhathal PS, Hughes NR, O'Brien PE. Nonalcoholic fatty liver disease: Improvement in liver histological analysis with weight loss. Hepatology. 2004;39(6): 1647-54. Epub 2004/06/09.

[36] Mummadi RR, Kasturi KS, Chennareddygari S, Sood GK. Effect of bariatric surgery on nonalcoholic fatty liver disease: systematic review and meta-analysis. Clin Gastroenterol Hepatol. 2008;6(12):1396-402. Epub 2008/11/07.

[37] Schwimmer JB, Behling C, Newbury R, Deutsch R, Nievergelt C, Schork NJ, et al. Histopathology of pediatric nonalcoholic fatty liver disease. Hepatology. 2005;42(3): 641-9. Epub 2005/08/24.

[38] Carter-Kent C, Yerian LM, Brunt EM, Angulo P, Kohli R, Ling SC, et al. Nonalcoholic steatohepatitis in children: a multicenter clinicopathological study. Hepatology. 2009;50(4):1113-20. Epub 2009/07/29.

[39] Roberts EA. Non-alcoholic steatohepatitis in children. Clin Liver Dis. 2007;11(1): 155-72, x. Epub 2007/06/05.

[40] Hsu E, Murray K. Is nonalcoholic Fatty liver disease in children the same disease as in adults? Clin Liver Dis. 2012;16(3):587-98. Epub 2012/07/25.

[41] Cuadrado A, Orive A, Garcia-Suarez C, Dominguez A, Fernandez-Escalante JC, Crespo J, et al. Non-alcoholic steatohepatitis (NASH) and hepatocellular carcinoma. Obes Surg. 2005;15(3):442-6. Epub 2005/04/14.

[42] Charatcharoenwitthaya P, Lindor KD. Role of radiologic modalities in the management of non-alcoholic steatohepatitis. Clin Liver Dis. 2007;11(1):37-54, viii. Epub 2007/06/05.

[43] Saadeh S, Younossi ZM, Remer EM, Gramlich T, Ong JP, Hurley M, et al. The utility of radiological imaging in nonalcoholic fatty liver disease. Gastroenterology. 2002;123(3):745-50. Epub 2002/08/29.

[44] Hamaguchi M, Kojima T, Itoh Y, Harano Y, Fujii K, Nakajima T, et al. The severity of ultrasonographic findings in nonalcoholic fatty liver disease reflects the metabolic

syndrome and visceral fat accumulation. Am J Gastroenterol. 2007;102(12):2708-15. Epub 2007/09/27.

[45] Park SH, Kim PN, Kim KW, Lee SW, Yoon SE, Park SW, et al. Macrovesicular hepatic steatosis in living liver donors: use of CT for quantitative and qualitative assessment. Radiology. 2006;239(1):105-12. Epub 2006/02/18.

[46] Mazhar SM, Shiehmorteza M, Sirlin CB. Noninvasive assessment of hepatic steatosis. Clin Gastroenterol Hepatol. 2009;7(2):135-40. Epub 2009/01/03.

[47] Cassidy FH, Yokoo T, Aganovic L, Hanna RF, Bydder M, Middleton MS, et al. Fatty liver disease: MR imaging techniques for the detection and quantification of liver steatosis. Radiographics. 2009;29(1):231-60. Epub 2009/01/27.

[48] Grandison GA, Angulo P. Can nash be diagnosed, graded, and staged noninvasively? Clin Liver Dis. 2012;16(3):567-85. Epub 2012/07/25.

[49] Reeder SB, Cruite I, Hamilton G, Sirlin CB. Quantitative assessment of liver fat with magnetic resonance imaging and spectroscopy. J Magn Reson Imaging. 2011;34(4): 729-49. Epub 2011/09/20.

[50] Adams LA, Feldstein AE. Non-invasive diagnosis of nonalcoholic fatty liver and nonalcoholic steatohepatitis. J Dig Dis. 2011;12(1):10-6. Epub 2010/11/26.

[51] Miller MH, Ferguson MA, Dillon JF. Systematic review of performance of non-invasive biomarkers in the evaluation of non-alcoholic fatty liver disease. Liver Int. 2011;31(4):461-73. Epub 2011/03/09.

[52] Poynard T, Ratziu V, Naveau S, Thabut D, Charlotte F, Messous D, et al. The diagnostic value of biomarkers (SteatoTest) for the prediction of liver steatosis. Comp Hepatol. 2005;4:10. Epub 2005/12/27.

[53] Bedogni G, Bellentani S, Miglioli L, Masutti F, Passalacqua M, Castiglione A, et al. The Fatty Liver Index: a simple and accurate predictor of hepatic steatosis in the general population. BMC Gastroenterol. 2006;6:33. Epub 2006/11/04.

[54] Palekar NA, Naus R, Larson SP, Ward J, Harrison SA. Clinical model for distinguishing nonalcoholic steatohepatitis from simple steatosis in patients with nonalcoholic fatty liver disease. Liver Int. 2006;26(2):151-6. Epub 2006/02/02.

[55] Feldstein AE, Lopez R, Tamimi TA, Yerian L, Chung YM, Berk M, et al. Mass spectrometric profiling of oxidized lipid products in human nonalcoholic fatty liver disease and nonalcoholic steatohepatitis. J Lipid Res. 2010;51(10):3046-54. Epub 2010/07/16.

[56] Shimada M, Kawahara H, Ozaki K, Fukura M, Yano H, Tsuchishima M, et al. Usefulness of a combined evaluation of the serum adiponectin level, HOMA-IR, and serum type IV collagen 7S level to predict the early stage of nonalcoholic steatohepatitis. Am J Gastroenterol. 2007;102(9):1931-8. Epub 2007/05/22.

[57] Younossi ZM, Jarrar M, Nugent C, Randhawa M, Afendy M, Stepanova M, et al. A novel diagnostic biomarker panel for obesity-related nonalcoholic steatohepatitis (NASH). Obes Surg. 2008;18(11):1430-7. Epub 2008/05/27.

[58] Poynard T, Ratziu V, Charlotte F, Messous D, Munteanu M, Imbert-Bismut F, et al. Diagnostic value of biochemical markers (NashTest) for the prediction of non alcoholo steato hepatitis in patients with non-alcoholic fatty liver disease. BMC Gastroenterol. 2006;6:34. Epub 2006/11/14.

[59] Angulo P, Hui JM, Marchesini G, Bugianesi E, George J, Farrell GC, et al. The NAFLD fibrosis score: a noninvasive system that identifies liver fibrosis in patients with NAFLD. Hepatology. 2007;45(4):846-54. Epub 2007/03/30.

[60] Nobili V, Alisi A, Vania A, Tiribelli C, Pietrobattista A, Bedogni G. The pediatric NAFLD fibrosis index: a predictor of liver fibrosis in children with non-alcoholic fatty liver disease. BMC Med. 2009;7:21. Epub 2009/05/05.

[61] Harrison SA, Oliver D, Arnold HL, Gogia S, Neuschwander-Tetri BA. Development and validation of a simple NAFLD clinical scoring system for identifying patients without advanced disease. Gut. 2008;57(10):1441-7. Epub 2008/04/09.

[62] Shah AG, Lydecker A, Murray K, Tetri BN, Contos MJ, Sanyal AJ. Comparison of noninvasive markers of fibrosis in patients with nonalcoholic fatty liver disease. Clin Gastroenterol Hepatol. 2009;7(10):1104-12. Epub 2009/06/16.

[63] Kruger FC, Daniels CR, Kidd M, Swart G, Brundyn K, van Rensburg C, et al. APRI: a simple bedside marker for advanced fibrosis that can avoid liver biopsy in patients with NAFLD/NASH. S Afr Med J. 2011;101(7):477-80. Epub 2011/09/17.

[64] Guha IN, Parkes J, Roderick P, Chattopadhyay D, Cross R, Harris S, et al. Noninvasive markers of fibrosis in nonalcoholic fatty liver disease: Validating the European Liver Fibrosis Panel and exploring simple markers. Hepatology. 2008;47(2):455-60. Epub 2007/11/27.

[65] Ratziu V, Giral P, Charlotte F, Bruckert E, Thibault V, Theodorou I, et al. Liver fibrosis in overweight patients. Gastroenterology. 2000;118(6):1117-23. Epub 2000/06/02.

[66] Ratziu V, Massard J, Charlotte F, Messous D, Imbert-Bismut F, Bonyhay L, et al. Diagnostic value of biochemical markers (FibroTest-FibroSURE) for the prediction of liver fibrosis in patients with non-alcoholic fatty liver disease. BMC Gastroenterol. 2006;6:6. Epub 2006/03/01.

[67] Cales P, Laine F, Boursier J, Deugnier Y, Moal V, Oberti F, et al. Comparison of blood tests for liver fibrosis specific or not to NAFLD. J Hepatol. 2009;50(1):165-73. Epub 2008/11/04.

[68] Yoneda M, Yoneda M, Mawatari H, Fujita K, Endo H, Iida H, et al. Noninvasive assessment of liver fibrosis by measurement of stiffness in patients with nonalcoholic fatty liver disease (NAFLD). Dig Liver Dis. 2008;40(5):371-8. Epub 2007/12/18.

[69] Palmeri ML, Wang MH, Rouze NC, Abdelmalek MF, Guy CD, Moser B, et al. Noninvasive evaluation of hepatic fibrosis using acoustic radiation force-based shear stiffness in patients with nonalcoholic fatty liver disease. J Hepatol. 2011;55(3):666-72. Epub 2011/01/25.

[70] Chen J, Talwalkar JA, Yin M, Glaser KJ, Sanderson SO, Ehman RL. Early detection of nonalcoholic steatohepatitis in patients with nonalcoholic fatty liver disease by using MR elastography. Radiology. 2011;259(3):749-56. Epub 2011/04/05.

[71] Yang HR, Kim HR, Kim MJ, Ko JS, Seo JK. Noninvasive parameters and hepatic fibrosis scores in children with nonalcoholic fatty liver disease. World J Gastroenterol. 2012;18(13):1525-30. Epub 2012/04/18.

[72] Torres DM, Harrison SA. Nonalcoholic steatohepatitis and noncirrhotic hepatocellular carcinoma: fertile soil. Semin Liver Dis. 2012;32(1):30-8. Epub 2012/03/16.

[73] Younossi ZM, Gorreta F, Ong JP, Schlauch K, Del Giacco L, Elariny H, et al. Hepatic gene expression in patients with obesity-related non-alcoholic steatohepatitis. Liver Int. 2005;25(4):760-71. Epub 2005/07/07.

[74] Sreekumar R, Rosado B, Rasmussen D, Charlton M. Hepatic gene expression in histologically progressive nonalcoholic steatohepatitis. Hepatology. 2003;38(1):244-51. Epub 2003/06/28.

[75] Cayon A, Crespo J, Guerra AR, Pons-Romero F. (Gene expression in obese patients with non-alcoholic steatohepatitis). Rev Esp Enferm Dig. 2008;100(4):212-8. Epub 2008/06/20. Expresion genica en pacientes obesos con enfermedad hepatica por deposito de grasa.

[76] Chalasani N, Guo X, Loomba R, Goodarzi MO, Haritunians T, Kwon S, et al. Genome-wide association study identifies variants associated with histologic features of nonalcoholic Fatty liver disease. Gastroenterology. 2010;139(5):1567-76, 76 e1-6. Epub 2010/08/17.

[77] Romeo S, Kozlitina J, Xing C, Pertsemlidis A, Cox D, Pennacchio LA, et al. Genetic variation in PNPLA3 confers susceptibility to nonalcoholic fatty liver disease. Nat Genet. 2008;40(12):1461-5. Epub 2008/09/30.

[78] Speliotes EK, Butler JL, Palmer CD, Voight BF, Hirschhorn JN. PNPLA3 variants specifically confer increased risk for histologic nonalcoholic fatty liver disease but not metabolic disease. Hepatology. 2010;52(3):904-12. Epub 2010/07/22.

[79] Griffin TJ, Aebersold R. Advances in proteome analysis by mass spectrometry. J Biol Chem. 2001;276(49):45497-500. Epub 2001/10/05.

[80] Kito K, Ito T. Mass spectrometry-based approaches toward absolute quantitative proteomics. Curr Genomics. 2008;9(4):263-74. Epub 2009/05/20.

[81] Younossi ZM, Baranova A, Ziegler K, Del Giacco L, Schlauch K, Born TL, et al. A genomic and proteomic study of the spectrum of nonalcoholic fatty liver disease. Hepatology. 2005;42(3):665-74. Epub 2005/08/24.

[82] Charlton M, Viker K, Krishnan A, Sanderson S, Veldt B, Kaalsbeek AJ, et al. Differential expression of lumican and fatty acid binding protein-1: new insights into the histologic spectrum of nonalcoholic fatty liver disease. Hepatology. 2009;49(4):1375-84. Epub 2009/03/31.

[83] Bell LN, Theodorakis JL, Vuppalanchi R, Saxena R, Bemis KG, Wang M, et al. Serum proteomics and biomarker discovery across the spectrum of nonalcoholic fatty liver disease. Hepatology. 2010;51(1):111-20. Epub 2009/11/04.

[84] Trak-Smayra V, Dargere D, Noun R, Albuquerque M, Yaghi C, Gannage-Yared MH, et al. Serum proteomic profiling of obese patients: correlation with liver pathology and evolution after bariatric surgery. Gut. 2009;58(6):825-32. Epub 2008/04/12.

[85] Cayon A, Crespo J, Mayorga M, Guerra A, Pons-Romero F. Increased expression of Ob-Rb and its relationship with the overexpression of TGF-beta1 and the stage of fibrosis in patients with nonalcoholic steatohepatitis. Liver Int. 2006;26(9):1065-71. Epub 2006/10/13.

[86] Kelly DP. Medicine. Irisin, light my fire. Science. 2012;336(6077):42-3. Epub 2012/04/12.

[87] Pedersen BK. A muscular twist on the fate of fat. N Engl J Med. 2012;366(16):1544-5. Epub 2012/04/20.

[88] Bostrom P, Wu J, Jedrychowski MP, Korde A, Ye L, Lo JC, et al. A PGC1-alpha-dependent myokine that drives brown-fat-like development of white fat and thermogenesis. Nature. 2012;481(7382):463-8. Epub 2012/01/13.

[89] Farrell GC, van Rooyen D, Gan L, Chitturi S. NASH is an Inflammatory Disorder: Pathogenic, Prognostic and Therapeutic Implications. Gut Liver. 2012;6(2):149-71. Epub 2012/05/10.

[90] Puri P, Wiest MM, Cheung O, Mirshahi F, Sargeant C, Min HK, et al. The plasma lipidomic signature of nonalcoholic steatohepatitis. Hepatology. 2009;50(6):1827-38. Epub 2009/11/26.

[91] Barr J, Vazquez-Chantada M, Alonso C, Perez-Cormenzana M, Mayo R, Galan A, et al. Liquid chromatography-mass spectrometry-based parallel metabolic profiling of human and mouse model serum reveals putative biomarkers associated with the progression of nonalcoholic fatty liver disease. J Proteome Res. 2010;9(9):4501-12. Epub 2010/08/06.

[92] Kalhan SC, Guo L, Edmison J, Dasarathy S, McCullough AJ, Hanson RW, et al. Plasma metabolomic profile in nonalcoholic fatty liver disease. Metabolism. 2011;60(3):404-13. Epub 2010/04/29.

[93] Ruiz AG, Casafont F, Crespo J, Cayon A, Mayorga M, Estebanez A, et al. Lipopolysaccharide-binding protein plasma levels and liver TNF-alpha gene expression in obese patients: evidence for the potential role of endotoxin in the pathogenesis of non-alcoholic steatohepatitis. Obes Surg. 2007;17(10):1374-80. Epub 2007/11/15.

[94] Crespo J, Cayon A, Fernandez-Gil P, Hernandez-Guerra M, Mayorga M, Dominguez-Diez A, et al. Gene expression of tumor necrosis factor alpha and TNF-receptors, p55 and p75, in nonalcoholic steatohepatitis patients. Hepatology. 2001;34(6):1158-63. Epub 2001/12/04.

Chapter 9

Liver Biopsy After Liver Transplantation

Alpna R. Limaye, Lisa R. Dixon and Roberto J. Firpi

Additional information is available at the end of the chapter

http://dx.doi.org/10.5772/52617

1. Introduction

Histological evaluation of liver allograft biopsies is an integral part of the management of liver transplant patients. From the time of donor hepatectomy onward, the allograft is susceptible to multiple insults, including warm and cold ischemia, complications related to surgical anastomoses, acute cellular rejection, and recurrence of underlying liver disease. It is often quite challenging to distinguish these various entities by their clinical presentation alone. In these situations, evaluation of a liver biopsy is frequently necessary to confirm the diagnosis, to stage recurrent fibrosis, or to monitor response to treatment.

2. Post-transplant liver biopsy techniques

Liver biopsies can be performed with various techniques, including a percutaneous approach (with marking by percussion/palpation, marking by ultrasound (US), or under real-time US or computed tomography (CT) guidance), a transjugular approach, or a surgical/laparoscopic approach. Although percutaneous liver biopsies on non-transplant patients can be done without the use of imaging, it is recommended that patients who have undergone any abdominal surgery (including liver transplantation) undergo biopsies aided by the use of US to avoid vascular or other structures [1]. While US marking followed by biopsy is sufficient in most post-transplant patients, in certain situations (such as split-liver recipients), biopsy under real-time US or CT guidance is preferred to avoid encountering intervening bowel loops. While specimens at least 1.5cm in length and containing at least 6-8 portal triads are considered adequate for the diagnosis of chronic liver disease [2,3], some advocate a minimum length of 2.0 cm and at least 11 complete portal tracts for accurate grading and staging of liver disease [4].

Percutaneous liver biopsy can be performed rapidly and safely in an outpatient setting with the appropriate monitoring equipment and staff availability [5]. After discharge, patients are typically instructed to avoid strenuous physical activity or driving for 24-48 hours, and are asked to contact the clinical provider in the event of concerning symptoms. In our institution, a review of over 3,000 liver biopsies (including liver transplant patients) demonstrated that the majority of complications were discovered within the first hour after percutaneous liver biopsy, and that shortening the recovery time to 1-2 hours did not impact the frequency of complications [6].

Percutaneous liver biopsy can be performed with suction needles (such as Jamshidi needle or Menghini needle), cutting needles (such as the Tru-Cut needle), or spring-loaded needle "guns". Specimens adequate for diagnosis, grading, and staging can usually be obtained by all of the biopsy needles used in current practice.

In patients with severe/uncorrectable coagulopathy, thrombocytopenia (typically platelet count < 50,000/mm^3), large ascites, morbid obesity, or an inability to cooperate, a transjugular liver biopsy (TJLB) is typically recommended [7]. In addition, TJLB is useful in patients for whom wedged hepatic venous pressure gradient (HVPG) measurement would be clinically useful. Miraglia et al reported on the safety of TJLB in liver transplant patients, with only one complication in 183 biopsies (0.5%) [8].

TJLB is typically performed with the use of automated needle systems, such as the Quick-Core needle and the Flexcore needle. It has been established that these automated needle systems often require multiple passes, and usually collect smaller core samples than those obtained by percutaneous liver biopsy [9]. Despite this fact, specimens obtained via TJLB are adequate for diagnosis, staging, and grading liver disease in greater than 90% of cases [10,11].

Surgical liver biopsies (either open liver biopsy or laparoscopic liver biopsy) are typically performed when patients require a surgical procedure for another indication. In liver transplant patients, this often involves repair of postoperative hernias. Biopsies in this setting can be performed with either automated needle systems or with a wedge resection, and the procedure provides the advantage of direct visualization of the liver and the ability to immediately diagnose and treat any bleeding which occurs.

3. Complications of liver biopsy

Although invasive, liver biopsy is a relative safe procedure, whether performed percutaneously or via the transvenous route. In a review of over 60,000 non-transplant patients, death within seven days directly related to liver biopsy occurred in 1 out of every 10,000 procedures, and all-cause mortality within seven days occurred in approximately 0.2% of patients [12]. Serious complications were similarly rare, with pain occurring in 2% of patients, hemoperitoneum occurring in 0.04%, and hemobilia occurring in 0.01% [12]. Similarly, studies of allograft liver biopsies demonstrate a mortality rate of up to 0.2%, and a rate of major complications between 0.2% and 1.8% [13]. While early studies suggested an increased risk of post-biopsy sepsis in patients with Roux-en-Y choledochojejunostomy, subsequent studies show that the risk is similar to patients with a duct-to-duct anastomosis [14].

4. Post-transplant liver enzyme abnormalities

Abnormalities in liver enzyme levels are often encountered in liver transplant patients, and can represent hepatocellular injury (reflected by the transaminases), biliary injury [reflected by alkaline phosphatase or gamma-glutamyl transferase (GGT)], or hepatic synthetic dysfunction (reflected by the albumin or by coagulation abnormalities). While the use of serum blood tests (such as viral or autoimmune serologies) and imaging techniques (such as ultrasound with Doppler, angiography, and magnetic resonance cholangiography) can be useful to determine the etiology of abnormal liver enzymes, liver biopsy is often necessary for a definitive diagnosis.

5. Early post-transplant liver enzyme abnormalities

The differential diagnosis of liver enzyme abnormalities varies with the amount of time which has passed since liver transplant. In the normal post-transplant course, liver enzymes typically rise immediately following transplant and become normal or near-normal within 3-5 days. If the enzymes fail to improve or normalize but soon rise again, it is likely that an early complication has occurred (Table 1). In the very early post-transplant period (within the first week), liver enzyme abnormalities can be related to primary graft nonfunction (PNF) or dysfunction, hepatic arterial insufficiency, small for size syndrome (SFSS), or portal venous thrombosis (PVT).

5.1. Primary graft dysfunction

PNF and primary graft dysfunction are associated with prolonged ischemia time [15], and it is likely that preservation and reperfusion injury play a role. PNF is heralded by a precipitous rise in hepatic transaminases in the second or third postoperative day accompanied by signs of hepatic failure (encephalopathy and coagulopathy). Once hepatic artery thrombosis (HAT) has been ruled out by imaging, a liver biopsy confirms the diagnosis. Biopsies in this setting typically show centrilobular hepatocyte dropout due to hepatocellular necrosis, with compensatory zone 2 hepatocyte proliferation and bile ductular proliferation [16].

5.2. Hepatic artery thrombosis

The clinical presentation of HAT is quite similar to that of PNF, with a dramatic increase in hepatic transaminases and bilirubin in the very early post-transplant period. A liver biopsy is typically not required, as the diagnosis can usually be confirmed with angiography. When performed, biopsies of patients with hepatic arterial insufficiency show hepatocyte foamy degeneration or necrosis and features of ischemic cholangitis [17].

Disease/ Complication	**Incidence**	**Time of presentation**	**Clinical presentation**	**Risk Factors**	**Histological Characteristics**
Preservation/ Reperfusion Injury	Up to 30% (2-7% severe) [15]	Within 3 days	Elevated transaminases, bilirubin, INR. Encephalopathy in severe injury	Prolonged cold or warm ischemia time, greater than 30% donor steatosis	Centrilobular hepatocyte dropout, zone 2 hepatocyte proliferation, bile duct proliferation [16]
Hepatic artery thrombosis	3-10% in adult transplant (up to 40% in pediatric transplant) [17]	Day 2 to 7 post-transplant	Severe elevation of transaminases, bilirubin, alkaline phosphatase/GGT	Technical/anastomotic complications	Foamy hepatocyte degeneration, features of ischemic cholangitis
Acute Cellular Rejection	24-80% by 6 months post-transplant [26]	Typically 2-3 weeks after transplant, up to 3 months post-transplant	Elevated transaminases, bilirubin, alkaline phosphatase. Possible recent history of inadequate immunosuppression	Younger recipient, older donor, history of autoimmune disorder, ? female recipient [17]	Portal inflammation, biliary inflammation, endothelitis
Portal vein thrombosis	Less than 1%	Early: within first week post-transplant Late: within first year post-transplant	Early: acute hepatic failure Late: ascites, variceal bleeding	Hypercoagulable state, prior history of PVT	Often normal, may show features of focal nodular hyperplasia [21, 22]
Small for size syndrome	Not well defined, but greatest when graft-to-recipient body weight ratio is less than 0.6 [18]	Sequelae of portal hypertension: 6 to 12 months post-transplant	Ascites, spontaneous bacterial peritonitis, variceal bleeding	Graft-to-recipient body weight ratio less than 0.6 [18, 19]	Centrilobular cholestasis and steatosis, interface bile duct inflammation [20]

Table 1. Differential diagnosis of early post-transplant liver enzyme abnormalities

http://dx.doi.org/10.5772/52617

5.3. Portal vein thrombosis

Early acute PVT presents clinically as acute hepatic failure and demonstrates histological features of hepatocyte necrosis. Occasionally, PVT presents later, in which case the features of portal hypertension dominate. In this situation, if a biopsy is performed, it can be normal or show features of nodular regenerative hyperplasia [18,19].

5.4. Small for size syndrome

Patients with SFSS present with dominant features of portal hypertension, such as ascites and variceal bleeding. This syndrome is the result of relative portal hyperperfusion compared to hepatic arterial blood flow, and often occurs when the transplanted liver (or liver segment) is less than 0.6- 0.8% of the recipient body weight [20,21]. The diagnosis is typically made clinically, with signs of portal hypertension such as ascites and variceal bleeding. If a liver biopsy is performed, the allograft typically shows centrilobular cholestasis, centrilobular steatosis, and interface ductular proliferation [22].

5.5. Acute cellular rejection

The most common cause of early allograft dysfunction is acute cellular rejection (ACR). Although most cases of ACR occur in the first three months post-transplant (most often in the second or third post-transplant week), late-onset ACR (occurring up to 10 years post-transplant) has been reported [23]. ACR typically presents as moderate to severe elevations in hepatic transaminases and alkaline phosphatase/GGT, with some degree of bilirubin elevation, often in patients with a recent history of inadequate immunosuppression. The "gold standard" for the diagnosis of ACR remains the liver biopsy, which typically shows variable degrees of mixed portal inflammation (often with increased eosinophils), bile duct inflammation, and endotheliitis (typically in the portal vein or central vein branches) (Figure 1). The Banff criteria are the most widely used to describe ACR, and give a score of 1-3 for each component. These scores are added to calculate the Rejection Activity Index (RAI), which ranges from 3-4 (mild ACR) up to greater than 7 (severe ACR) [24]. It should be noted that late-onset ACR often appears quite different histologically, with a greater likelihood of lobular inflammation, less prominent bile duct inflammation, and a tendency towards monotypic portal inflammation [25]. A follow-up liver biopsy after 3-7 days of increased immunosuppression is occasionally used to confirm response to treatment.

5.6. Late post-transplant liver enzyme abnormalities

Beyond three months post-transplant, the differential of liver enzyme abnormalities changes. Broadly, the diagnoses can be categorized as chronic rejection, native disease recurrence, de novo infectious complications, toxic complications, de novo hepatitis, or vascular complications (Table 2).

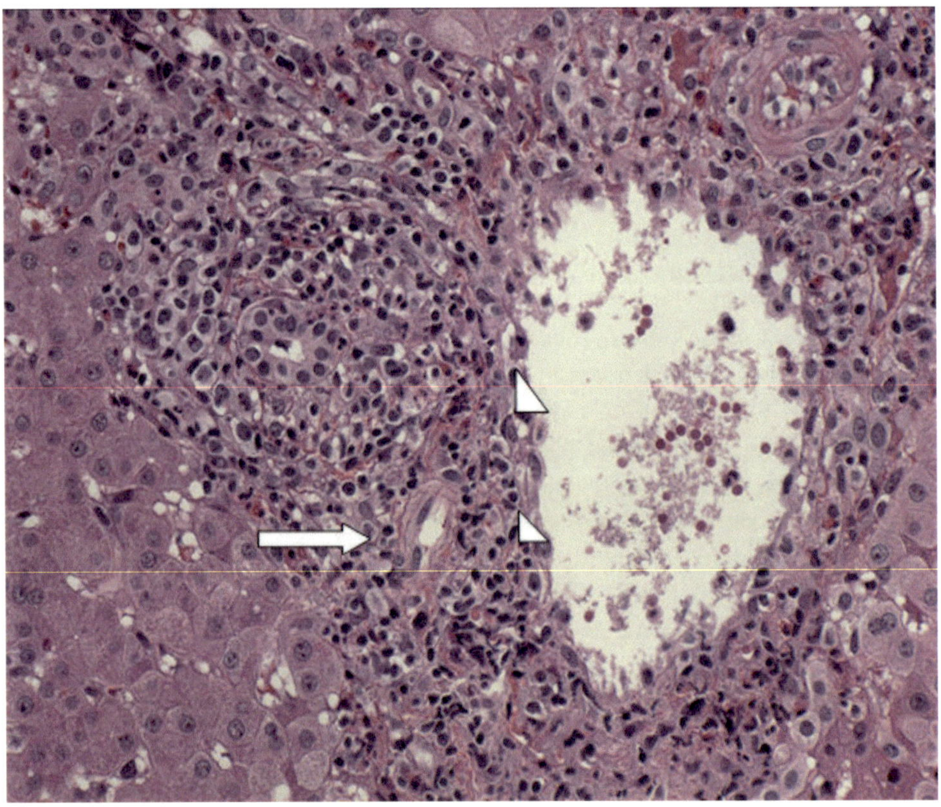

Figure 1. Acute rejection, with endotheliitis (arrowhead), bile duct destruction (arrow), and mixed portal inflammation (40x, H&E)

http://dx.doi.org/10.5772/52617

Disease/ Complication	**Incidence**	**Time of presentation**	**Clinical presentation**	**Risk Factors**	**Histological Characteristics**
Chronic rejection	3-5%	3-12 months after transplant	Rising alkaline phosphatase/GGT, late elevation in bilirubin	Inadequate immunosuppression, history of multiple episodes of or ongoing acute cellular rejection [17]	Bile duct atrophy/loss, foamy arteriopathy [26]
Recurrent HCV	Near-universal	Re-infection within 72 hours; histological recurrence within 1-2 weeks; clinically significant recurrence within 3 years (within 1 year for FCH) [27]	Elevated transaminases in typical recurrent HCV FCH: jaundice, marked elevation of alkaline phosphatase/GGT, extremely high HCV viral load	FCH: excessive immunosuppression	Portal inflammation, interface hepatitis, lobular activity [28-30] FCH: cholestasis, fibrosis [35]
Recurrent HBV	Less than 10% with adequate prophylaxis [36]	Typical recurrent HBV: 6-12 months post-transplant FCH: within 1 month post-transplant	Elevated transaminases, elevated HBV viral load	Inadequate prophylaxis	Lymphoplasmacytic portal inflammation, Kupffer cell hypertrophy, lobular disarray; ground-glass hepatocytes; positive immunostaining for hepatitis B surface antigen and core antigen [37]
Recurrent AIH	Up to 40% [38]	Variable	Slow progression of transaminase elevation	Inadequate immunosuppression, native type II AIH	Lymphoplasmacytic portal infiltrate, prominent interface activity [29]
CMV infection	5-8% with prophylaxis	1-12 months post-transplant	CMV hepatitis: Elevated transaminases Extrahepatic CMV: gastroenteritis, colitis, pneumonitis	Graft from CMV-antibody-positive donor into CMV-antibody-negative recipient	Portal inflammation, hepatocytes with CMV inclusions, focal bile duct damage [29]
EBV infection	Up to 80% of patients who are EBV-antibody-negative at time of transplant	6-12 or more months post-transplant	EBV hepatitis: usually asymptomatic PTLD: lymphoma-like presentation	Primary infection: EBV-antibody-negative recipient Progression to PTLD: excessive immunosuppression, preceding CMV infection [43]	EBV hepatitis: portal and sinusoidal infiltrates with atypical lymphocytes, +EBER PTLD: immunoblasts, with varying degrees of architectural distortion [45]

Table 2. Differential diagnosis of late post-transplant liver enzyme abnormalities

5.7. Chronic rejection

Chronic rejection involves immune-mediated injury to the hepatic arterial endothelium and bile duct epithelium. It is most commonly seen in patients who have experienced repeated bouts of significant ACR and/or have a recent history of inadequate immunosuppression. The typical clinical presentation is a slow rise in alkaline phosphatase/GGT, often followed by a rise in bilirubin. Procurement of an adequate biopsy sample (with at least ten complete portal triads) is crucial in the histologic diagnosis of chronic rejection [26]. The minimal criteria for diagnosis of chronic rejection, as defined by the 2000 Banff recommendations, are (1) bile duct atrophy/pyknosis affecting a majority of bile ducts (with or without bile duct loss); (2) foam cell obliterative arteriopathy (Figure 2); or (3) bile duct loss in greater than half of the portal tracts [26].

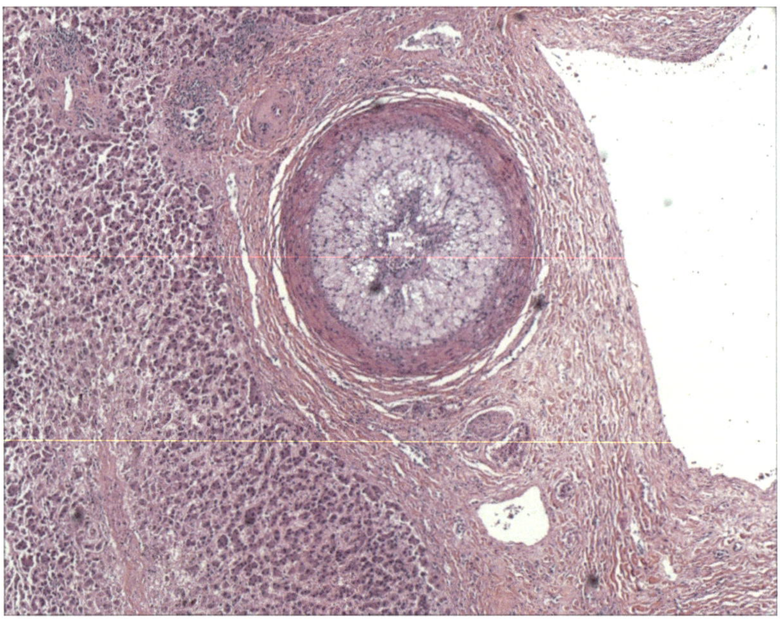

Figure 2. Foamy arteriopathy in the setting of chronic rejection (H&E 10x)

In the months and early years following liver transplant, recurrence of the underlying disease which led to transplant becomes a common problem. Disease recurrence can be viral (most commonly hepatitis B or C), immunological (such as autoimmune hepatitis, primary sclerosing cholangitis [PSC], or primary biliary cirrhosis [PBC]), metabolic (such as non-alcoholic fatty liver disease [NAFLD]), malignant (hepatocellular carcinoma or cholangiocarcinoma), or idiopathic. The diagnosis of recurrent PSC, PBC, NAFLD, and malignancy is relatively straightforward and is therefore not discussed further. However, the degree of clinical and histological overlap between entities such as rejection, recurrent viral hepatitis, and autoimmune hepatitis can create diagnostic conundrums without close clinicopathological correlation.

http://dx.doi.org/10.5772/52617

5.8. Recurrent hepatitis C

Recurrent hepatitis C (HCV) infection is a universal phenomenon after liver transplantation, and exhibits an accelerated progression to advanced liver disease [27]. Particularly in the early months after transplant, the differential diagnosis of abnormal liver enzymes in HCV patients includes both ACR and recurrent HCV. These entities are usually distinguished histologically. Histologically established recurrent HCV demonstrates portal inflammation, often with lymphoid aggregates, interface hepatitis, and lobular disarray [28-30] (Figure 3). There is often a component of ductular reaction, which is uncommon in HCV in native livers [30]. While endotheliitis was traditionally considered specific to rejection, recent data demonstrate portal branch endothelitis in biopsies of native HCV livers [31,32]. It does appear that moderate to severe central vein branch endotheliitis remains fairly specific for rejection. In a prospective analysis of biopsies from 48 HCV transplant patients, Demetris et al described strict criteria to avoid overdiagnosis of ACR: (1) inflammatory bile duct injury in at least 50% of portal tracts, and/or (2) mononuclear perivenular inflammation with hepatocyte necrosis in at least 50% of terminal hepatic venules [33]. In cases where the differentiation of ACR and recurrent HCV is not clear, the use of an immune function assay can be a useful adjunct [34]. Occasionally, recurrent HCV presents aggressively, in an entity known as fibrosing cholestatic hepatitis (FCH). The risk of FCH increases with aggressive immunosuppression, such as that used to treat ACR. Histologically, FCH is distinguished by a prominent component of cholestasis and fibrosis [35].

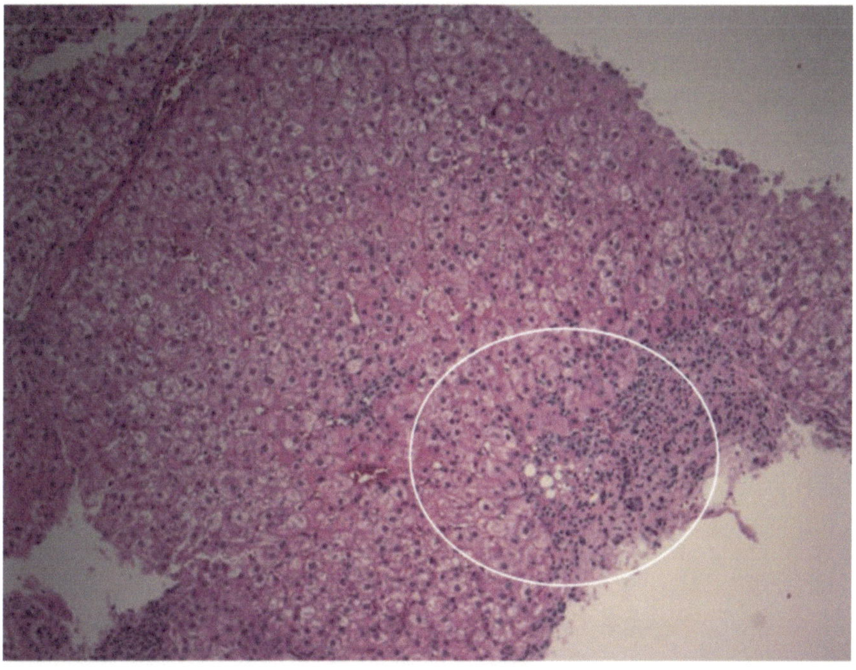

Figure 3. Recurrent HCV, with chronic portal inflammation (ellipse), and interface as well as lobular activity (H&E,10x)

5.9. Recurrent hepatitis B

Recurrent hepatitis B (HBV) infection was common in the era before combination prophylaxis with hepatitis B immunoglobulin and oral antiviral agents. The current rate of recurrent HBV (less than 10%) is attributed to a lack of prophylaxis for various reasons [36]. Histologically, recurrent HBV demonstrates lymphoplasmacytic portal inflammation, Kupffer cell hypertrophy, and lobular disarray [37]. Ground glass cells containing HBV surface antigen are often seen. Immunostaining demonstrates HBV surface antigen in hepatocyte cytoplasm and HBV core antigen in hepatocyte nuclei. Recurrent HBV can also cause FCH, characterized by cholestasis, perisinusoidal fibrosis, and swollen hepatocytes with immunoreactivity for HBV core antigen [37]. In patients without demonstrable HBV core antigen staining, other causes of hepatic dysfunction should be sought.

5.10. Recurrent and *de novo* autoimmune hepatitis

Recurrence of autoimmune hepatitis (AIH) can occur in up to 40% of patients, but the course is typically slowly progressive [38]. The biochemical/serological diagnosis of AIH [39] can be difficult in post-transplant patients, and therefore a liver biopsy is often required for a definitive diagnosis. In the chronic phase, recurrent AIH demonstrates lymphoplasmacytic portal infiltrate with prominent interface activity, perivenular activity and variable degrees of lobular necroinflammatory activity [29] (Figure 4). In patients without a pre-transplant history of AIH, the findings of lymphoplasmacytic infiltrate and perivenular activity, the differential diagnosis includes recurrent HCV, rejection, and de novo AIH. This distinction relies on close clinicopathological correlation which takes into account the timing of onset, the immunosuppressive state, and the degree of perivenular damage [40].

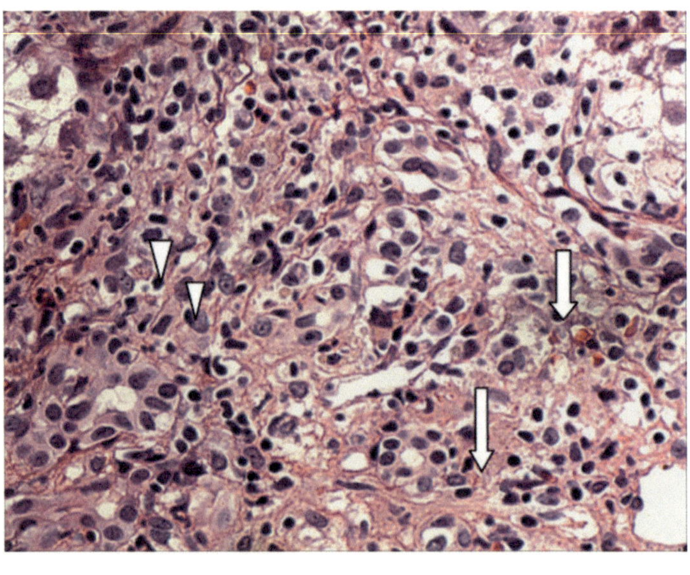

Figure 4. Portal area with interface hepatitis, numerous plasma cells (arrowhead) and scattered eosinophils (arrow) (H&E, 40x)

Liver transplant patients are also at risk of de novo infections due to their immunosuppressed state. While the diagnosis of most of these infections is fairly straightforward, post-transplant cytomegalovirus (CMV) and Epstein-Barr virus (EBV) infection can be more difficult.

5.11. CMV infection

CMV is the most common clinically significant viral infection after solid organ transplantation, with an incidence of up to 30% prior to the use of routine prophylaxis [41]. The risk of post-transplant CMV infection is greatest in CMV-antibody-negative recipients who receive a graft from a CMV-antibody-positive donor. Clinically, CMV infection can present with fever, myelosuppression, and/or organ involvement (such as gastritis, colitis, hepatitis, or pneumonitis). While detection of CMV in the serum can provide a rapid diagnosis, a liver biopsy is often required to distinguish CMV from allograft rejection or demonstrate that both entities are present [42]. Typically, CMV hepatitis is characterized by mononuclear or mixed portal inflammation, focal bile duct damage, and hepatocytes with CMV inclusions (large eosinophilic nuclear inclusions surrounded by a clear halo [29] (Figure 5). Although some features similar to allograft rejection (portal lymphocytic inflammation, mild endotheliitis) can be seen in CMV hepatitis, immunostaining for CMV antigens and/or the presence of CMV inclusions confirms that CMV is the driving force behind the hepatic dysfunction.

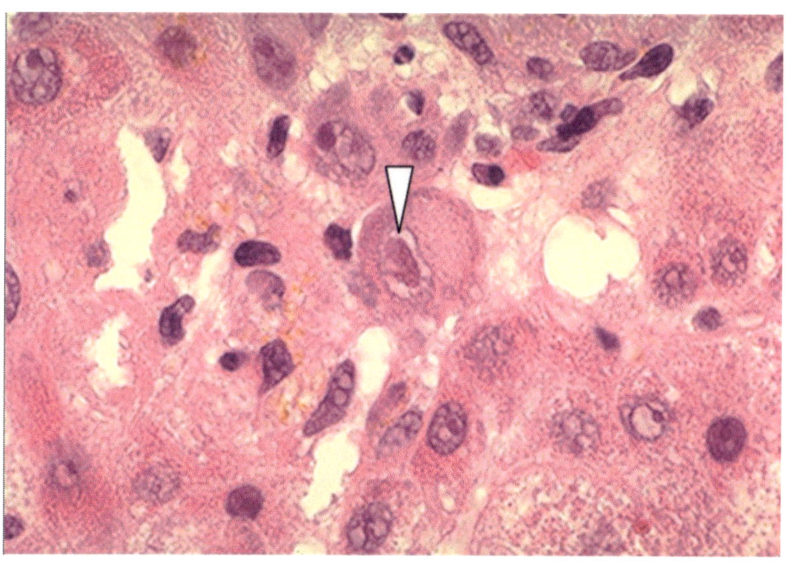

Figure 5. Hepatocyte with intranuclear CMV inclusion (arrowhead) (H&E, 100x)

5.12. EBV infection and post-transplant lymphoproliferative disorder

The clinical presentation of EBV infection can vary from asymptomatic hepatitis to post-transplant lymphoproliferative disorder (PTLD). Patients without pre-transplant immunity to EBV are at the greatest risk of infection. Patients with primary post-transplant EBV infection, those with previous symptomatic CMV infection, and those with recent excessive immunosuppression are at the highest risk for progression to PTLD [43]. EBV hepatitis typically demonstrates portal and sinusoidal infiltrates consisting of atypical lymphocytes. Often the lymphocytes are arranged in a single-file pattern within sinusoids [29]. Another histological pattern which can be seen in EBV hepatitis consists of mixed periportal and sinusoidal infiltrates with large atypical mononuclear cells and immunoblasts, mild bile duct damage, and hepatic lobular activity [44]. The finding of EBV-encoded RNAs (EBERs) is confirmatory in most cases.

PTLD is a heterogeneous lymphoproliferative disease divided into three main categories: early lesions, polymorphic PTLD, and monomorphic PTLD [45]. Early lesions demonstrate plasmacytic hyperplasia, and may or may not have prominent immunoblasts [29,45]. Polymorphic PTLD is characterized by mixed infiltrates of monoclonal or polyclonal plasma cells, immunoblasts, and destruction of the underlying lymphoid architecture [45]. In monomorphic PTLD, most cases arise from B cell populations which demonstrate invasion, architectural effacement, and cellular atypia [29]. A fourth category, Hodgkin's lymphoma-like PTLD, is sometimes described [46], and appears histologically like Hodgkin's lymphoma which occurs in non-transplant patients. PTLD patients with positive EBER results may represent relatively better histopathological features than patients with EBER-negative PTLD [47].

6. Indication and protocol liver biopsies

The majority of post-transplant liver biopsies are performed in response to changes in liver enzyme levels and/or abnormal imaging findings. Particularly in the early post-transplant period, these so-called "indication" biopsies are usually diagnostic and often result in a change in management. However, as patient and graft survival continues to improve, it has become clear that normal histology is rarely seen in the long-term liver graft [48]. What is not clear, however, is whether the histologic abnormalities seen in most late allograft biopsies correlate to clinically-significant disease, and whether the routine use of so-called "protocol" liver biopsies (performed at regular time points despite normal liver enzyme levels) is clinically justified. In our institution, we no longer perform annual protocol biopsies on patients with alcoholic liver disease, non-alcoholic fatty liver disease, or cryptogenic liver disease. The use of annual or semi-annual protocol biopsies in patients with AIH, PSC, or PBC is left to the discretion of the treating provider and/or the desires of the patient. In all HCV patients, protocol biopsies are performed at four months post-transplant, at one year post-transplant, and annually thereafter for at least the first five years. In contrast, an informal survey of 35 transplant centers found that only 65% of centers perform protocol liver biopsies for HCV patients, and only 25% of centers perform protocol biopsies for other post-transplant patients [13].

The rationale for protocol biopsies is the detection of those patients with severe dysfunction in the hopes that early treatment and/or change in immunosuppression might improve graft survival. However, the evidence of the clinical utility of these biopsies is conflicted. In studies of long-term protocol biopsies in non-viral hepatitis transplant patients, it does appear that histological abnormalities in the setting of normal liver enzymes likely are not clinically significant [49,50]. The rationale for the use of protocol liver biopsies in HCV patients is the identification of those with severe HCV recurrence in the hopes that prompt treatment could improve graft survival [51]. This appears to be justified, as several studies have demonstrated the clinical utility of protocol biopsies in HCV patients, even as long as 20 years post-transplant [52-54]. It is notable, however, that the vast majority of patients with recurrent HCV (and all patients with severe recurrent HCV) had abnormal liver enzymes at the pre-determined time of protocol biopsy.

A separate but equally important factor in long-term patient survival is the avoidance of extrahepatic complications of chronic immunosuppression, including renal insufficiency, the development of diabetes mellitus, and infectious complications. In this regard, another utility of protocol liver biopsy is the identification of those patients in whom immunosuppression can be safely lowered. A retrospective study of patients with various liver diseases found that protocol biopsy results led to a change in immunosuppression in almost on third of patients [55]. Recently, an international working group developed recommendations for protocol biopsy monitoring in patients in whom minimizing or weaning immunosuppression is being considered [56].

7. Summary

The liver allograft is susceptible to a broad range of insult and injury from the time that it is removed from the donor. While some complications are easily diagnosed by the clinical presentation and advanced imaging, the majority of conditions display overlapping clinical features. As the treatment of these various conditions can be radically different, a definitive diagnosis is crucial. To that end, post-transplant liver biopsy continues to play a key role in the evaluation of liver transplant patients with hepatic dysfunction. While the role of protocol biopsies in patients with no biochemical evidence of hepatic dysfunction has begun to fall out of favor (especially in non-HCV patients), the use of biopsy in immunosuppression-weaning protocols could promote a renewed interest in this methodology. The current data support the use of protocol biopsies in HCV patients (particularly in the first few years post-transplant). Areas for future investigation include non-invasive alternatives to liver biopsy such as immune assays and advanced imaging, and the use of routine protocol biopsies in weaning of immunosuppression.

Author details

Alpna R. Limaye[1], Lisa R. Dixon[2] and Roberto J. Firpi[1*]

*Address all correspondence to: roberto.firpi@medicine.ufl.edu

1 Section of Hepatobiliary Diseases, Division of Gastroenterology, Hepatology, and Nutrition, Department of Medicine, University of Florida, Gainesville, FL, USA

2 Department of Pathology, Immunology, and Laboratory Medicine, University of Florida, Gainesville, FL, USA

References

[1] Rockey DC, Caldwell SH, Goodman ZD, Nelson RC, Smith AD; American Association for the Study of Liver Diseases. Liver biopsy. Hepatology. 2009 Mar;49(3): 1017-44.

[2] Chan J, Alwahab Y, Tilley C, Carr N. Percutaneous medical liver core biopsies: correlation between tissue length and the number of portal tracts. J Clin Pathol. 2010 Jul; 63(7):655-6.

[3] Bravo AA, Sheth SG, Chopra S. Liver Biopsy. N Engl J Med. 2001 Feb 15;344(7): 495-500.

[4] Colloredo G, Guido M, Sonzogni A, Leandro G. Impact of liver biopsy size on histological evaluation of chronic viral hepatitis: the smaller the sample, the milder the disease. J Hepatol. 2003 Aug;39(2):239-44.

[5] Jacobs WH, Goldberg SB. Statement on outpatient percutaneous liver biopsy. Dig Dis Sci. 1989 Mar;34(3):322-3.

[6] Firpi RJ, Soldevila-Pico C, Abdelmalak MF, Morelli G, Judah J, Nelson DR. Short recovery time after percutaneous liver biopsy: should we change our current practices? Clin Gastroenterol Hepatol. 2005 Sep;3(9):926-9.

[7] Van Ha TG. Liver biopsy in liver transplant recipients. Semin Intervent Radiol. 2004 Dec;21(4):271-4.

[8] Miraglia R, Maruzzelli L, Minervini MI, Volpes R, Vissini G, Gruttadauria S, Caruso S, Luca A, Gridelli B. Transjugular liver biopsy in liver transplant patients using an 18-gauge automated core biopsy needle. Eur J. Radiol. 2011 Dec;80(3):e269-72.

[9] De Hoyos A, Loredo ML, Martinez-Rios MA, Gil MR, Kuri J, Cardenas M. Transjugular liver biopsy in 52 patients with an automated Trucut-type needle. Dis Dis Sci 1999;44:177-80.

[10] Cholongitas E, Quaglia A, Samonakis D, Senzolo M, Triantos C, Patch D, Leandro G, Dhillon AP, Burroughs AK. Transjugular liver biopsy: how good is it for accurate histological interpretation? Gut. 2006 Dec;55(12):1789-94.

[11] Cholongitas E, Senzolo M, Standish R, Marelli L, Quaglia A, Patch D, Dhillon AP, Burroughs AK. A systematic review of the quality of liver biopsy specimens. Am J Clin Pathol. 2006 May;125(5):710-21.

[12] West J, Card TR. Reduced mortality rates following elective percutaneous liver biopsies. Gastroenterology. 2010 Oct;139(4):1230-7.

[13] Mells G, Neuberger J. Protocol liver allograft biopsies. Transplantation. 2008 Jun 27;85(12):1686-92.

[14] Ben-Ari Z, Neville L, Rolles K, Davidson B, Burroughs AK. Liver biopsy in liver transplantation: no additional risk of infections in patients with choledochojejunostomy. J Hepatol. 1996 Mar;24(3):324-7.

[15] Sirivatanauksorn Y, Taweerutchana V, Limsrichamrern S, Kositamongkol P, Mahawithitwong P, Asavakarn S, Tovikkai C, Sanphasitvong V. Analysis of donor risk factors associated with graft outcomes in orthotopic liver transplantation. Transplant Proc. 2012 Mar;44(2):320-3.

[16] Kakizoe S, Yanaga K, Starzl TE, Demetris AJ. Evaluation of protocol before transplantation and after reperfusion biopsies from human orthotopic liver allografts: considerations of preservation and early immunological injury. Hepatology. 1990 Jun;11(6):932-41.

[17] Gao Z. Seeking beyond rejection: an update on the differential diagnosis and a practical approach to liver allograft biopsy interpretation. Adv Anat Pathol. 2009;16:97-117.

[18] Wang JT, Zhao HY, Liu YL. Portal vein thrombosis. Hepatobiliary Pancreat Dis Int. 2005 Nov;4(4):515-8.

[19] Shimamatsu K, Wanless IR. Role of ishchemia in causing apoptosis, atrophy, and nodular hyperplasia in human liver. Hepatology. 1997 Aug;26(2):343-50.

[20] Selzner M, Kashfi A, Cattral MS, Selzner N, Greig PD, Lilly L, McGilvray ID, Therapondos G, Adcock LE, Ghanekar A, Levy GA, Renner EL, Grant DR. A graft to body weight ratio less than 0.8 does not exclude adult-to-adult right-lobe living donor liver transplantation. Liver Transpl. 2009 Dec;15(12):1776-82.

[21] Alves RC, Fonseca EA, Mattos CA, Abdalla S, Goncalves JE, Waisberg J. Predictive factors of early graft loss in living donor liver transplantation. Arg Gastroenterol. 2012 Jun;49(2):157-61.

[22] Demetris AJ, Kelly DM, Eghtesad B, Fontes P, Wallis Marsh J, Tom K, Tan HP, Shaw-Stiffel T, Boig L, Novelli P, Planinsic R, Fung JJ, Marcos A. Pathophysiologic observations and histopathologic recognition of the portal hyperperfusion or small-for-size syndrome. Am J Surg Pathol. 2006 Aug;30(8):986-93.

[23] Nakanishi C, Kawagishi N, Sekiguchi S, Akamatsu Y, Sato K, Miyagi S, Takeda I, Hukushima K, Aiso T, Sato A, Fujimori K, Satomi S. Steroid-resistant late acute rejection after a living donor liver transplantation: case report and review of the literature. Tohuko J Exp Med. 2007 Feb;211(2):195-200.

[24] No authors listed. Banff schema for grading liver allograft rejection: an international consensus document. Hepatology. 1997 Mar;25(3)658-63.

[25] Demetris AJ, Adeyi O, Bellamy CO, Clouston A, Charlotte F, Czaja A, Daskal I, El-Monayeri MS, Fontes P, Fung J, et al; Banff Working Group. Liver biopsy interpretation for causes of late liver allograft dysfunction. Hepatology. 2006;44:489-501.

[26] Demetris A, Adams D, Bellamy C, Blakolmer K, Clouston A, Dhillon AP, Fung J, Gouw A, Gustafsson B, Haga H, Harrison D, Hart J, et al. Update of the International Banff Schema for Liver Allograft Rejection: working recommendations for the histopathologic staging and reporting of chronic rejection. An International Panel. Hepatology. 2000 Mar;31(3):792-9.

[27] Limaye AR, Firpi RJ. Management of recurrent hepatitis C infection after liver transplantation. Clin Liver Dis. 2011 Nov;15(4);845-58.

[28] Gane EJ. The natural history of recurrent hepatitis C and what influences this. Liver Transpl. 2008;14(Suppl 2):S36-S44.

[29] Adeyi O, Fischer SE, Guindi M. Liver allograft pathology: approach to interpretation of needle biopsies with clinicopathological correlation. J Clin Pathol. 2010;63:47-74.

[30] Moreira RK. Recurrent hepatitis C and acute allograft rejection: clinicopathologic features with emphasis on the differential diagnosis between these entitities. Adv Anat Pathol. 2011 Sep;18(5):393-405.

[31] Souza P, Prihoda TJ, Hoyumpa AM, Sharkey FE. Morphologic features resembling transplant rejection in core biopsies of native livers from patients with Hepatitis C. Hum Pathol. 2009 Jan;40(1):92-7.

[32] Yeh MM, Larson AM, Tung BY, Swanson PE, Upton MP. Endotheliitis in chronic viral hepatitis: a comparison with acute cellular rejection and non-alcoholic steatohepatitis. Am J Surg Pathol. 2006 Jun;30(6):727-33.

[33] Demetris AJ, Eghtesad B, Marcos A, Ruppert K, Nalesnik MA, Randhawa P, Wu T, Krasinskas A, Fontes P, Cacciarelli T, Shakil AO, Murase N, Fung JJ, Starzl TE. Recurrent hepatitis C in liver allografts: prospective assessment of diagnostic accuracy, identification of pitfalls, and observations about pathogenesis. Am J Surg Pathol. 2004 May;28(5):658-69.

[34] Cabrera R, Ararat M, Soldevila-Pico C, Dixon L, Pan JJ, Firpi R, Machicao V, Levy C, Nelson DR, Morelli G. Using an immune functional assay to differentiate acute cellular rejection from recurrent hepatitis C in liver transplant patients. Liver Transpl. 2009 Feb;15(2);216-22.

[35] Dixon LR, Crawford JM. Early histologic changes in fibrosing cholestatic hepatitis C. Liver Transpl. 2007 Feb;13(2):219-26.

[36] Laryea MA, Watt KD. Immunoprophylaxis against and prevention of recurrent viral hepatitis after liver transplantation. Liver Transpl. 2012 May;18(5):514-23.

[37] Thung SN. Histologic findings in recurrent HBV. Liver Transpl. 2006 Nov;12(11 Suppl 2):S50-53.

[38] Ayata G, Gordon FD, Lewis WD, Pomfret E, Pomposelli JJ, Jenkins RL, Khettry U. Liver transplantation for autoimmune hepatitis: a long-term pathologic study. Hepatology. 2000 Aug;32(2):185-92.

[39] Hennes EM, Zeniya M, Czaja AJ, Pares A, Dalekos GN, Krawitt EL, Bittencourt PL, Porta G, Boberg KM, Hofer H, Bianchi FB, et al; International Autoimmune Hepatitis Group. Simplified criteria for the diagnosis of autoimmune hepatitis. Hepatology. 2008 Jul;48(1):169-76.

[40] Demetris AJ, Sebagh M. Plasma cell hepatitis in liver allografts: Variant of rejection or autoimmune hepatitis? Liver Transpl. 2008 Jun;14(6):750-5.

[41] Lee SO, Razonable RR. Current concepts on cytomegalovirus infection after liver transplantation. World J Hepatol. 2010 Sep 27;2(9):325-36.

[42] Razonable RR. Cytomegalovirus infection after liver transplantation: current concepts and challenges. World J Gastroenterol. 2008 Aug 21;14(31);4849-60.

[43] Knight JS, Tsodikov A, Cibrik DM, Ross CW, Kaminski MS, Blayney DW. Lymphoma after solid organ transplantation: risk, response to therapy, and survival at a transplantation center. J Clin Oncol. 2009 Jul 10;27(20):3354-62.

[44] Randhawa P, Blakolmer K, Kashyap R, Raikow R, Nalesnik M, Demetris AJ, Jain A. Allograft liver biopsy in patients with Epstein-Barr virus-associated posttransplant lymphoproliferative disease. Am J Surg Pathol. 2001 Mar;25(3):324-30.

[45] Harris NL, Jaffe ES, Diebold J, Flandrin G, Muller-Hermelink HK, Vardiman J, Lister TA, Bloomfield CD. The World Health Organization classification of the hematopoietic and lymphoid tissues: report of the Clinical Advisory Committee meeting—Airlie House, Virginia, November, 1997. Hematol J. 2000;1(1):53-66.

[46] Jagadeesh D, Woda BA, Draper J, Evens AM. Post transplant lymphoproliferative disorders: risk, classification, and therapeutic recommendations. Curr Treat Options Oncol. 2012 Mar;13(1);122-36.

[47] Izadi M, Taheri S. Significance of in situ hybridization results for EBV-encoded RNA in post-transplantation lymphoproliferative disorder setting: report from the PTLD.Int Survey. Ann Transplant. 2010 Oct-Dec;15(4):102-9.

[48] Ekong UD. The long-term liver graft and protocol biopsy: do we want to look? What will we find? Curr Opin Organ Transplant. 2011 Oct;16(5):505-8.

[49] Maor-Kendler Y, Batts KP, Burgart LJ, Wiesner RH, Krom RA, Rosen CB, Charlton MR. Comparative allograft histology after liver transplantation for cryptogenic cirrhosis, alcohol, hepatitis C, and cholestatic liver diseases. Transplantation. 2000 Jul 27;70(2):292-7.

[50] El-Masry M, Gilbert CP, Saab S. Recurrence of non-viral liver disease after orthotopic liver transplantation. Liver Int. 2011 Mar;31(3):291-302.

[51] Firpi RJ, Clark V, Soldevila-Pico C, Morelli G, Cabrera R, Levy C, Machicao VI, Chaoru C, Nelson DR. The natural history of hepatitis C cirrhosis after liver transplantation. Liver Transpl. 2009 Sep;15(9):1063-71.

[52] Berenguer M, Rayon JM, Prieto M, Aguilera V, Nicolas D, Ortiz V, Carrasco D, Lopez-Andujar R, Mir J, Berenguer J. Are posttransplantation protocol liver biopsies useful in the long term? Liver Transpl. 2001 Sep;7(9):790-6.

[53] Firpi RJ, Abdelmalek MF, Soldevila-Pico C, Cabrera R, Shuster JJ, Theriaque D, Reed AI, Hemming AW, Liu C, Crawford JM, Nelson DR. One-year protocol liver biopsy can stratify fibrosis progression in liver transplant recipients with recurrent hepatitis C infection. Liver Transpl. 2004 Oct;10(10):1240-7.

[54] Sebagh M, Samuel D, Antonini TM, Coilly A, Degli Esposti D, Roche B, Karam V, Dos Santos A, Duclos-Vallee JC, Roque-Afonso AM, Ballott E, Guettier C, Blandin F, Saliba F, Azoulay D. Twenty-year protocol liver biopsies: invasive but useful for the management of liver recipients. J Hepatol. 2012 Apr;56(4):840-7.

[55] Mells G, Mann C, Hubscher S, Neuberger J. Late protocol liver biopsies in the liver allograft: a neglected investigation? Liver Transpl. 2009 Aug;15(8):931-8.

[56] Adeyi O, Alexander G, Baiocchi L, Balasubramanian M, Batal I, OC BC, Bhan A, Bridges N, Bucuvalas J, Charlotte F, et al; The Banff Working Group on Liver Allograft Pathology. Importance of liver biopsy findings in immunosuppression management: Biopsy monitoring and working criteria for patients with operational tolerance (OT). Liver Transpl. 2012 May 29. [Epub ahead of print].

Section 3

Non-Invasive Alternatives of Liver Biopsy

Chapter 10

Non-Invasive Evaluation of Liver Steatosis, Fibrosis and Cirrhosis in Hepatitis C Virus Infected Patients Using Unidimensional Transient Elastography (Fibroscan®)

Monica Lupsor, Horia Stefanescu, Diana Feier and Radu Badea

Additional information is available at the end of the chapter

http://dx.doi.org/10.5772/52621

1. Introduction

1.1. The importance of non-invasive evaluation of liver steatosis and fibrosis in virus C infected patients

Chronic conditions of the liver represent an important public health issue. Whatever the nature of the aggression against the liver, it seems that it always follows the same pattern: inflamation -> necrosis -> healing (fibrosis) -> regeneration (cirrhosis) -> dysplasia -> hepatocellular carcinoma. An important link in this course of events is represented by fibrogenesis. On the other hand, there are more and more evidence that, in patients with chronic hepatitis C, steatosis is a risk factor independently associated with necroinflammatory activity and fibrosis progression.

At the moment, the gold standard in the evaluation of both liver fibrosis and steatosis is represented by liver biopsy (LB), an invasive method with possible side effects. As a result, most of the research done worldwide is focused towards developing other alternative, non-invasive diagnosis methods, that would be capable to evaluate fibrosis and steatosis as accurately as possible.

Therefore, the following pages will present an evaluation of unidimensional transient elastography (TE) performance in the assessment of liver fibrosis and steatosis in patients suffering from chronic viral hepatitis type C (HCV).

2. Liver biopsy – An imperfect gold standard

Liver biopsy was performed by P Ehrlich in 1883 and became a common exploration method in 1958, when G Menghini introduced the first biopsy technique with a needle that was named after him [1].

Liver biopsy provides a lot of information [2-6]:

- it represents the gold standard for a positive and differential diagnosis of diffuse liver diseases;
- provides important etiology data;
- allows for the evaluation of the necroinflammatory activity, evolutive stage (fibrosis) and confirms if cirrhosis is present or not;
- helps establish the prognosis;
- identifies concomitent morphological alterations that may influence therapy response and its evaluation (steatosis, iron overload, etc);
- it can determine treatment efficiency.

At the same time, one can not ignore the fact that liver biopsy has significant limitations: possible complications, including mortality; important sampling errors; high cost; subjective appreciations that may be due to important intra and interobserver variations.

Biopsy complications may vary in magnitude and frequency depending on the subjacent liver pathology. Among these can be listed: pain (epigastric area, right shoulder, right hypocondrium); vagal response; hemorrhagic accidents (hemoperitoneum, hemobilia, liver hematoma); bile peritonitis, bilioma; bacteremia; infections and abscesses; pneumothorax and/or pleural reactions; hemothorax; arteriovenous fistula; subcutaneous emphysema; adverse reactions caused by the anesthetic; breaking of the biopsy needle; penetration of other organs: lung, kidney, colon. The mortality associated with this technique is low, but it is possible in 0.0088-0.3% of the cases [7-11].

The most significant problem encountered when interpreting a biopsy is represented by samplig error. Considering the fact that the tissue sample obtained through liver biopsy represents approximately 1/50.000-1/100.000 of the liver volume, it can be inadequate for the diagnosis of diffuse liver conditions, as the histopathological changes may be spread unevenly [5]. Even though liver biopsy is considered the standard exploration in the evaluation of liver diseases, it has an accuracy of only 80% in staging fibrosis and it can miss cirrhosis in 30% of the cases [12]. For example, Ragev reported that in HCV patients, there is a discrepancy of at least 1 stage between the right and left lobe in 33% of the patients [13]. At the same time, Siddique observed that a difference of at least one stage between 2 samples (15 mm long) cut from the same area occurs in 45% of the cases [14].

Considering all these observations, the results of the studies performed to validate a non-invasive diagnosis method must be interpreted with caution, since they are compared with an imperfect „gold standard".

Because of the limitations and invasive nature of liver biopsy, other non-invasive means are being tested for the evaluation of diffuse hepatopathies, and implicitly of fibrosis and steatosis as major prognosis factors in the evolution of the hepatopathy. Therefore, there is interest in developing other methods, either serological or imaging, which are all non-invasive, in order to determine the presence and degree of fibrosis, as well as of steatosis. One of these methods is unidimensional transient elastography (Fibroscan).

3. The principle of unidimentional transient elastography

The divice consists of a special transducer, that is placed in the axis of a mechanical vibrator. The vibrator generates pain-free vibrations that produce a train of elastic waves that will be transmited through the skin and subcutaneous tissue to the liver. At the same time with activating the vibration, the probe performs a number of ultrasound acquisitions (the same process of emision-reception used in conventional ultrasonography), with a frequency of 4 kHz. Reports on the tissues deformation caused by elastic wave transmission can be formulated by comparing the succesive ultrasound (US) signals acquired in this manner. The time necessary for the train of waves to propagate along the area of interest, as well as propagation velocities are being measured. This way liver stiffness can be determined using the following formula: $E = 3\varrho Vs_2$ (E – elasticity module, ϱ – density, a constant of the material; Vs – propagation velocity within the liver parenchyma). The more rigid the material, the higher the velocity of propagation [15-17].

During the examination, the patient is lying down, face-up, with his right arm placed in hyperextension and above the head for an adequate exposure of his right hypocondrium. The probe is placed in contact with the patient's skin, at the level of an intercostal space, in an area of full liver dullness and avoiding any large vessels.

When the button on the probe is pushed, the vibration that will be transmitted through the liver is activated. By analyzing tissue deformation report, the software of the equipment will measure the liver stiffness (LS). The results are given in kiloPascals (kPa) and correspond to a median value of 10 valid measurements. The machine can determine values between 2.5 and 75 kPa.

The monitor of the machine will display data regarding the patient's identity, diagnosis, name of the examining physician, the instantaneous value of liver stiffness (CS), the median stiffness resulted from 10 valid measurements, the success rate (SR), as well as the variation of the 10 values compared with the median value (IQR).

To be in agreement with the recommendations of the producer, the success rate must be at least 60% and IQR must not exceed 30% of the median liver stiffness [16], even though it seems that the best concordance with liver biopsy is obtained when this value does not exceed 20% of the median [18].

There are no studies that especially focus on the issue of the variability of LS measurements and therefore the interpretation of the results is done according to the experience of the examiner and the recommandations of the producer [19]. It is not known whether this variability is encountered only in the diseased liver or whether it is present in the healthy liver as well and to what degree this affects the interpretation of the results. The cause of this problem can be an inadequate technique or the liver pathology itself (for example, in macronodular cirrhosis, liver stiffness can be different in different areas of the liver). When there is a high variability of the results, it is important to check whether the probe is placed perfectly perpendicular on the thoracic wall, if the transmited vibration does not encounter the ribs and if the waves are transmited vertically, strictly between the ribs. If the generated wave is large, bifid or angulated, than the software of the machine will reconstruct the velocity curve in different points of the wave and therefore lead to variations of the acquired values. In order to obtain an accurate elastogram the transducer must be placed in the middle area of the right lobe, avoiding contact with the ribs that may lead to vibration distorsion and absorbtion [19].

The technique measures the stiffness of a volume that is equivalent with that of a cilinder of 1 cm in diameter and 4 cm in length (the measurement can be performed on a distance of 25 to 45 cm from the skin). This volume, representing about 1/500 of the liver volume, is at least a 100 times larger than the one obtained through liver biopsy and it is therefore more representative for the whole liver parenchyma [20, 21].

The examination can be performed by a technician following a short period of training (approximately 100 cases) [22-23], while the clinical interpretation of the results must always be done by an expert who would consider the demographic data, the etiology of the disease and the biochemical profile of the patient at the moment of the examination [21].

A multivariate analysis of the relationship between liver stiffness and fibrosis, necroinflammatory activity and steatosis Showed, in some studies, that there is a significant correlation with fibrosis, but no correlation with necroinflammatory activity and steatosis [16, 24]. Nevertheless, the authors of the initial concept acknowledged, following in vitro studies, that it is unlikely that a single physical parameter (liver stiffness) would describe entirely a complex biological system in which fibrosis is only a part [15].

A prospective assessment of the role of the histopathological parameters seen in LB in explaining the variance of liver stiffness was performed on 345 chronic hepatitis C patients that all underwent liver biopsy [25]. First, LS correlated highly with the degree of fibrosis assessed by liver biopsy,, but we also found a weak correlation with hepatic iron deposition and steatosis and a mild correlation with activity. In multiple regression analysis, fibrosis, activity, and steatosis independently influenced LSM. Iron deposition does not seem to influence the liver stiffness in CHC patients. Fibrosis, activity, and steatosis together explained 62.4% of the variance of the LS. The three significant parameters uniquely explained 45.95% of the amount of LS, with fibrosis making the most unique contribution (44.49%); the difference of 16.25% (62.4%-45.95%) was accounted for by the joint contribution of the three parameters. The size and the direction of the relationships suggest that higher LS values are obtained for patients with advanced fibrosis, increased necroinflammatory activity and increased steatosis. Among these three, however, the stage of fibrosis is the single most important predictor, as suggested by the squared partial correlation [25].

http://dx.doi.org/10.5772/52621

The prediction model computed from this study [25] can be expressed as follows:

Liver stiffness (log-transformed) = 0.493 + 0.180*fibrosis stage +0.034*steatosis + 0.033*activity grade.

Therefore, our studies showed that fibrosis is indeed the main predictor of liver stiffness, but the activity and steatosis cannot be neglected, and may explain the LS variability within the same fibrosis stage.

4. Performance of TE for the noninvasive evaluation of liver fibrosis HCV patients

The first condition that benefited from unidimensional transient elastography was chronic hepatitis type C [21, 26].

4.1. The diagnosis of liver fibrosis stages

Studies performed on a large number of HCV patients indicate that the LS value is highly correlated with the stage of fibrosis. The practical utility of the method is based on establishing cutoff values for each stage of fibrosis. A diagnosis of stage F ≥2, F ≥3 and F4 (cirrhosis) is based on measurements of liver stiffness that vary, according to some studies, from 6.2 to 8.8 Kpa, 7.7 to 10.8 kPa and from 11 to 14.8 kPa (Table 1) [24, 26-30].

There are some meta-analyses addressing the issue of diagnosis performance of TE. Fifty studies were included in the analysis performed by Friedrich Rust et al. The mean AUROC for the diagnosis of significant fibrosis, severe fibrosis, and cirrhosis were 0.84, 0.89 and 0.94, respectively [31]. In Stebbing's meta-analysis, a total of 22 studies were selected, comprising 4430 patients, most of them suffering from a virus C liver infection. The pooled estimates for significant fibrosis (≥F2) measured 7.71 kPa (LSM cutoff value) with a sensitivity of 71.9% and a specificity of 82.4%, whereas for cirrhosis (F4) the results showed a cutoff of 15.08 kPa with a sensitivity of 84.45% and a specificity of 94.69% [32].

It must be underlined that, in spite of the very good areas under the ROC curves, overlaps of the stiffness values were registered in adjacent stages, especially for early fibrosis [33]. The increase of liver stiffness is higher between stage F2 (6.6 kPa) and F3 (10.3 kPa) of fibrosis than between F1 (5.5 kPa) and F2 (6.6 kPa), a fact that is in agreement with the morphological data according to which the increase in fibrotic tissue is more significant from F2 to F3 than from F1 to F2 [12].

The diagnosis accuracy of TE is much better in predicting cirrhosis. In Friedrich-Rust metaanalysis [31], the AUROC mean for the diagnosis of cirrhosis was 0.94 and the performance estimated by Talwalkar [34] was also very good: sensitivity 87%, specificity 91%, positive probability rate 11.7, and negative probability rate 0.14 (95% CI 0.10-0.20).

Fibrosis Stage	Author	Cutoff (kPa)	Se(%)	Sp(%)	PPV(%)	NPV(%)	+LR	-LR	AUROC
F≥1	Ziol [24]	-	-	-	-	-	-	-	-
	Castera [26]	-	-	-	-	-	-	-	-
	Sporea [27]	-	-	-	-	-	-	-	-
	Nitta [28]	-	-	-	-	-	-	-	-
	Arena [29]	-	-	-	-	-	-	-	-
	Kim SU [30]	-	-	-	-	-	-	-	-
F≥2	Ziol [24]	8.8	56	91	56	88	0.63	0.48	0.79
	Castera [26]	7.1	67	89	48	95	6.09	0.37	0.83
	Sporea [27]	6.8	59.6	93.3	98	30.1	-	-	0.773
	Nitta [28]	7.1	82.8	80.3	86	73.6	4.1		0.88
	Arena [29]	7.8	83	82	83	79	4.58	0.20	0.91
	Kim SU [30]	6.2	76	97.5	97.4	80	30.4	0.3	0.909
F≥3	Ziol [24]	9.6	86	85	93	71	5.76	0.16	0.91
	Castera [26]	9.5	73	91	81	87	8.11	0.29	0.90
	Sporea [27]	-	-	-	-	-	-	-	-
	Nitta [28]	9.6	87.7	82.4	72.5	92.7	5	-	0.90
	Arena [29]	10.8	91	94	92	73	11.27	0.07	0.99
	Kim SU [30]	7.7	100	95.7	87.5	100	0	23.3	0.993
F4	Ziol [24]	14.6	86	96	97	78	23.05	0.14	0.97
	Castera [26]	12.5	87	91	95	77	9.66	0.14	0.95
	Sporea [27]	-	-	-	-	-	-	-	-
	Nitta [28]	11.6	91.7	78	41.5	98.2	4.2	-	0.90
	Arena [29]	14.8	94	92	73	98	11.27	0.07	0.98
	Kim SU [30]	11	77.8	93.9	58.3	97.5	12.8	0.2	0.970

Table 1. Liver stiffness cutoff values for staging liver fibrosis using TE in HCV patients. Sensibility (Se), specificity (Sp), positive predictive value (PPV) and negative predictive value (NPV) for each fibrosis stage (using Metavir scorring system).

But it must not be forgotten that the cutoff values for predicting the stages of fibrosis were chosen using the ROC curves in such a way that the sum of sensitivity and specificity is maximum. The country where the study was performed was among the factors that influenced the diagnosis performance of TE [31]. Therefore, even though the cutoff values defined for a certain population may be relevant, they may not be applicable in another population where the incidence of fibrosis is different. Because of this, it is indicated that each centre establishes its own cutoff values, in agreement with the prevalence of fibrosis stages in that particular population, and calculates the performance of the method in relation with those cutoff values. According to our experience on a number of 1138 HCV patients that underwent liver biopsy, the predictive cutoff values for stages F1, F2, F3 and F4 are: 5.1kPa, 7.5kPa, 9.1kPa and 13,2kPa, with an AUROC of 0.836, 0.826, 0.933 and 0.973, and diagnosis accuracy between 77 and 92.8% [35]. In table 2 are presented the liver stiffness cutoff values that predict each stage of fibrosis for the Romanian patients suffering from viral C chronic hepatitis. The table also presents the sensitivity (Se), specificity (Sp), positive predictive value (PPV) and negative predicting value (NPV), false positive (FPR) and false negative rate (FNR) the area under the ROC curve (AUROC) as well as the diagnosis accuracy (DA) of these cutoff values. In our study, the adjusted AUROC according to the prevalence of each individual stage of fibrosis did not significantly differ from the observed ones (0.847 for F≥1, p=1.00; 0.893 for F≥2, p=0.06; 0.945 for F≥3, p=0.34; 0.983 for F4, p=0.312), therefore the cutoff values that we obtained may have a large applicability.

4.2. Monitoring disease progression

4.2.1. Diagnosis of liver cirrhosis. Prediction of portal hypertension and related complications

TE has a very good diagnosis accuracy in predicting cirrhosis (stage F4 Metavir), with areas under ROC varying from 0.90 to 0.99 and cutoff values between 9-26.6 kPa [31], but there is a high interest to determine whether the use of the machine's entire specter of measurements (up to 75 kPa) can predict the clinical events characteristic to the evolution of cirrhosis. Some authors [36] indicated, with a negative predictive value of over 90%, that the suggestive values for predicting the presence of various complications are: 27.5 kPa for large esophageal varices; 37.5 kPa for Child B and C cirrhosis; 49.1 kPa for ascites; 53.7 kPa for hepatocarcinoma and 62.7 kPa for bleeding esophageal varices.

Portal hypertension is the main characteristic of liver cirrhosis, and the hepatic venous portal gradient (HVPG) is the best surrogate marker to assess its presence.

A positive strong correlation between liver stiffness and HVPG was reported in HCV patients [37] and, afterwards, independently confirmed in another group of patients with severe fibrosis (Metavir F3-F4) [38]. The correlation was excellent for HVPG values lower than 10 or 12 mm Hg, but the linear regression analysis did not reveal exceptional results for HVPG values >10 mm Hg or >12 mm Hg. This means that, even though TU may detect a progressive elevation of the portal pressure, mainly because of an increase in intrahepatic vascular resistance caused by the accumulation of extracellular fibrillar matrix, this method can not entirely determine the extremely complex hemodynamic alterations that characterize the delayed phase of portal hypertension [39]. As a result, some authors believe it is unlikely that elastography can be useful in monitoring the hemodynamic therapeutic response, as the effect of the treatment is mainly mediated by the splanchnic circulatory changes [40].

	≥ F1; F0vsF1234	≥ F2; F01vsF234	≥ F3; F012vsF34	F4; F0123vsF4
Liver stiffness cutoff value (kPa)	5.1	7.5	9.1	13.2
Se (%)	85.09	74.27	86.99	93.59
Sp (%)	65.45	82.95	88.51	92.71
+LR	2.46	4.36	7.57	12.84
-LR	0.23	0.31	0.15	0.07
PPV (%)	97.9	88.8	83.2	83.4
NPV (%)	18.7	63.9	91.2	97.4
FPR (%)	36.36	17.30	12.23	7.41
FNR (%)	13.86	25.59	12.55	6.41
Diagnosis accuracy (%)	85.01	77.34	87.63	92.87
Observed AUROC	0.836	0.860	0.933	0.973
Adjusted AUROC according to the prevalence of the fibrosis stages	0.847	0.893	0.945	0.983
p (difference between obs vs adj AUROC)	1.00	0.06	0.34	0.312

Table 2. Diagnostic performance of different cutoff values of liver stiffness in staging liver fibrosis in HCV Romanian patients [35].

Regarding the relationship between liver stiffness and the presence of esophageal varices, the area under the ROC curve for predicting the presence of varices varied between 0.76 and 0.84 [38, 41, 42]. Using cutoff values of 13.9 kPa, 17.6 kPa and 21.3 kPa, the sensitivity for varices prediction was high (95%, 90% and 79%), but the specificity was relatively low (43%, 43% and 70%) [38, 41, 42]. There are studies that demonstrated a relationship between the value of liver stiffness and the size of the varices [41, 42, 43], while other studies were not able to demonstrate this correlation [38]. Using cutoff values of 19 and 30.5 kPa, the sensitivity of TE for varices prediction was higher, but the specificity and the positive predictive value were modest [41, 42]. TE did not provide better results than the serological markers (like prothrombin time, thrombocytes [44] or FibroTest [45]), neither for varice detection (regardless of their grade), nor for the diagnosis of significant varices [41]. Yet, a predictive role of liver stiffness in anticipating variceal bleeding cannot be excluded [43, 46].

These contradicting results may be caused by the heterogeneity of the studied populations, the variable prevalence of varices (in general, but also of the large ones), the lack of prospective validation (all the cited studies were cross-sectional studies) and the variability of the cutoff values [47]. In conclusion, the evaluation of liver stiffness is not safe enough for the detection and grading of esophageal varices in such a manner that it may replace upper digestive tract endoscopy in patients with cirrhosis, since the specificity and positive predictive value reported until now are too low to allow for a regular use of the method in clinical practice.

The literature data available on this topic are synthetized in table 3

Author	etiology	prev EV	cutoff (kPa)			Se	Sp	VPP	VPN	AUROC
			HVPG	VE	VEM					
Carion[37]	HCV	-	8.7[a]	-	-	90	81	90	81	0.92
Bureau[43]	toate	-	21[b]	-	-	90	93	91	90	0.94
Lemoine [48]	HCV	-	20.5[b]	-	-	63	70	35	88	0.76
	-OH		34.9[b]	-	-	90	88	64	98	0.94
Vizutti [38]	HCV	66%	17.6[c]	-	-	94	81	91	86	0.92
			-	17.6	-	90	43	66	77	0.76
Kazemi [42]	toate	45%	-	13.9	-	95	43	91	57	0.84
			-	-	19	91	60	95	48	0.83
Castera [41]	HCV	36%	-	21.5	-	76	78	84	68	0.82
			-	-	30.5	77	85	92	54	0.85

HCV = hepatits C virus; -OH = etanol; EV = esophageal varices; LEV =large esophageal varices; Se = sensibility; Sp = specificity; P/NPV =positive/negative predictive value; AUROC = area under the ROC curve; HVPG = Hepatic venous pressure gradient ([a] HVPG ≥ 6 mm Hg; [b] HVPG ≥ 10 mm Hg; [c] HVPG ≥ 12 mm Hg).

Table 3. TE performance in EV diagnosis and HVPG prediction in liver cirrhosis patiens.

The huge potential of TE for cirrhosis patients was acknowledged ever since the method was introduced, as it can serve as a fast and non-invasive screening toll in the assessment of actual complications, it can estimate the long term risk and thus place the patient in a certain risk category [49]. The first signs of this possibility were the outcome of a retrospective study which found that the risk of a patient with hepatitis C for developing hepatocellular carcinoma is 5 times higher in patients with a LS value above 25 kPa, at the moment of the diagnosis [50]. Even more, a recent prospective study [51], that evaluated the role of liver stiffness in predicting complications related to portal hypertension in cirrhosis patients, demonstrated that a LS value < 21.1 kPa at diagnosis was as valuable as a HVPG<12 mmHg in the selection of the patients who will not experiment clinical events.

4.2.2. *Optimization of liver stiffness performance in the diagnosis of liver cirrhosis or its complications*

Based on the principle enounced by Pinzani et al, which states that a concordance between two distinct noninvasive tests is needed for an accurate diagnosis [52], an association between LS and serum noninvasive tests for liver fibrosis was used to improve the diagnostic accuracy. Such an algorithm was proposed by the Bordeaux group [53] and it is based on the concordance between FibroScan and FibroTest. Using this approach, cirrhosis could be diagnosed with an accuracy of 93% and liver biopsy could be avoided for the diagnosis of cirrhosis in almost 80% of cases.

On the other hand, our group managed to demonstrate that the Lok Score and LS used together as part of a noninvasive algorithm (see figure 1) can improve (78% diagnostic accuracy) the noninvasive estimation of large esophageal varices in cirrhotic patients [54].

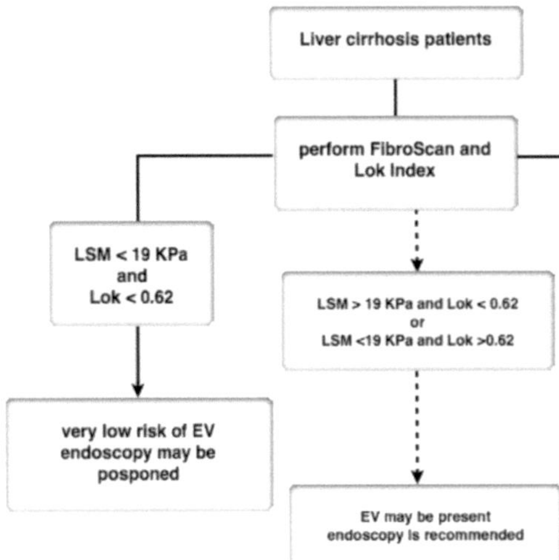

Figure 1. Proposition for a non-invasive algorithm for the assessment of esophageal varices in patients with liver cirrhosis.

4.2.3. TE efficacy in hepatocellular carcinoma risk assessment

Early detection of hepatocellular carcinoma (HCC) in HCV patients represents an emerging health problem. As a common practice, alpha-fetoprotein (AFP) is widely used for the diagnosis of HCC, despite its low sensitivity and specificity [55]. Tateyama et al report AFP above normal levels as a risk factor for the development of hepatocellular carcinoma in patients infected with hepatitis C virus [56].

Besides AFP, it has been proven that LS values increase as the liver disease progresses, the highest values being specific for cirrhotic patients with associated HCC [36]. The evidence prove that the individual role of increased LS measurements and serological markers are predictive biomarkers of HCC [57, 58]. The first risk evaluation of HCC development in HCV patients using TE was first performed by Foucher et al in 2006, reporting a cut-off value of 53.7 kPa [36]. Also, according to Akima T et al [59] liver stiffness as measured by TE is a good predictor of HCC development in viral hepatitis, with serum total bilirubin ≥1.0 mg/dL significantly correlated with tumor development. The latest published results report good diagnostic accuracy of LS in HCC prediction, for cut-off values ranging between 12.5 and 53.7 kPa [57,59,60]. However none of these studies have been designed to evaluate the accuracy of more predictive parameters, others than LS. On the other hand, adding biomarkers and other variables (such as variance) to LS measurement could represent confounding factors in the assessment of patients with liver cirrhosis and HCC [61]. This may lead to an over- or under-estimation of the risk assessed by TE, so a new accuracy testing is

http://dx.doi.org/10.5772/52621

needed. Nevertheless, increased LS seems to be a determinant of advanced cirrhosis, being associated with decompensating episodes (high grade esophageal varices, bleeding, development of ascites) as well as with the presence of HCC [62], proving that increased LS alone cannot be a good predictor of HCC.

On the other hand, Japanese studies also suggest that TE could be used as an indicator for the development of hepatocellular carcinoma in patients with virus C hepatitis [58, 63], the risk being 5 times higher in patients with a liver stiffness of over 25 kPa. Yet, these results must be confirmed in prospective studies performed on larger groups of patients, in order to see whether liver stiffness can trully predict complication development in patients with compensated cirrhosis [21]. If this fact is confirmed, elastography may serve as a non-invasive, quick screening modality which could place the cirrhosis patient in a certain risk category [64].

4.2.4. Hepatitis C infection recurrence after liver transplant

ETU is useful in the appreciation of the severity of hepatitis C recurrence after transplantation, thus reducing the number of liver biopsies [65]. In Carrion's study, for a cutoff value of 8.5 kPa, the sensitivity, specificity, negative predictive value and positive predictive value in anticipating significant fibrosis were 90%, 81%, 79% and 92%. The important thing is that none of the patients with a liver stiffness below that value presented severe fibrosis (F3), cirrhosis (F4) or significant portal hypertension (HVPG ≥10 mm Hg). Furthermore only 6 (10%) out of the 62 patients, having LS below the established threshold limit value,, did develop portal hypertension, but in all cases it was a mild hypertension.

In Rigamonti's study [66], during the follow-up after transplantation, in 40 patients with double biopsies (at 6 and 21 months), the liver stiffness changed in parallel with the stage of fibrosis, having a sensitivity of 86 % and a specificity of 92% in predicting an increase in the stage of fibrosis.

A recently published meta-analysis [67] showed that in patients undergoing transplantation for HCV-related disease, TE appears to be a reliable diagnostic test for the exclusion of liver cirrhosis. Furthermore, low TE values can reliable exclude cirrhosis in patients with recurrent HCV after liver transplantation and liver biopsy may even be avoided in these situations. Among the studies that evaluated significant fibrosis due to a recurrent HCV infection after liver transplantation, the pooled estimates were 83% for sensitivity, 83% for specificity, 4.95 for the positive likelihood ratio, 0.17 for negative likelihood ratio and 30.5 for diagnostic odds ratio. For the studies that assessed cirrhosis, the pooled estimates were 98% for sensitivity, 84% for specificity, 7 for positive likelihood ratio, 0.06 for negative likelihood ratio, and 130 for diagnostic odds ratio[67].

5. Confounding factors influencing the interpretation of liver stiffness values

Since the liver is self-contained in the non extensible Glisson's capsule, stiffness is definitively influenced by pressure that can be either hydrostatic or osmotic [68]. There are a few conditions that may determine false results in situations where other factors, except from fibrosis, are influencing liver stiffness.

Necroinflammatory activity proved to influence liver stiffness in patients with viral hepatitis, causing an increase in stiffness in parallel with the grade of histological activity [29, 69, 70]. In agreement with these results, the risk of overestimating the stage of fibrosis may occur in patients with acute hepatitis or reactivated chronic hepatitis, if just the value of liver stiffness is considered. Recent studies demonstrated that tissue alterations associated with acute hepatitis in a patient with no liver disease history produce a significant growth of liver stiffness, sometimes reaching cirrhosis values; this is due either to cellular intumescence or to severe cholestasis [71]. The contribution of these non-fibrotic changes upon liver stiffness was demonstrated by the progressive reduction of liver stiffness parallel with the decrease of the transaminases [72, 73].

On the other hand, in patients with reactivated chronic hepatitis (therefore with preexisting fibrosis), the increased stiffness is not caused by fibrosis alone, but also by the added cellular intumescence [74].

From a practical perspective, it is important that the values of liver stiffness in patients with acute hepatitis or in those with reactivated chronic hepatitis must be interpreted carefully, within the patient's clinical and biochemical context [75]. In these patients, a certain diagnosis of severe fibrosis or cirrhosis cannot be established. The right management in these cases is to wait until the transaminases come back to normal and only when the potential involvement of inflammation is removed, the real status of fibrosis can be determined; it can thus be established whether the event was an acute hepatitis on a diseased liver or a chronic hepatitis with pre-existing fibrosis that was reactivated [76].

At the same time, in patients with acute hepatitis, the evaluation of liver stiffness at various time intervals, can indicate the evolutive pattern of the condition, that may be characterized either by evolution towards fulminant hepatitis (significant increase in LS), or by remission (decrease in LS) [77].

Liver steatosis. The influence of steatosis on liver stiffness remains controversial. In some studies, steatosis did not have a significant impact on liver stiffness, even after adjusting for fibrosis stage [16, 24, 28]. Still, in these studies, the proportion of patients with severe steatosis was too low to reliably quantify a possible influence and therefore further studies are necessary to clarify this aspect.

We noticed from our experience that, after performing a stratified analysis of liver stiffness for each stage of fibrosis, for the same grade of necroinflammatory activity (moderate-severe), the presence of steatosis lead to a significant increase in LS from 5.89 ± 1.64 kPa to 7.15 ± 2.67 kPa for those with stage F1 Metavir ($p=0.004$), and from 7.23 ± 2.74 to 8.55 ± 4.67 kPa for those with stage F2 ($p=0.04$) [78]. Besides, our studies have demonstrated that fibrosis is indeed the main predictor of liver stiffness, but activity and steatosis cannot be neglected and may explain the LS variability within the same fibrosis stage [25]. Afterwards, Ziol et al, using computer analysis of the microscopic image on a group of 152 patients, confirmed that steatosis clearly influences liver stiffness independently from fibrosis, an influence that is insignificant in patients with cirrhosis, but important in non-cirrhosis patients [79].

http://dx.doi.org/10.5772/52621

Extra-hepatic cholestasis. The impact of extrahepatic cholestasis on liver stiffness was recently demonstrated by Milloning [80] by evaluating cholestasis before endoscopic retrograde cholangiopancreatography as well as 3 and 12 days after the procedure, in a study group of patients with cholestasis caused mainly by a neoplastic invasion of the biliary tree. If initially liver stiffness had values close to cirrhosis values (a mean of 15.2 kPa), after drainage, the LS decreased as low as 7 kPa, in parallel with a decrease in values of bilirubin of 2.8-2.9 mg/dl. In all patients that underwent biliary drainage, the decrease of liver stiffness correlated with that of the bilirubin values, with a mean of decrease of 1.2 ±0.56 kPa for a reduction of the bilirubin of 1g/dl. The relationship between liver stiffness and cholestasis was afterwards reproduced in the same study on an animal model that underwent ligation of the biliary duct. This resulted in an elevation of liver stiffness from 4.6 kPa to 8.8 kPa in the first 120 minutes after ligation and a decrease in stiffness to 6.1 kPa within the first 30 minutes after decompression. In conclusion, it is indicated that before an interpretation of the stiffness measurements is performed, an eventual extrahepatic cholestasis must be excluded using imaging investigations and lab tests.

Congestive heart failure may lead to an increased liver stiffness, with values similar to cirrhosis, because of the elevated blood content of the liver, in 60% of the patients [80-84]. In the context of cardiopulmonary conditions, TE may be relevant for the evaluation of treatment efficacy, as liver stiffness decreases once cardiac compensation is achieved.

6. Optimizing the non-invasive diagnosis of portal hypertension using spleen stiffness measurements

Splenomegaly is a common finding in liver cirrhosis that should determine changes in spleen density as well, because of tissue hyperplasia and fibrosis [85, 86], and/or because of portal and splenic congestion due to the splanchnic hyper-dynamic state [87]. These changes might be quantified by elastography. Until recently, only magnetic resonance elastography (MRE) was used with encouraging results in this respect [88]. The preliminary data showed a highly significant correlation between liver and spleen sti ▪ ness in patients with portal hypertension, but, according to the authors, the validity of spleen stiffness as noninvasive measure of portal venous pressure is not reliable enough [89].

6.1. Principle of TE for Spleen Stiffness Measurements (SSM) and technique assessment

Our group proposed for the first time the use of FibroScan® for spleen stiffness measurement (SSM) [90]. For the measurement itself we proposed the same procedure as for the liver stiffness measurement, with the sole exception that the patient had his left arm in maximum abduction and the transducer was placed in the left intercostal spaces, usually on the posterior axillary line. For better locating the splenic parenchyma, we also used ultrasound guidance, so that we could choose the best location for performing the analysis.

6.2. Efficacy of spleen stiffness measurements for the evaluation of the presence and the grade of esophageal varices

In the above mentioned study, we demonstrated that spleen stiffness can be assessed using transient elastography, the sole factor influencing the measurement being the spleen size. Spleen stiffness increases as the liver disease worsens, from normal to chronic hepatitis and to liver cirrhosis (figure 2).

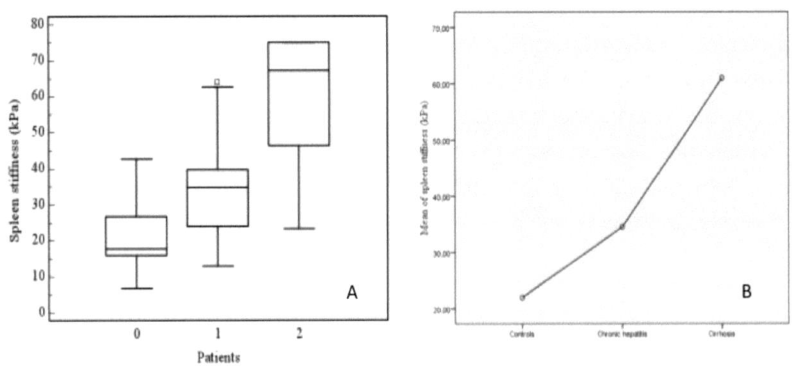

Figure 2. A - Box plots of spleen stiffness values for controls (0), chronic hepatitis (1) and cirrhosis patients (2). The top and the bottom of the boxes are the first and third quartiles, respectively. The length of the box thus represents the interquartile range within which 50% of the values were located. The line through the middle of each box represents the median. The error shows the minimum and maximum values (range); B - Graphic representation of the significant increase of SSM in healthy controls and patients with chronic hepatitis and liver cirrhosis, respectively.

In liver cirrhosis patients, the spleen stiffness measurement, can predict the presence, but not the grade of esophageal varices. Therefore, for a cutoff value of 46.4 kPa, we managed to predict the presence of esophageal varices with a diagnostic accuracy of 80.45% and an AUROC of 0.781 (figure 3).

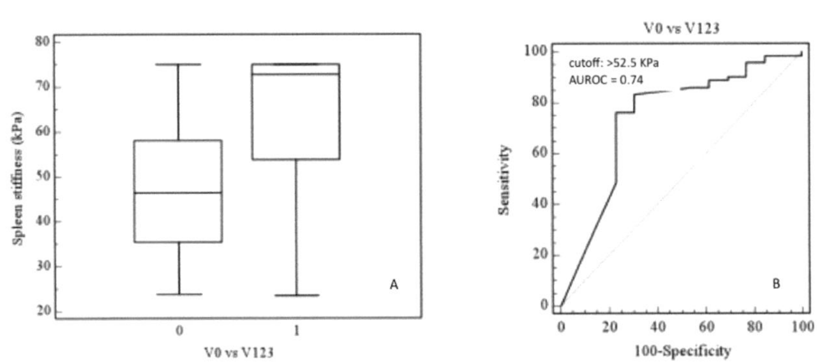

Figure 3. A - Box plots showing the increase of SSM in liver cirrhosis patients with esophageal varices as compared with those without; B - ROC curve representation of SSM in distinguishing LC patients with or without EV.

http://dx.doi.org/10.5772/52621

In another more recent study [91], another group demonstrated that SSM also correlates with HVPG values, suggesting that this new elastographic technique may become a valuable noninvasive method for liver cirrhosis patients

6.3. Improving diagnostic accuracy for esophageal varices by modifying the SSM calculation algorithm

Regarding the spleen stiffness measurement itself, we observed that the results seem to be influenced by the intrinsic characteristics of the machine (FibroScan). Regardless of the variceal status of the patients, or the grade of the varices, SSM reached the maximum value that can be measured by the machine (75 KPa). This is an important drawback, because we have to face a significant interpolation between the patients groups. If the FibroScan had been able to determine values beyond 75 KPa, we may have obtained better figures. In order to overcome this situation, we cooperated with the manufacturer of the device for developing a new calculation algorithm, not available on the commercial device, which allows stiffness measurements of up to 150 kPa. In a validation study [54], using the new calculation algorithm, we could differentiate between any classes of esophageal varices, except V1 vs V2 ($p<0.005$) and could select patients with V3 (V012 vs V3 = 63.49 vs 116.08 kPa, $p<0.005$), the ones that are at higher risk for bleeding (figure 4).

7. Noninvasive evaluation of liver steatosis using Controlled Attenuation Parameter (CAP)

Even though liver stiffness provides an alternative to liver biopsy for fibrosis staging, it can identify very important histologic features such as macrovesicular steatosis, ballooned hepatocytes, inflammation, etc [68].

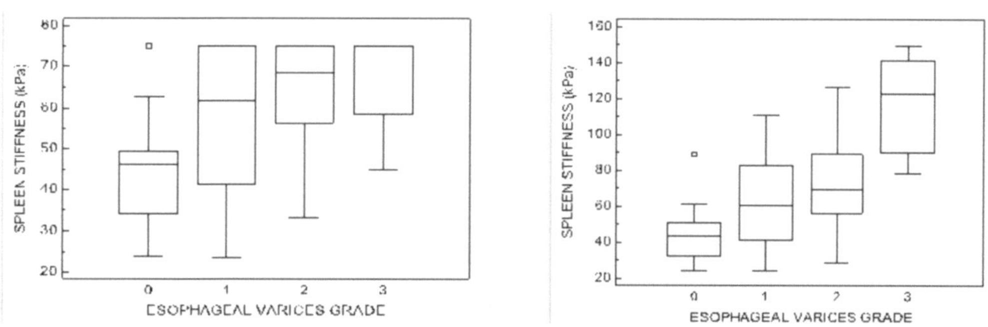

Figure 4. Boxplots representing mean SSM values according to the esophageal varices grade using the original (A) or the modified (B) calculation algorithm.

Knowing that fat interferes with ultrasound propagation, a novel attenuation parameter has been developed to detect and quantify liver steatosis. This parameter is based on the ultrasonic properties of the radio-frequency back propagated signals acquired by the Fibroscan [92]. It is called controlled attenuation parameter (CAP). This ultrasonic attenuation coefficient is an estimate of the total ultrasonic attenuation (go-and-return path) at the central frequency of the regular or M Fibroscan® probe, i.e. at 3.5 MHz, and is expressed in dB.m^{-1}. CAP is evaluated using the same radio-frequency data and the same region of interest, as the region used to assess the LSM. CAP is only appraised if the acquisition is "valid". Therefore, CAP is guided by vibration-controlled transient elastography (VCTE), which ensures that the operator automatically obtains an ultrasonic attenuation value of the liver [92, 93]. The device is used to assess, at the same time, LS (which is related to liver fibrosis) and CAP (which is related to liver steatosis).

Even though relatively few studies have been published on this topic [92, 93, 94,95] the preliminary results showed that CAP is a promising non-invasive tool to detect steatosis in CHC patients.

In the study conducted by Sasso et al, the CAP performance was appraised on 115 patients, taking the histological grade of steatosis as reference. CAP was significantly correlated to steatosis with an AUROC equal to 0.91 and 0.95 for the detection of more than 10% and 33% of steatosis, respectively.

A study performed recently on 615 HCV patients, who underwent both Fibroscan (®) and liver biopsy showed in multivariate analysis, that CAP was related to steatosis, independently of fibrosis stage (which was related to LS. The AUROCs of the were 0.80, 0.86 and 0.88 respectively, for predicting a fatty overload of more than 11%, 33%, and 66%, respectively. CAP also exhibited a good ability to differentiate steatosis grades (Obuchowski measure = 0.92) [96].

CAP is evaluated using the same radio-frequency data and the same region of interest, as the region used to assess the liver stiffness for fibrosis quantification. Preliminary studies performed in our department have found significantly different CAP values for different steatosis grades and AUROCs of 0.830 and 0.85 respectively, for the prediction of a hepatic fat content over 33% and 66%, respectively [97].

8. The advantages of TE in liver steatosis, fibrosis and cirrhosis diagnosis

Compared with other diagnosis indicators or predictive models based on lab tests, the evaluation of fibrosis using elastography has some important advantages [98,99]:

- It is easy to use; noninvasive; pain-free; does not require anesthesia or hospitalization and is therefore easily accepted by the patient;
- It is quick, the time needed for the examination being very short;
- It is not influenced by concomitant conditions;
- It is operator independent;

- The liver volume used to evaluate fibrosis is 150-400 times higher than the volume obtained through liver biopsy.

As far as the evaluation of liver steatosis is concerned, in comparison to other modalities, CAP is non-invasive, quantitative, non-ionizing, and inexpensive. Furthermore, the procedure is easy to perform, even by an operator who does not have any radiological skills and provides immediate results. The procedure is also machine-independent and does not require corrections to be made for gain, frequency, focusing or beam diffraction, and is also not subject to operator interpretation. In addition, CAP has been shown to efficiently detect steatosis at a level of ≥ 10%, which is more sensitive than other imaging modalities. Compared to a liver biopsy, CAP is less prone to sampling error as it explores a liver volume ~100 times larger [92, 93].

9. Limitations of TE

Liver fibrosis can not be evaluated by TE in 5-8 % of the cases. Some of the possible causes for this are listed below [16]:

- obesity (an ultrasound machine may be used in order to find the best window and thus increase the ability to measure liver stiffness in overweight patients);
- a narrow intercostal space;
- ascites (vibrations are not transmitted through fluid);
- the quality of the liver parenchyma and other liver structures;
- large vascular structure present in the acquisition window (may lead to false results).

The failure of TE varies according to different authors from 2.4% to 9.4% [16, 21, 24, 36, 74, 64, 100]. In a study performed on 2114 patients [101], liver stiffness could not be determined in 4.5% of the cases and multivariate analysis showed that the only element associated with measurement failure is a body mass index over 28. Yet, with more experience, one may realize that a thick thoracic wall is more likely to be a limiting factor for a failed measurement than the growth of the body mass index in itself [102].

Technical solutions regarding the design of the probe were investigated lately, in order to overcome these limitations. Recently a new probe became available, that was specially designed for obese patients, with a central frequency of 2.5% MHz (compared with the 5MHz probe that is usually used), and that is able to determine liver stiffness on a distance of 35-75 mm from the skin (while the normal probe is able to do that on distance of 25 to 45 cm). With the help of this new transducer, it was possible to obtain valid measurements in 49% of the patients with a BMI ≥30 kg/m2, in which the usual probe failed to determine the LS [103].

As far as predicting steatosis in HCV patients is concerned, CAP has further validation in larger populations and by independent teams, since there are rather few studies published until now. Another important limitation is that CAP cannot be used with measurements taken from the XL probe, which is a novel probe designed to assess liver stiffness in overweight and obese patients [75,76]. Thus, CAP needs to be developed to work with the XL probe.

10. Conclusions

The possibility of concomitant assessment of liver fibrosis (using liver stiffness measurement) and of steatosis (using CAP) makes Fibroscan a promising non-invasive tool for assessing and quantifying both fibrosis and steatosis, that may broaden the spectrum of non-invasive methods used for the investigation and follow-up of patients with chronic hepatitis C. But it is important that interpretation of the liver stiffness values be done by an experienced physician and always within the clinical and biochemical context of the patient.

Acknowledgments

This material is part of the research project no 27020/ 6/ 15.11.2011, entitled "The non-invasive evaluation of fibrosis and steatosis in diffuse liver diseases by unidimensional transient elastography – Fibroscan" from "Iuliu-Hatieganu" University of Medicine and Pharmacy, Cluj-Napoca.

Author details

Monica Lupsor[1], Horia Stefanescu[2], Diana Feier[1] and Radu Badea[1]

*Address all correspondence to: monica.lupsor@umfcluj.ro

1 Medical Imaging Department, Regional Institute of Gastroenterology and Hepatology Prof Dr Octavian Fodor, "Iuliu Hatieganu" University of Medicine and Pharmacy, Cluj-Napoca, Romania

2 Hepatology Department, Regional Institute of Gastroenterology and Hepatology Prof Dr Octavian Fodor, "Iuliu Hatieganu" University of Medicine and Pharmacy, Cluj-Napoca, Romania

References

[1] Menghini G. One-second needle biopsy of the liver. Gastroenterology 1958; 35(2): 190-199.

[2] Maharaj B, Maharaj RJ, Leary WP, et al. Sampling variability and its influence on the diagnostic yield of percutaneous needle biopsy of the liver. Lancet. 1986; 1(8480): 523-525.

[3] Poynard T, Ratziu V, Benmanov Y, Di Martino V, Bedossa P, Opolon P. Fibrosis in patients with chronic hepatitis C: detection and significance. Semin Liver Dis. 2000; 20(1): 47-55.

[4] Desmet VJ. Liver tissue examination. J Hepatol. 2003; 39(1): S43-49.

[5] Guido M, Rugge M. Liver biopsy sampling in chronic viral hepatitis. Semin Liver Dis. 2004; 24(1): 89-97.

[6] Kleiner DE. The liver biopsy in chronic hepatitis C: a view from the other side of the microscope. Semin Liver Dis. 2005; 25(1): 52-64.

[7] Buscarini E, Di Stasi M. Biopsy of the liver. In:Buscarini E, di Stasi M (eds). Complications of abdominal interventional ultrasound. Poletto Edizioni 1996, 34-50.

[8] Nazarian LN, Feld RI, Herrine SK, et al. Safety and efficacy of sonographically guided random core biopsy for diffuse liver disease. J Ultrasound Med 2000;19(8): 537-541.

[9] Farrell R, Smiddy PF, Pilkington RM, et al. Guided versus blind liver biopsy for chronic hepatitis C: clinical benefits and costs. J Hepatol 1999; 30: 580-587.

[10] Schiff ER, Schiff L. Needle biopsy of the liver. In: Schiff ER, Schiff L. Diseases of the liver J.B.Lippincott Company, 1993, 216-225.

[11] McGill DB., Rakela J. A 21-year experience with major hemorrage after percutaneous liver biopsy. Gastroenterology 1990; 99: 1396-1400.

[12] Bedossa P, Dargere D, Paradis V. Sampling variability of liver fibrosis in chronic hepatitis C. Hepatology. 2003; 38(6): 1449-1457.

[13] Regev A, Berho M, Jeffers LJ, Sampling error and intraobserver variation in liver biopsy in patients with chronic HCV infection. Am J Gastroenterol. 2002; 97(10): 2614-2618.

[14] Siddique I, El-Naga HA, Madda JP, Memon A, Hasan F. Sampling variability on percutaneous liver biopsy in patients with chronic hepatitis C virus infection. Scand J Gastroenterol. 2003; 38(4): 427-432.

[15] Yeh WC, Li PC, Jeng YM, et al. Elastic modulus measurements of human liver and correlation with pathology. Ultrasound Med Biol. 2002; 28(4): 467-474.

[16] Sandrin L, Fourquet B, Hasquenoph JM, et al. Transient elastography: a new noninvasive method for assessment of hepatic fibrosis. Ultrasound Med Biol. 2003; 29(12): 1705-1713.

[17] Carstensen EL, Parker KJ, Lerner RM. Elastography in the management of liver disease. Ultrasound Med Biol. 2008; 34(10): 1535-1546.

[18] Lucidarme D, Foucher J, Le Bail B, et al. Factors of accuracy of transient elastography (Fibroscan) for the diagnosis of liver fibrosis in chronic hepatitis C. Hepatology. 2008; 49(4): 1083-1089.

[19] Del Poggio P, Colombo S. Is transient elastography a useful tool for screening liver disease? World J Gastroenterol. 2009; 15(12): 1409-1414.

[20] Nguyen-Khac E, Capron D. Noninvasive diagnosis of liver fibrosis by ultrasonic transient elastography (Fibroscan). Eur J Gastroenterol Hepatol. 2006; 18(12): 1321-1325.

[21] Castera L, Forns X, Alberti A. Non-invasive evaluation of liver fibrosis using transient elastography. J Hepatol. 2008; 48(5): 835-847.

[22] Kettaneh A, Marcellin P, Douvin C, et al. Features associated with success rate and performance of FibroScan measurements for the diagnosis of cirrhosis in HCV patients: a prospective study of 935 patients. J Hepatol. 2007; 46(4): 628-634.

[23] Boursier J, Konate A, Guilluy M, et al. Learning curve and interobserver reproducibility evaluation of liver stiffness measurement by transient elastography. Eur J Gastroenterol Hepatol. 2008; 20(7): 693-701.

[24] Ziol M, Handra-Luca A, Kettaneh A, et al. Noninvasive assessment of liver fibrosis by measurement of stiffness in patients with chronic hepatitis C. Hepatology. 2005; 41(1): 48-54.

[25] Lupsor M, Badea R, Stefanescu H, et al. Analysis of histopathological changes that influence liver stiffness in chronic hepatitis C. Results from a cohort of 324 patients. J Gastrointestin Liver Dis. 2008;17(2):155-63.

[26] Castera L, Vergniol J, Foucher J, et al. Prospective comparison of transient elastography, Fibrotest, APRI, and liver biopsy for the assessment of fibrosis in chronic hepatitis C. Gastroenterology. 2005; 128(2): 343-350.

[27] Sporea I, Sirli R, Deleanu A, et al. Comparison of the liver stiffness measurement by transient elastography with the liver biopsy. World J Gastroenterol. 2008; 14(42): 6513-6517.

[28] Nitta Y, Kawabe N, Hashimoto S, et al. Liver stiffness measured by transient elastography correlates with fibrosis area in liver biopsy in patients with chronic hepatitis C. Hepatol Res. 2009; 39(7): 675-684.

[29] Arena U, Vizzutti F, Abraldes J, et al. Reliability of transient elastography for the diagnosis of advanced fibrosis in chronic hepatitis C. Gut. 2008; 57(9): 1288-1293.

[30] Kim SU, Jang HW, Cheong JY, et al. The usefulness of liver stiffness measurement using FibroScan in chronic hepatitis C in South Korea: a multicenter, prospective study. J Gastroenterol Hepatol. 2011; 26(1): 171-178.

[31] Friedrich-Rust M, Ong MF, Martens S, et al. Performance of transient elastography for the staging of liver fibrosis: a meta-analysis. Gastroenterology. 2008; 134(4): 960-974.

[32] Stebbing J, Farouk L, Panos G, et al. A meta-analysis of transient elastography for the detection of hepatic fibrosis. J Clin Gastroenterol. 2010; 44(3): 214-9.

[33] Castera L. Assessing liver fibrosis. Expert Rev Gastroenterol Hepatol. 2008; 2(4): 541-552.

[34] Talwalkar JA, Kurtz DM, Schoenleber SJ, West CP, Montori VM. Ultrasound-based transient elastography for the detection of hepatic fibrosis: systematic review and meta-analysis. Clin Gastroenterol Hepatol. 2007; 5(10): 1214-1220.

[35] Lupsor M, Badea R, Stefanescu H, Sparchez Z, Serban A, Feier D. The diagnosis performance of ultrasonic transient elastography for noninvasive assessment of liver fibrosis in 1138 chronic hepatitis C patients. Ultrasound in Medicine and Biology 2011; 37 (8S): S81.

[36] Foucher J, Chanteloup E, Vergniol J, et al. Diagnosis of cirrhosis by transient elastography (FibroScan): a prospective study. Gut. 2006; 55(3): 403-408.

[37] Carrion JA, Navasa M, Bosch J, Bruguera M, Gilabert R, Forns X. Transient elastography for diagnosis of advanced fibrosis and portal hypertension in patients with hepatitis C recurrence after liver transplantation. Liver Transpl. 2006; 12(12): 1791-1798.

[38] Vizzutti F, Arena U, Romanelli RG, et al. Liver stiffness measurement predicts severe portal hypertension in patients with HCV-related cirrhosis. Hepatology 2007; 45(5): 1290-1297.

[39] Lim JK, Groszmann RJ. Transient elastography for diagnosis of portal hypertension in liver cirrhosis: Is there still a role for hepatic venous pressure gradient measurement? Hepatology 2007; 45(5): 1087-1090.

[40] Castera L, Forns X, Alberti A. Non-invasive evaluation of liver fibrosis using transient elastography. J Hepatol. 2008; 48(5): 835-847.

[41] Castera L, Le Bail B, Roudot-Thoraval F, et al. Early detection in routine clinical practice of cirrhosis and oesophageal varices in chronic hepatitis C: Comparison of transient elastography (FibroScan) with standard laboratory tests and non-invasive scores. J Hepatol 2009; 50(1): 59-68.

[42] Kazemi F, Kettaneh A, N'kontchou G, et al. Liver stiffness measurement selects patients with cirrhosis at risk of bearing large oesophageal varices. J Hepatol. 2006; 45(2): 230-235.

[43] Bureau C, Metivier S, Peron JM, et al. Transient elastography accurately predicts presence of significant portal hypertension in patients with chronic liver disease. Aliment Pharmacol Ther 2008; 27(12): 1261-1268.

[44] Sanyal AJ, Fontana RJ, Di Bisceglie AM, et al. The prevalence and risk factors associated with esophageal varices in subjects with hepatitis C and advanced fibrosis. Gastrointest Endosc. 2006;64(6): 855-864

[45] Thabut D, Trabut JB, Massard J et al. Non-invasive diagnosis of large oesophageal varices with FibroTest in patients with cirrhosis: a preliminary retrospective study. Liver International 2006; 26(3):271-278

[46] de Franchis R. Noninvasive diagnosis of esophageal varices: is it feasible? Am J Gastroenterol 2006; 101(11): 2520-2522

[47] Bosch J. Predictions from a hard liver. J Hepatol. 2006; 45(2): 174-177

[48] Lemoine M, Katsahian S, Ziol M, et al. Liver stiffness measurement as a predictive tool of clinically significant portal hypertension in patients with compensated hepatitis C virus or alcohol-related cirrhosis. Aliment Pharmacol Ther. 2008; 28(9): 1102-1110

[49] Pinzani M. Non-invasive evaluation of hepatic fibrosis: don't count your chickens before they're hatched. Gut. 2006; 55(3): 310-312

[50] Masuzaki R, Tateishi R, Yoshida H, et al. Prospective risk assessment for hepatocellular carcinoma development in chronic hepatitis C patients by transient elastography. Hepatology 2009; 49(6): 1954–1961

[51] Robic MA, Procopet B, Métivier S, Péron JM, Selves J, Vinel JP, Bureau C. Liver stiffness accurately predicts portal hypertension related complications in patients with chronic liver disease: a prospective study. J Hepatol. 2011; 55(5): 1017-1024.

[52] Pinzani M, Vizzutti F, Arena U, Marra F. Technology Insight: noninvasive assessment of liver fibrosis by biochemical scores and elastography. Nat Clin Pract Gastroenterol Hepatol. 2008; 5(2): 95-106.

[53] Castera L, Vergniol J, Foucher J, et al. Prospective comparison of transient elastography, Fibrotest, APRI, and liver biopsy for the assessment of fibrosis in chronic hepatitis C. Gastroenterology 2005; 128(2): 343-350.

[54] Stefanescu H, Grigorescu M, Lupsor M, et al. A New and Simple Algorithm for the Noninvasive Assessment of Esophageal Varices in Cirrhotic Patients Using Serum Fibrosis Markers and Transient Elastography. J Gastrointestin Liver Dis 2011; 20(1): 57-64

[55] Zhang G, Ha SA, Kim HK, et al. Combined analysis of AFP and HCCR-1 as an useful serological marker for small hepatocellular carcinoma: A prospective cohort study. Dis Markers 2012; 32: 265-271.

[56] Tateyama M, Yatsuhashi H, Taura N et al. Alpha-fetoprotein above normal levels as a risk factor for the development of hepatocellular carcinoma in patients infected with hepatitis C virus. J Gastroenterol 2011; 46: 92-100.

[57] Nahon P, Kettaneh A, Lemoine M et al. Liver stiffness measurement i n patients with cirrhosis and hepatocellular carcinoma: a case-control study. Eur J Gastroenterol Hepatol 2009;21:214-9.

[58] Masuzaki R, Tateishi R, Yoshida H, et al. Prospective risk assessment for hepatocellular carcinoma development in patients with chronic hepatitis C by transient elastography. Hepatology 2009; 49: 1954-1961.

[59] Akima T, Tamano M, Hiraishi H. Liver stiffness measured by transient elastography is a predictor of hepatocellular carcinoma development in viral hepatitis. Hepatol Res 2011; 41: 965-970.

[60] Kuo YH, Lu SN, Hung CH. Liver stiffness measurement in the risk assessment of hepatocellular carcinoma for patients with chronic hepatitis. Hepatol Int 2010; 4: 700-706.

[61] Castéra L, Foucher J, Bernard PH et al. Pitfalls of liver stiffness measurement: a 5-year prospective study of 13,369 examinations. Hepatology. 2010; 5: 828-835.

[62] Tapper EB, Cohen EB, Patel K, et al. Levels of Alanine Aminotransferase Confound Use of Transient Elastography to Diagnose Fibrosis in Patients with Chronic HCV Infection. Clin Gastroenterol Hepatol 2012; DOI: 10.1016/j.cgh.2012.01.015.

[63] Masuzaki R, Tateishi R, Yoshida H, et al. Risk assessment of hepatocellular carcinoma in chronic hepatitis C patients by transient elastography. J Clin Gastroenterol. 2008; 42(7): 839-843.

[64] Pinzani M. Non-invasive evaluation of hepatic fibrosis: don't count your chickens before they're hatched. Gut. 2006; 55(3): 310-312.

[65] Carrion JA, Navasa M, Bosch J, Bruguera M, Gilabert R, Forns X. Transient elastography for diagnosis of advanced fibrosis and portal hypertension in patients with hepatitis C recurrence after liver transplantation. Liver Transpl. 2006; 12(12): 1791-1798.

[66] Rigamonti C, Donato MF, Fraquelli M, et al. Transient elastography predicts fibrosis progression in patients with recurrent hepatitis C after liver transplantation. Gut 2008; 57(6): 821-827.

[67] Adebajo CO, Talwalkar JA, Poterucha JJ, Kim WR, Charlton MR. Ultrasound-based transient elastography for the detection of hepatic fibrosis in patients with recurrent hepatitis C virus after liver transplantation: a systematic review and meta-analysis. Liver Transpl. 2012; 18(3): 323-331. doi: 10.1002/lt.22460.

[68] Sandrin L, Oudry J, Bastard C, Fournier C, Miette V, Mueller S. Non-Invasive Assessment of Liver Fibrosis by Vibration-Controlled Transient Elastography (Fibroscan®). Intech: p293-414.

[69] Fraquelli M, Rigamonti C, Casazza G, et al. Reproducibility of transient elastography in the evaluation of liver fibrosis in patients with chronic liver disease. Gut 2007; 56(7): 968-973.

[70] Chan HL, Wong GL, Choi PC, et al. Alanine aminotransferase-based algorithms of liver stiffness measurement by transient elastography (Fibroscan) for liver fibrosis in chronic hepatitis B. J Viral Hepat. 2009; 16(1): 36-44.

[71] Kim SU, Han KH, Park JY, et al. Liver stiffness measurement using FibroScan is influenced by serum total bilirubin in acute hepatitis. Liver Int. 2009; 29(6): 810-5.

[72] Arena U, Vizzutti F, Corti G, et al. Acute viral hepatitis increases liver stiffness values measured by transient elastography. Hepatology. 2008; 47(2): 380-384.

[73] Sagir A, Erhardt A, Schmitt M, Häussinger D. Transient elastography is unreliable for detection of cirrhosis in patients with acute liver damage. Hepatology. 2008; 47(2): 592-595.

[74] Coco B, Oliveri F, Maina AM, et al. Transient elastography: a new surrogate marker of liver fibrosis influenced by major changes of transaminases. J Viral Hepat. 2007; 14(5): 360-369.

[75] Cobbold JF, Taylor-Robinson SD. Transient elastography in acute hepatitis: All that's stiff is not fibrosis. Hepatology. 2008; 47(2): 370-372.

[76] Lupşor M, Badea R, Stefănescu H. Noninvasive evaluation of chronic liver disseases using transient elastography (Fibroscan®). In: Present and perspectives in infectios diseases. Conference proceedings, July 4-7, 2008.

[77] Panos G, Holmes P, Valero S, Anderson M, Gazzard B, Nelson M. Transient elastography, liver stiffness values, and acute hepatopathy. Hepatology. 2008; 47(6): 2140.

[78] Lupsor M. New ultrasound techniques for non-invasive evaluation of chronic liver diseases. The added value of elastography and computed imaging techniques. Ph thesis, University of Medicine and Pharmacy Cluj-Napoca. 2009.

[79] Ziol M, Kettaneh A, Ganne-Carrié N, Barget N, Tengher-Barna I, Beaugrand M. Relationships between fibrosis amounts assessed by morphometry and liver stiffness measurements in chronic hepatitis or steatohepatitis. Eur J Gastroenterol Hepatol. 2009; 21(11): 1261-1268.

[80] Millonig G, Reimann FM, Friedrich S, et al. Extrahepatic cholestasis increases liver stiffness (FibroScan) irrespective of fibrosis. Hepatology. 2008; 48(5): 1718-1723.

[81] Pozzoni P, Prati D, Berzuini A, et al. Liver stiffness values measured by transient elastography are increased in patients with acutely decompensated heart failure. Dig Liver Dis. 2009; 41(3): A39.

[82] Lebray P, Varnous S, Charlotte F, Varaut A, Poynard T, Ratziu V. Liver stiffness is an unreliable marker of liver fibrosis in patients with cardiac insufficiency. Hepatology. 2008; 48(6): 2089.

[83] Bioulac-Sage P, Couffinhal T, Foucher J, Balabaud CP. Interpreting liver stiffness in the cirrhotic range. J Hepatol. 2009; 50(2): 423-424.

[84] Hopper I, Kemp W, Porapakkham P, et al. Impact of heart failure and changes to volume status on liver stiffness: non-invasive assessment using transient elastography. Eur J Heart Fail. 2012; 14(6): 621-627

[85] Bolognesi M, Boscato N. Spleen and liver cirrhosis: relationship between spleen enlargement and portal hypertension in patients with liver cirrhosis. In TM Chen. New Developments in Liver Cirrhosis Research. Nova Science Publishers 2006, pp 49-67.

[86] Bolognesi M, Merkel C, Sacerdoti D, Nava V, Gatta A. The role of spleen enlargement in cirrhosis with portal hypertension. Dig Liver Dis 2002; 34:144-150.

[87] Kuddus RH, Nalesnik MA, Subbotin VM, Rao AS, Gandhi CR. Enhanced synthesis and reduced metabolism of endothelin 1 (ET-1) by hepatocytes – an important mechanism of increased endogenous levels of ET-1 in liver cirrhosis. J Hepatol 2000; 33: 725-732.

[88] Yin M, Talwalkar JA, Glaser KJ. A Preliminary Assessment of Hepatic Fibrosis with Magnetic Resonance Elastography. Clin Gastroenterol Hepatol. 2007; 5(10): 1207–1213

[89] Talwalkar J. Evaluation of Fibrosis and Portal Hypertension: Non-Invasive Assessment. Oral presentation abstract, Procedings of EASL Monothematic Conference Portal Hypertension: Advances in Knowledge, Evaluation and Management, Budapest, 2009, p47.

[90] Stefanescu H, Grigorescu M, Lupsor M, Procopet B, Maniu A, Badea R. Spleen stiffness measurement using fibroscan for the noninvasive assessment of esophageal varices in liver cirrhosis patients. J Gastroenterol Hepatol 2011; 26: 164-170.

[91] Colecchia A, Montrone L, Scaioli E, et al. Measurement of Spleen Stiffness to Evaluate Portal Hypertension and the Presence of Esophageal Varices in Patients With HCV-Related Cirrhosis. Gastroenterology 2012; 143(3): 646-654.

[92] Sasso M, Beaugrand M, de Ledinghen V, et al. Controlled attenuation parameter (CAP): a novel VCTE™ guided ultrasonic attenuation measurement for the evaluation of hepatic steatosis: preliminary study and validation in a cohort of patients with chronic liver disease from various causes. Ultrasound Med Biol. 2010; 36(11): 1825-1835.

[93] Sasso M, Miette V, Sandrin L, Beaugrand M. The controlled attenuation parameter (CAP): a novel tool for the non-invasive evaluation of steatosis using Fibroscan. Clin Res Hepatol Gastroenterol. 2012; 36(1): 13-20.

[94] de Lédinghen V, Vergniol J, Foucher J, Merrouche W, le Bail B. Non-invasive diagnosis of liver steatosis using controlled attenuation parameter (CAP) and transient elastography. Liver Int. 2012; 32(6) :911-918.

[95] Myers RP, Pollett A, Kirsch R, et al. Controlled Attenuation Parameter (CAP): a noninvasive method for the detection of hepatic steatosis based on transient elastography. Liver Int. 2012; 32(6): 902-910.

[96] Sasso M, Tengher-Barna I, Ziol M, et al. Novel controlled attenuation parameter for noninvasive assessment of steatosis using Fibroscan(®): validation in chronic hepatitis C. J Viral Hepat. 2012; 19(4): 244-253.

[97] Lupsor M, Badea R, Stefanescu H, Feier D, Tamas A, Sparchez Z. The performance of controlled attenuation parameter (CAP) for the non-invasive evaluation of steatozis using Fibroscan. Preliminary results. J Hepatolol 2012: 56: S514.

[98] Blanc JF, Bioulac-Sage P, Balabaud C, Desmouliere A. Investigation of liver fibrosis in clinical practice. Hepatol Res. 2005; 32(1): 1-8.

[99] Kelleher TB, Afdhal N. Noninvasive assessment of liver fibrosis. Clin Liver Dis. 2005; 9(4): 667-683.

[100] Ganne-Carrie N, Ziol M, de Ledinghen V, et al. Accuracy of liver stiffness measurement for the diagnosis of cirrhosis in patients with chronic liver diseases. Hepatology 2006; 44(6): 1511-1517.

[101] Foucher J, Castera L, Bernard PH, et al. Prevalence and factors associated with failure of liver stiffness measurement using FibroScan in a prospective study of 2114 examinations. Eur J Gastroenterol Hepatol. 2006; 18(4): 411-412.

[102] Castera L. Non-invasive diagnosis of steatosis and fibrosis. Diabetes Metab. 2008; 34(6 Pt 2): 674-679.

[103] De Ledinghen V, Fournier C, Foucher J, et al. New Fibroscan probe for obese patients. A pilot study of feasibility and performances in patients with BMI≥30 kg/m2. J Hepatol 2009; 50(1): S359.

Chapter 11

Computer Image Analysis of Liver Biopsy Specimens in Patients with Heroin Abuse and Coinfection (Tuberculosis, HCV, HIV)

Ivan B. Tokin, Ivan I. Tokin and Galina F. Filimonova

Additional information is available at the end of the chapter

http://dx.doi.org/10.5772/52971

1. Introduction

The computer morphometry in histopathology is one of the most perspective directions in contemporary medicine including the hepatopathology. The potential advantages of measurement in histopathology have been recognized for many years [1]. The quantitative estimation has several advantages over conventional visual assessment such as objectivity and reproducibility [2]. The employment of modern optical equipment and special computer programs creates the possibilities for significant acceleration of quantitative analysis.

At present the computer morphometry has been rather intensively used to study liver changes of the patients with chronic viral hepatitis. The quantitative assessment of the fibrosis was performed mainly in chronic virus hepatitis C [3, 4, 5, 6, 7. 8, 9].

Many investigators considered that the quantitative evaluation of hepatic fibrosis was mostly useful for assessing the origin, location and the stage of fibrosis. Using the morphometric analysis is also very important for the correct evaluation of repeated biopsies [10]. Some investigators studied the changes in liver fibrosis after the interferon therapy [11, 12, 13]. This technique can be used in future for therapeutic trials by the estimation of the agents inhibiting the fibrosis progression [7].

Rates of fibrosis progression differ markedly in patients with HIV/HCV co-infection [14, 15, 16]. The natural history of hepatitis C virus infection in tuberculosis and in human immunodeficiency virus-infected patients has never been studied with the use of the computer morphometric analysis of liver fibrosis progression. In this chapter the changes of liver biopsies in patients with heroin abuse and infected by hepatitis C virus (HCV), human immunodeficiency virus (HIV), pulmonary tuberculosis (TB) were studied by the morphological and computer morphometric analysis.

2. Patients and methods

2.1. Patients

13 male patients with co-infection of pulmonary tuberculosis (TB), chronic viral hepatitis C (HCV) and human immunodeficiency virus (HIV) were investigated during the study. All the patients used also the injections of heroin (Table 1).

The patients started their history as a rule from heroin using (mean duration – 9.5 years) and later all of them acquired HCV (mean duration – 7.1 years), HIV (mean duration – 4.7 years) and TB at last (the duration of TB infection of the most part of patients was less than 1 year).

The diagnosis was established after careful examination of the patients: the anamneses of diseases and life, laboratory analyses, virological and morphological studies. Serum level of alanine aminotransferase (ALT) and aspartate aminotransferase (AST) was expressed. The upper limit of normal (ULN) of ALT was 41 U/L, AST – 31 U/L.

2.2. Histological evaluation

To refine the diagnosis as well as for detection of the activity of pathological processes in the liver, aspiration biopsy was taken from all the patients. All liver biopsies were performed to the routine medical follow up program, using the standard Menghini procedure [17, 18]. Criteria for adequacy of the biopsy specimens included a core length of 10 mm and at least 5-6 portal tracts. So, only 9 biopsy specimens were used for further histological evaluation. Four biopsy specimens were fragmented and weren't used (Table 1). Samples were formalin-fixed and paraffin-embedded. Serial paraffin sections were cut at 5 mcm. Hematoxylin-eosin and tolluidine blue stains were used.

Each biopsy for necro-inflammatory activity and fibrosis was assessed by two hepatologists. Knodell Histology Activity Index (HAI) was used to grade histopathological lesions [19]. HAI was graded as minimal (scores 1–3), mild (scores 4–8), moderate (scores 9–12), or severe hepatitis (scores 13–18). METAVIR group scoring system was used for detecting the stage of fibrosis [20]. Fibrosis was staged on the scale from F0 to F4, as follows: F0 = no fibrosis, F1 = portal fibrosis without septa, F2 = few septa, F3 = numerous septa without cirrhosis, F4 = cirrhosis. Only single patient showed any signs of cirrhosis. Fibrosis was also staged by Ishak scoring system[21]. In the Ishak scoring system interface hepatitis (piecemeal necrosis), focal necrosis in the lobule, portal inflammation were scored from 0 to 4, incomplete cirrhosis (bridging necrosis with occasional nodules) and cirrhosis were scored from 5 to 6.

Patient number	Sex	Age (years)	Biopsy number in next tables	Duration of infections (years)			Duration of heroin abuse (years)
				TB	HCV	HIV	
1	male	26	1	1	8	1	7
2	male	26	fragment	1	11	11	11
3	male	27	7	1	1	1	3
4	male	31	8	1	5	5	8
5	male	31	fragment	1	2	2	4
6	male	32	fragment	10	1	8	17
7	male	33	9	12	9	13	15
8	male	33	3	1	1	1	8
9	male	34	6	3	18	3	unknown
10	male	34	2	1	7	8	11
11	male	36	fragment	8	13	1	13
12	male	37	4	5	1	1	10
13	male	39	5	1	16	6	16

Table 1. Characteristics of patients with heroin abuse and co-infection of TB, HCV, HIV. The patients are arranged according to their age.

2.3. Computer digital analysis

Quantitative morphometric analysis was performed using an image analysis system consisting of a microscope (Leica DM 2500) with attached digital camera (Leica DFC 320 R2) and a computer. Serial pictures of biopsy slices of patients with co-infection were photographed by light microscope and were saved electronically. Serial microphotographs of biopsies were made by an objective x20. The further process was performed with the computer program Adobe Photoshop CS 5.0. Serial microphotographs were mounted to receive the general picture of liver biopsy (Figure 1). The digital image was converted into a binary image. The two-dimensional patterns were measured by direct pixels counting on the binary images under simultaneous visual control of the light microscopy.

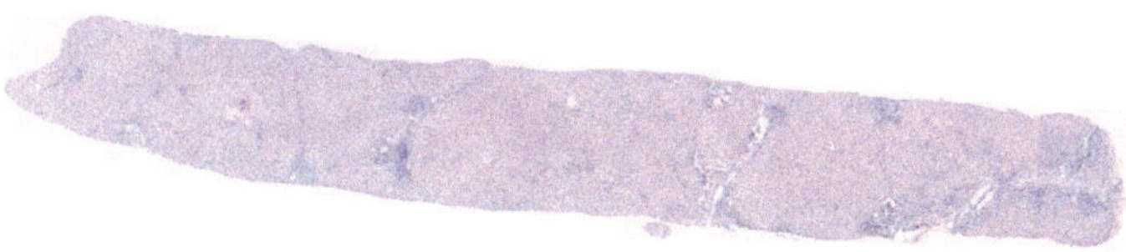

Figure 1. General picture of the liver biopsy composed by computer microscopy (Obj. x20) using Adobe Photoshop CS 5.0. Total area of the biopsy is 11449177 pixels

Three main parameters were used for quantitative evaluation: the total area of portal zones, the total area of intralobular infiltrates and necroses, as well as the total area of hepatic vessels (central and sublobular veins). We considered the total amount of these main parameters as non-parenchymal elements. Liver plates and sinusoids were attributed to the hepatic parenchyma.

The measurement of portions (in percentages) of portal area, foci of intralobular necroses, and vessels was estimated.

2.4. Statistical analysis

Statistical analysis was performed by tabulated processor Microsoft Excel 2003 and STATISTIKA 9.0.

3. Results

3.1. Features of histopathological structure of biopsies

Morphological analysis of liver biopsies of the patients – heroin addicts with tuberculosis (TB) and virus (HCV, HIV) co-infection showed that the extension of portal zones, the damage of limiting plates of liver cells and the formation of piecemeal and bridging necroses took place practically in all biopsies (Figure 2).

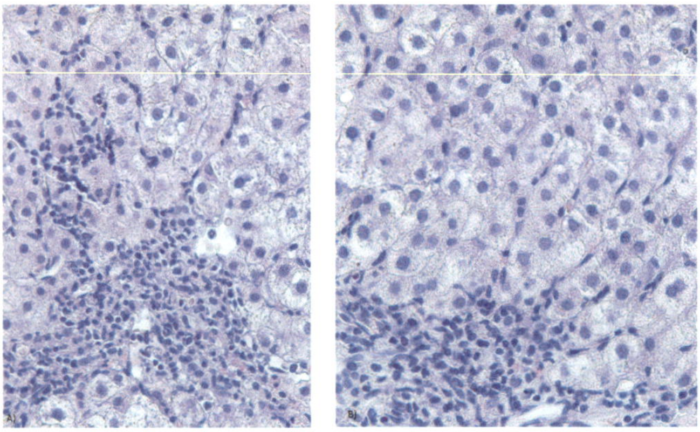

Figure 2. Subfigure with two images. Section of the liver biopsy specimen of a patient with co-infection (TB, HCV, HIV) and heroin abuse. Variants (a, b) of the development of interface hepatitis with piecemeal necrosis at the peripheral zone of portal tract. Hematoxylin-eosin. Obj. x40

The peripheral regions of the portal zones were usually densely infiltrated by lymphocytes and mononuclear histiocytes (Figure 2). Sometimes the lymphoid aggregates adjacent to the damaged bile ducts were formed. Dense connective tissue elements developed more often around the portal vessels (portal veins and hepatic arteries).

The appearance of focal lymphohistiocyte infiltrates and the formation of numerous intralobular necroses, containing hepatocytes, surrounded by lymphocytes (encircled hepatocytes) were typical to peripheral and middle zones of liver lobules (Figure 3).

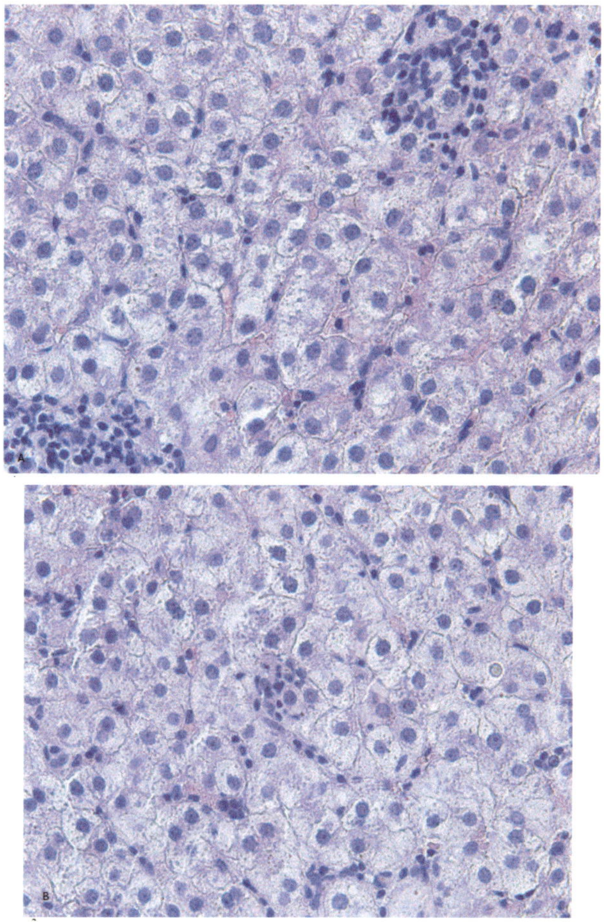

Figure 3. Subfigure with two images. Section of the liver biopsy specimen of a patient with co-infection (TB, HCV, HIV) and heroin abuse. Variants (a, b) of the development of intralobular necroses containing encircled hepatocytes at the middle part of liver lobule. Hematoxylin-eosin. Obj. x40

In the liver parenchyma the narrowing of sinusoids, as without of inflammatory infiltration signs and with the elements of lymphohistiocyte infiltration and chains of lymphocytes inside of them, was predominated (Figure 4).

There were features of moderate protein and vacuole dystrophia in all biopsies. In two cases some hepatocytes contained large lipid inclusions (Figure 5). Disturbance of the lobular architecture was observed only in one biopsy (Figure 6).

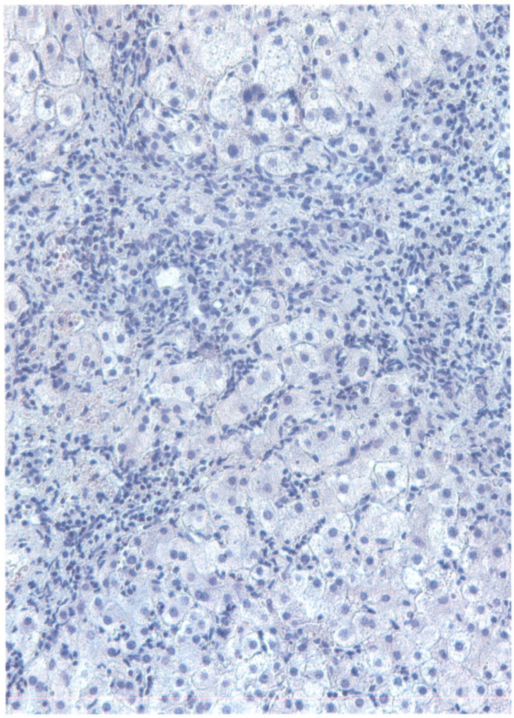

Figure 4. Section of the liver biopsy specimen of a patient with co-infection (TB, HCV, HIV) and heroin abuse. Severe infiltration of intralobular sinusoids by lymphocytes and histiocytes at the peripheral zone of liver lobule. Hematoxylin-eosin. Obj. x20

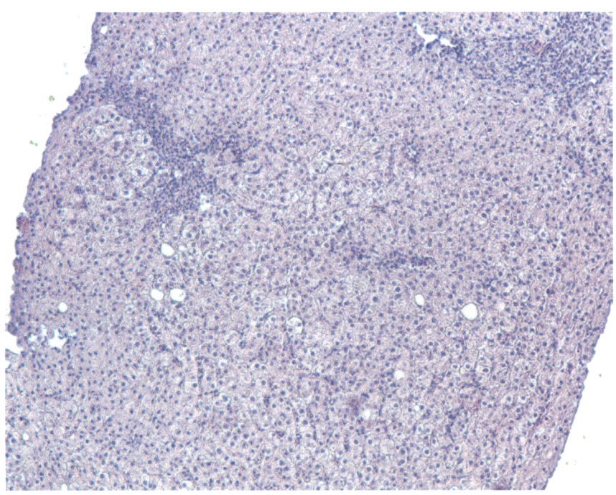

Figure 5. Section of the liver biopsy specimen of a patient with co-infection (TB, HCV, HIV) and heroin abuse. Expansion and infiltration of portal areas, presence of intralobular necroses at the middle zone of liver lobules, deposition of lipid droplets were in some hepatocytes. Hematoxylin-eosin. Obj. x10

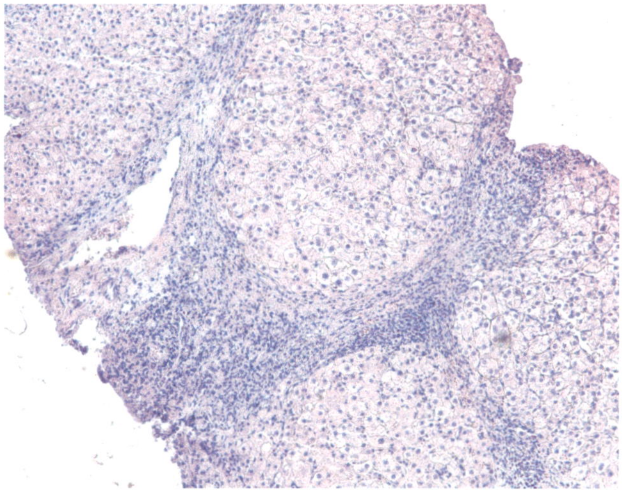

Figure 6. Section of the liver biopsy specimen of a patient with co-infection (TB, HCV, HIV) and heroin abuse. Strong development of bridging fibroses and disturbance of the lobular architecture. Hematoxylin-eosin. Obj. x10

3.2. Quantitative image analysis for evaluation of pathological changes in liver biopsy structure

Quantitative computer image morphometric analysis included three indexes. We calculated separately the square (in pixels) occupied by portal zones, the square of intralobular focal infiltrates and necroses and the square of hepatic vessels (central and sublobular veins).

The portal areas were divided into two groups: the portal zones with primary formation of piece-meal necroses and the portal zones with primary formation of bridging necroses. We took into account the calculation of portal zones fragments and septa. We also subdivided the intralobular damages in liver in two groups: the focal lymphohistiocyte infiltrates without hepatocytes and the intralobular piecemeal necroses with encircled hepatocytes.

As for hepatic vein, we separately considered terminal hepatic veins (central veins) and sublobular veins. In each case we estimated the relative square of the above-mentioned indexes in pixels and then calculated the specific parts in percents to the total square of biopsy.

We assigned the total sum of a specific part of portal zones, the specific part of intralobular focal infiltrates and necroses and the specific part of the hepatic veins as non-parenchymal elements. Respectively, the hepatic plates and sinusoids were remained in the composition of the parenchyma.

Then we calculated the parenchyma indexes as the relation of non-parenchymal elements to the parenchyma; these indexes characterized a certain degree of the replacement of the functioning hepatic tissue.

The data obtained were summarized in the Tables 2, 4, 5, 6 and 7. The samples of biopsies were arranged in sequence of increasing of non-parenchymal elements in bioptats.

The control group included the analysis of cohort of the patients with the monoinfection of chronic virus hepatitis C (Table 3). The morphometric analysis of liver structure of the patients belonging to given group was made earlier with the use of the method of the stereometric point morphometry [8].

3.2.1. The general characterization of morphometric data

The analysis showed that the specific part of non-parenchymal elements strongly varied in the group of the patients with co-infection and heroin abuse: from 2.65% to 27.43% (Table 2). Mean value of non-parenchymal elements was 12.08±2.38. The specific part of non-parenchymal elements varied in cases of monoinfection of hepatitis C with the different degree of activity from 2.16% до 11.93%, the mean value was 6.94±0.77. Thus, the mean value of non-parenchymal elements of liver biopsy of the patients – heroin addicts with co-infection exceeded the mean value of non-parenchymal elements in liver biopsy of the patients with monoinfection of hepatitis C (HCV) in 1.74 times. The maximal value of the specific part of non-parenchymal elements in case of co-infection was in 2.29 times higher than in cases of monoinfection HCV (Tables 2 and 3).

Biopsy number	Parenchymal elements, %	Non-parenchymal elements, %	Ratio of non-parenchymal elements	Total area of portal zones, %	Total area of spotty infiltrates , %	Total area of hepatic veins, %	Chains of lymphocytes (absent or present)
1	97,35	2,65	0,03	1,86	0,52	0,27	-
2	93,39	6,71	0,07	5,80	0,74	0,17	+
3	93,07	6,93	0,07	6,43	0,21	0,27	-
4	90,73	9,27	0,10	7,59	1,33	0,35	+
5	90,52	9,48	0,10	7,93	0,46	1,08	-
6	88,87	11,13	0,13	10,41	0,37	0,35	+
7	83,72	16,28	0,19	14,52	1,53	0,53	+
8	81,19	18,81	0,23	17,99	0,75	0,07	+
9	72,57	27,43	0,38	27,16	0,31	0	+

Table 2. Quantitative characteristics of liver biopsy specimens of patients with heroin abuse and co-infection of TB, HCV and HIV by computer morphometric analysis

http://dx.doi.org/10.5772/52971

Biopsy number	ALT activity (U/L)	Total area of morphometry (points of intersections)	Total number of microscopic fields(SU) (x400)	Parenchymal elements, %	Non-parenchymal elements, %	Ratio of non-parenchymal elements	Total area of portal area, %	Total area of spotty infiltrates ,%	Total area of hepatic veins, %	Chains of lymphocytes (absent or present)
1	15,	29450	95	97,84	2,16	0,02	1,79	0,05	0,32	-
2	20	18910	61	97,54	2,46	0,03	2,00	0,25	0,21	-
3	57	37690	126	96,49	3,51	0,04	2,30	0,46	0,75	-
4	14	17980	58	96,40	3,60	0,04	3,18	0,01	0,42	-
5	26	46190	149	95,70	4,30	0,04	3,15	0,12	1,02	-
6	104	70060	226	95,37	4,63	0,05	3,25	0,30	1,09	-
7	15	86800	280	95,30	4,70	0,05	2,91	0,02	1,77	-
8	42	37820	122	94,94	5,06	0,05	3,81	0,26	1,00	-
9	35	80290	259	94,82	5,18	0,05	3,93	0,84	0,41	+
10	441	89900	290	93,36	6,64	0,07	3,29	2,02	1,32	+
11	214	54560	176	91,33	8,67	0,09	7,24	0,89	0,55	-
12	187	70680	228	90,54	9,46	0,10	7,57	1,76	0,13	+
13	333	47720	152	90,32	9,68	0,11	7,51	1,17	1,00	-
14	107	32860	106	90,29	9,71	0,11	8,32	1,02	0,37	-
15	38	53514	193	89,44	10,56	0,12	6,23	2,61	1,71	+
16	122	49600	160	89,11	10,89	0,12	9,07	1,27	0,54	+
17	596	75330	243	88,24	11,76	0,13	9,26	1,56	0,94	+
18	162	60760	196	88,07	11,93	0,14	11,49	0,44	0,00	+

Table 3. Quantitative characteristics of liver biopsy specimens of the patients with monoinfection of chronic hepatitis C by stereometric point morphometry

We made the comparative analysis of histopathological changes in liver biopsy structure in the group of the patients – heroin addicts and co-infected using the standard semi quantitative methods of the Ishak score evaluation (Table 4).

We determined the histological activity index HAI according to Knodell [19]. The stages of the fibrosis development were defined by two ways: with the use of the research group French METAVIR [20] recommendations and with Ishak method [21]. Under the METAVIR system we evaluated the fibroses using five indexes where the maximal evaluation was 4 scores (F4 – cirrhosis). It consisted 6 scores (F6 – cirrhosis) according the Ishak system.

Standard semi quantitative analysis methods for the most part of biopsies (6 patients from 9) made possible to determine the same fibrosis stage: F3 according to the Ishak system and F2 according to the METAVIR system (Table 4).

Biopsy number	Non-parenchymal elements, %	HAI by score Knodell	Stage of fibrosis by score Ishak	Stage of fibrosis by score METAVIR
1	2,65	8	F3	F2
2	6,71	8	F3	F2
3	6,93	8	F3	F2
4	9,27	9	F3	F2
5	9,48	10	F3	F2
6	11,13	12	F3	F2
7	16,28	15	F4	F3
8	18,81	11	F3	F2
9	27,43	16	F5	F4

Table 4. Comparative characteristics of non-parenchymal elements specific parts, grading of histopathological lesions (HAI) and the stages of fibrosis in liver biopsy specimens of the patients with heroin abuse and co-infection of TB, HCV and HIV by computer morphometry and semi quantitative evaluation

At that time the quantitative computer image morphometric analysis showed (Table 2) that among studied biopsies the specific parts of non-parenchymal elements differed significantly in various biopsies at the same fibrosis stages.

The minimal value of the specific part of non-parenchymal elements was 2.65%. These values were 6.71% и 6.93% (two biopsy specimens), 9.27% and 9.48% (two other specimens of biopsy) and 11.13% (one biopsy specimen). Thus, in this case the methods of the semi quantitative score evaluation reflected only common regularities of the process of the fibrosis development. Meanwhile, the quantitative value of fibrosis was very essential for decision making of the medical treatment tactic and the estimation of the medical treatment effectiveness.

The quantitative value of fibrosis is especially important in the process of repeated studies for the determination of positive or negative dynamics of the fibrosis development. The histological activity index HAI according to Knodell proved to be more informative. HAI increased gradually from 8 to 16 points in accordance with the increasing of specific parts of non-parenchymal elements in biopsies.

http://dx.doi.org/10.5772/52971

3.2.2. Computer image analysis of portal zones

The majority of non-parenchymal elements were situated in portal zones. Therefore these indexes were analyzed in details (Table 5).

Biopsy number	Total area of non-parenchymal elements, %	Total area of portal zones		Portal area with piecemeal necroses				Portal area with bridging necroses			
		%	Number per biopsy	Total area, %	Number per biopsy	Minimal size, %	Maximal size, %	Total area, %	Number per biopsy	Minimal size, %	Maximal size, %
1	2,65	1,86	5	0,00	0	0	0	1,86	5	0,14	0,99
2	6,71	5,80	13	2,98	5	0,10	0,86	2,82	8	0,10	1,23
3	6,93	6,43	7	0,18	2	0,06	0,12	6,25	5	0,01	3,93
4	9,27	7,59	9	4,94	4	0,16	2,38	2,65	5	0,14	0,97
5	9,48	7,93	8	4,89	4	0,90	1,45	3,04	4	0,37	1,35
6	11,13	10,41	12	0,62	2	0,19	0,42	9,79	10	0,16	2,92
7	16,28	14,52	12	1,13	2	0,47	0,66	13,39	10	0,12	4,51
8	18,81	17,99	5	7,92	4	1,17	3,37	10,07	1	0,01	10,07
9	27,43	27,16	18	11,17	8	0,25	2,39	15,96	10	0,17	4,34

Table 5. Quantitative characteristics of portal zones in liver biopsy specimens of the patients with heroin abuse and co-infection of TB, HCV and HIV by computer morphometric analysis

The amount of portal zones studied in each biopsy varied from 5 to 18. It depended on the total biopsy volume. The mean value of the portal zones number was 9.8 9±1.34. The amount of portal zones with piecemeal necroses varied from 2 to 8 (mean value was 3.44±0.72). The amount of portal zones with the septa and bridging necroses was more significant, it changed from 1 to 10 (mean value was 6.44±1.01).

In one case (biopsy specimen № 8) the portal zone included several portal tracts forming the extensive confluent bridging necrosis.Thus, the amount of portal zones with bridging necroses (6.44) exceeded in 1.87 times the amount of portal zones with piecemeal necroses (3.44).

The total specific part of portal zones varied from 1.86% to 27.16% (mean value was 11.08±2.42) (Table 5).

The specific part of portal zones with piecemeal necroses varied from 0.18% to 11.17% (mean value was 3.76±1.21). The minimal size of such portal zones characterized mainly its fragment, it changed from 0.06% to 0.9% (mean value is 0.37±0.13). The maximal sizes of such portal zones characterized in general the degree of the portal zone extension, they changed from 0.12% to 3.37% (mean value was 1.29±0.37).

The specific part of the portal zones with bridging necroses (Table 5) changed from1.86% to 15.96% (mean value was 7.31±1.63). Thus, the specific part of portal zones with bridging necroses was practically in 2 times (1.94) more than the specific part of portal zones with piecemeal necroses.

The minimal size of portal zones with bridging necroses characterized in general the septa fragments, it changed from 0.01% to 0.37% (mean value was 0.13±0.03). The maximal size reflected more correctly the specific part of the portal zones with bridging necroses, it changed from 0.97% to 10.07% (mean value was 3.37±0.91).

The quantitative computer image morphometric analysis showed that the significant extension of portal zones with the destruction of the limiting plate and the development of piecemeal or bridging necroses took place in all bioptats of this patients group. In addition the specific part of portal zones with bridging necroses exceeded considerably (in 1.9 times) the specific part of portal zones with piecemeal necroses.

For comparison: the total specific part of portal zones changed from 1.79% to 11.49% (mean value was 5.35±0.68) at chronic hepatitis C monoinfection (Table 3).

Thus, the specific part of portal zones of liver biopsies of the patients – heroine addicts with tuberculosis and virus (HCV, HIV) co-infection was 2.07 times higher than the specific part of portal zones of liver biopsies of the patients with the monoinfection HCV.

Moreover the bridging and piecemeal necroses were absent in the liver of the patients with monoinfection HCV under minimal and low activity. Their appearance was noticed only if

the value of specific parts of non-parenchymal elements exceeded 4.7%.

We have not observed any difference between the amounts of piecemeal and bridging necroses in biopsy specimens with monoinfection HCV.

3.2.3. Computer image analysis of intralobular infiltrates and necroses

We analyzed the morphometric indexes of intralobular infiltrates and necroses (Table 6).

Intralobular necroses presented in all biopsies, their number varied from 6 to 38 (mean value was 16.33±3.42). The amount of focal intralobular lymphohistiocyte infiltrates was significantly less in comparison with the intralobular necroses containing encircled hepatocytes.

The total number of focal intralobular infiltrates varied in different biopsies from 1 to 11 (mean value was 3.67±1.09), whereas the total number of intralobular piecemeal necroses varied from 4 to 28 (mean value was 12.78±2.5).

The relation between piecemeal necroses and focal intralobular infiltrates was especially demonstrative (Table 6). The number of piecemeal necroses in each biopsy was in several times more (up to 10 times) than the number of focal necroses. The total number of intralobular piecemeal necroses was 115, whereas the number of focal intralobular infiltrates was only 33, i.e. in 3.48 times less.

Biopsy number	Total area of non-parenchymal elements, %	Total area of intralobular necroses, %	Total number of intralobular necroses per biopsy	Focal lymphohistiocyte infiltrates				Intralobular necroses with encircled hepatocytes (piecemeal necroses)			
				Total area ,%	Total number per biopsy	Minimal size, %	Maximal size, %	Total area, %	Total number per biopsy	Minimal size, %	Maximal size, %
1	2,65	0,52	8	0,01	1	0,01	0,01	0,51	7	0,04	0,18
2	6,71	0,74	22	0,03	6	0	0,01	0,71	16	0,02	0,11
3	6,93	0,21	6	0,05	2	0,02	0,04	0,16	4	0,02	0,08
4	9,27	1,33	28	0,09	6	0,01	0,02	1,24	22	0,02	0,25
5	9,48	0,46	10	0,01	1	0,01	0,01	0,45	9	0,02	0,12
6	11,13	0,37	16	0,03	3	0,01	0,01	0,34	13	0,01	0,06
7	16,28	1,53	38	0,10	11	0,01	0,08	1,52	28	0,01	0,36
8	18,81	0,75	10	0	0	0	0	0,75	10	0,06	0,11
9	27,43	0,31	9	0,04	3	0,01	0,02	0,28	6	0,03	0,06

Table 6. Quantitative characteristics of intralobular necroses in the liver biopsy specimens of the patients with heroin abuse and co-infection of TB, HCV and HIV by computer morphometric analysis

The total specific part of intralobular necroses varied from 0.21% to 1.53% (mean value was 0.69±0.14). The specific part of the focal intralobular infiltrates varied from 0.01% to 0.1% (mean value was 0.04±0.01). The size of the minimal infiltrate was only 0.01%, the size of the maximal infiltrate was 0.08% (mean value was 0.02±0.01).

The total specific part of intralobular piecemeal necroses varied from 0.16% to 1.52% (mean value was 0.66±0.14). The minimal size of the specific part of intralobular piecemeal necroses was 0.01% (mean value was 0.03±0.01), whereas their maximal size was 0.36 % (mean value was 0.15±0.02).

The analysis of the total biopsy specimen (Figure 1) allowed attributing the topography of the intralobular necroses distribution. Thus, under the middle degree of the parenchyma injury (HAI according to Knodell system up to 10 points) the small lymphohistiocyte infiltrates dominated in periportal zones of lobules. Under the high activity of the process (HAI according to Knodell scoring system exceeded 10 points) the large piecemeal necroses dominated, they arranged mainly in the middle zones of lobules.

Hepatocytes surrounded by lymphocytes were well noticeable in large piecemeal necroses (Figure 3b); it is perhaps connected with hepatocytes death, mediated by lymphocytes.

It is typically that the inflammatory infiltration of sinusoids and the formation "chains" of lymphocytes in them are mostly expressed in large piecemeal necroses (Figure 4).

So, the histological activity index HAI according to Knodell reached 15 points, the total number of intralobular necroses reached 38 (28 from them were referred to piecemeal necroses) in the biopsy № 7 (Tables 4 and 6). Remarkably that during the cirrhosis development (biopsy № 9, fibrosis stage according to the METAVIR system scale was F4 – cirrhosis) the total number of intralobular necroses considerably reduced (6 piecemeal necroses and 3 focal infiltrates in one large biopsy; see Figure 6).

3.2.4. Computer image analysis of hepatic vessels

The amount of venous vessels in biopsy samples varied from 2 to 7 (mean value was 3.33±0.63). The central veins with endothelium which are often damaged predominated in all biopsies (Table 7).

Biopsy number	**Total area of non-parenchymal elements, %**	**Total area of hepatic vessels, %**	**Total number of hepatic vessels per biopsy**	**Terminal hepatic veins (central veins)**				**Sublobular veins**			
				Total area ,%	Number per biopsy	Minimal size , %	Maximal size, %	Total area, %	Number per biopsy	Minimal size, %	Maximal size, %
1	2,65	0,27	4	0,27	4	0,09	0,11	0	0	0	0
2	6,71	0,17	2	0,17	2	0,03	0,14	0	0	0	0
3	6,93	0,27	3	0,27	3	0,03	0,18	0	0	0	0
4	9,27	0,35	4	0,35	4	0,07	0,11	0	0	0	0
5	9,48	1,08	5	0,13	4	0,02	0,05	0,95	1	0,95	0,95
6	11,13	0,35	7	0,35	7	0,01	0,11	0	0	0	0
7	16,28	0,53	3	0	0	0	0	0,53	3	0,04	0,31
8	18,81	0,07	2	0,07	2	0,03	0,04	0	0	0	0
9	27,43	0	0	0	0	0	0	0	0	0	0

Table 7. Quantitative characteristics of hepatic vessels in liver biopsy specimens of the patients with heroin abuse and co-infection of TB, HCV and HIV by computer morphometric analysis

Sublobular veins were observed only in two biopsies, perhaps they did not get into biopsies because of large sizes in comparison with central veins.

The total specific part of the hepatic vessels varied from 0.07% to 1.08% (mean value was 0.34±0.1). The specific part of the central veins varied from 0.17% to 0.35% (mean value was 0.18±0.04). The minimal size of the central vein was 0.01% (mean value was 0.03±0.01), the maximal size was 0.18% (mean value was 0.08±0.02). The specific part of sublobular veins reached 1.48%, maximal size – 0.95%.

On the whole it is possible to note the tendencies to the stable extension of vessels and the damage of its internal walls. In addition, the sharp narrowing of intralobular sinusoids adjacent to above mentioned vessels, took part in the contribution of the impairment of the processes of the microcirculation inside of liver lobules. Perhaps the worsening of microcirculation lead to the bypass ways of the circulation, this may be one of the reasons of bridging necroses development.

3.3. Investigation of activity of alanin aminotransferase (ALT) and aspartate aminotransferase (AST)

The measurement of liver enzyme activities (serum ALT and AST) are important for diagnosis and assessment of liver diseases in clinical practice. However, ALT levels fluctuate in chronic HCV infection and may fall into the normal range [22].The use of many medications have been associated with elevated ALT levels [23]. In chronic hepatocellular injury, ALT increasing is more typical than AST. However, when the fibrosis progresses, ALT activity typically declines, and the ratio of AST to ALT gradually increases [24], especially during the development of cirrhosis [25,26].

We observed the increasing of the ALT and AST levels practically among all the patients (Table 8).

Biopsy number	Activity of ALT (U/L)	Activity of AST (U/L)	Ratio of AST/ALT
1	90	48	0,53
2	36	32	0,88
3	45	42	0,93
4	140	90	0,64
5	162	179	1,10
6	48	39	0,81
7	90	68	0,75
8	88	93	1,05
9	106	84	0,79

Table 8. Activity of serum alanine aminotransferase (ALT) and aspartate aminotransferase (AST) in liver biopsy specimens of the patients with heroin abuse and co-infection of TB, HCV and HIV

So, the ALT level changed from 36 to 162 points (mean value was 89.4±13.45). The AST level varied from 32 to179 points (mean value was 75±14.25). The AST/ALT ratio varied from 0.53 to 1.10 points (mean value was 0.83±0.06).

The mostly expressed increase of ALT and AST levels was discovered in the patients with the samples of biopsy having the specific part of non-parenchymal elements up to 10% (Table 8, samples of biopsies № 4 and № 5). As a rule the ferment activity rather reduced under the fibrosis intensification. The AST/ALT ratio was increased in 3 patients. In other cases it was closer to the upper border of the normal level.

We have not discovered any direct interconnections between the ferment activity levels and the sizes of the specific parts of intralobular necroses. The intralobular piecemeal necroses were dominant in this group of the patients; perhaps, the hepatocytes destruction was caused by the special mechanism of the cell death (apoptosis).

4. Discussion

Detailed information about natural history of HIV/HCV co-infection is discussed in special review article [27]. Some studies have suggested that human immunodeficiency infection modifies the natural history of hepatitis C virus infection accelerating the progression of fibrosis and the development of cirrhosis [28, 29, 30, 31].

Co-infection HCV/HIV is very often discovered among injecting drug users [32, 33]. Thus, it was shown that about 90% drug users (consumers of heroin) are infected by hepatitis C virus [34]. Intravenous heroin abuse induces significant morphological changes in liver tissue (vesicular changes, fatty changes, chronic hepatitis, cirrhosis), and the severity of these changes increases with years of heroin abuse [35]. Authors supposed that worsening of morphological changes in the liver happens mostly often because of a significantly reduced detoxification functions of the liver.

Espinal, Peréz, Baéz, Hénriguez et al. [36] analyzed the clinical aspects of the co-infection HIV and tuberculosis. Tuberculosis remains an important public health problem in the world that has been exacerbated by HIV epidemic, resulting in increased morbidity and mortality [37, 38]. The pathogenesis and mechanisms of inflammation and accelerated fibrosis in co-infected patients are still poorly understood [28, 39].

At present investigation the peculiarities of patients with heroin abuse and co-infection (TB, HCV and HIV) were analyzed (see Table 1). All the patients were males of the age from 26 to 39 years (mean value was 32.2 years). The heroin abuse was the longest (mean value was 13.6 years). Patients with HCV-infection occupied the second position of disease duration (mean value was 7.1 years), than there were the patients with HIV-infection (mean value was 4.7 years) and finally the patients with TB-infection (mean value was 3.5 years). At last case the tuberculosis was discovered for the first time of 7 patients from 13 patients. It is characteristic that *Mycobacterium tuberculosis* was not discovered in phlegm of any patients under repeated analyses.

We could not detect any interconnections between the quantitative parameters of biopsy specimen getting with the use of computer microscopy and for the duration of above-mentioned observations.

Moreover the tendency to the diseases heaviness increasing is evident. The good example of this tendency is the biopsy specimen № 9: the duration of heroin abuse in this case com-

http://dx.doi.org/10.5772/52971

posed 15 years, HIV – 13 years, TB – 12 years and HCV – 9 years. In accordance with it the cirrhosis developed in the liver of this patient (see Figure 6) and the segment of non-parenchymal elements reached 27.43%. Among them the specific part of portal zones was prevalent (27.16%).

The other peculiarity was the presence of the same stage of fibrosis (namely fibrosis F2 by METAVIR scoring) and F3 (by Ishak scoring) in liver of the majority of the patients.

At that time the segment of non-parenchyma elements in liver of these patients varied from 2.65% to 11.13%, and the specific part of the portal zones changed from 1.86% to 10.41%. The detailed information about discussion questions and interpretation of liver biopsy assessment by grading and staging systems was presented in recent works [40, 41].

The typical changes included the destruction of limiting plate, the expansion of portal areas and the development of interface hepatitis, formation of short septa or bridging necroses. The image analysis allows calculating of portal zones areas and intralobular infiltrates in different fields of biopsy vision. The expansion of portal zones took place especially during the development of interface hepatitis. As a rule, intensive lymphohistiocyte infiltration predominates in such a type of portal zones.

The region of intralobular infiltrates strongly varies. Our investigation showed that intralobular infiltrates developed as a result of lymphocyte-mediated death of hepatocytes (apoptosis).

Earlier we studied the apoptosis in liver biopsy specimens of the patients with HCV with the use of the TUNEL method [42, 43]. TUNEL-marked cells looked as small groups similar to intralobular piecemeal necroses. All morphometric parameters were significantly higher in comparison with monoinfection HCV [8].

5. Conclusion

Morphometric image analysis gives a possibility to evaluate quantitative parameters of necro-inflammatory and fibrosis changes in liver biopsy of patients with mixed infections and heroin abuse.

It is characteristic that the combination of different infections leads to the progression of liver inflammation and the increasing of the portion of non-parenchymal elements as a total sum of portal areas, intralobular infiltrates and distended hepatic vessels.

The investigation showed significant intensification of necroinflammatory lesions. Lymphohistiocyte infiltration was typical both for portal zones and intralobular areas. These morphological indications could be connected with the change of the immune state of patients as a result of combine effect of bacterial, viral infections and heroin abuse. So, numerous factors have been associated with an increased risk of fibrosis progression in liver of such type of patients.

Of course, it is necessary for more correct analysis to study the biopsies of the patients of several control groups with the sequential cut-off of the definite factors. We plan to carry out such investigation in future.

Quantitative analysis of digital images of total biopsies is indispensable to study the effectiveness of treatment tactics testing as the effect of therapy can be calculated as the percentage of morphological changes in biopsy.

Author details

Ivan B. Tokin[1*], Ivan I. Tokin[2] and Galina F. Filimonova[1,2*]

*Address all correspondence to: ivan.tokin@rambler.ru

1 St.-Petersburg State University, Russia

2 North-Western State Medical University named after I.I.Mechnikov, Russia

References

[1] Koss, L. G. (1982). Analytical and Quantitative Cytology. A Historical Perspectives. *Analytical and Quantitative Cytology and Histolology*, 4, 251-256.

[2] Hamilton, P., & Allen, D. (1995). Morphometry in Histopathology. *Journal of Pathology*, 175(4), 369-379.

[3] Pilette, S., Rousselet, M., Bedossa, P., Chappard, D., Óberti, F., Rifflet, H., Maiga, M., Gallois, Y., & Calès, P. (1998). Histopathological Evaluation of Liver Fibrosis: Quantitative Analysis vs Semi-Quantitative Scores. Comparison with Serum Markers. *Journal of Hepatology*, 28(3), 439-446.

[4] O` Brien., N., Keating, N., Elderiny, S., Cerda, S., Keaveny, A., Afdhal, N., & Nunes, D. (2000). An assessment of Digital Image Analysis to Measure Fibrosis in Liver Biopsy Specimen of Patients with Chronic Hepatitis C. *American Journal of Clinical Pathology*, 114(5), 712-718.

[5] Zaituon, A., Mardini, H., Awad, S., Ukabam, S., Makadisi, S., & Record, C. (2001). Quantitative Assessment of Fibrosis and Steatosis in Liver biopsies from Patients with Chronic Hepatitis C. *Journal of Clinical Pathology*, 54(6), June, 461-465.

[6] Goodman, Z., Becker, R., Pockros, P., & Afdhal, N. (2007). Progression of Fibrosis in Advanced Chronic Hepatitis C: Evaluation by Morphometric Image Analysis. *Hepatology*, 45(3), 886-894.

[7] Goodman, Z., Stoddard, A., Bonkovsky, H., Fontana, R., Ghany, M., Morgan, T., Wright, E., Brunt, E., Kleiner, D., Shiffmann, M., Everson, G., Lindsay, K., Dienstag,

J., Morishima, C., & the HALT-C Trial Group. (2009). Fibrosis Progression in Chronic Hepatitis C: Morphometric Image Analysis in the HALT-C Trial. *Hepatology,* 50(6), 1738-1749.

[8] Filimonova, G., Tokin, I. I., Tokin, I. B., & Hussar, P. (2010). An Assessment of Morphometric Analysis in Liver Biopsy Specimens with Chronic Hepatitis C. *Papers on Anthropology. Tartu, Estonia,* XIX, 69-80.

[9] Tokin, I. B., Tokin, I. I., & Filimonova, G. F. (2011). Quantitative Morphometric Analysis of Liver Biopsy: Problems and Perspectives. *In: Liver Biopsy. Ed. By Hirokazu Takahashi, INTECHWEB.ORG,* 137-154.

[10] Kage, M., Shimamatu, K., Nakashima, E., Kojiro, M., Inoue, O., & Yano, M. (1997). Long-Term Evolution of Fibrosis from Chronic Hepatitis to Cirrhosis in Patients with Hepatitis C: Morphometric Analysis of Repeated Biopsies. Hepatology April , 25(4), 1028-1031.

[11] Manabe, N., Chevallier, M., Chossegross, P., Causse, X., Guerret, S., & Trepo, Grimaud. G. (1993). Interferon-alfa 2b Therapy Reduces Liver Fibrosis in Cronic A, Non-B Hepatitis: A Quantitative Histological Evaluation. *Hepatology,* December , 18(6), 1344-1349.

[12] Duchatelle, V., Marcellin, P., Giostra, E., Bregeaud, L., Pouteau, M., Boyer, N., Auperin, A., Guerret, S., Erlinger, S., Henin, D., & Degott, C. (1998). Changes in Liver Fibrosis at the End of Alfa Interferon Therapy and 6 to 18 Months Later in Patients with Chronic Hepatitis C: Quantitative Assessment by a Morphometric Method. *Journal of Hepatology,* 29(1), 20-28.

[13] Caballero, T., Pérez-Milena, A., Masserolli, M., O`, Valle. F., Salmerón, F., Del Moral, R., & Sánches-Salgado, G. (2001). Liver Fibrosis Assessment with Semiquantitative Indexes and Image Analysis Quantification in Sustained-Responder and Non-Responder Interferon-treated Patients with Chronic Hepatitis C. *Journal of Hepatology,* 34(1), 740-747.

[14] Benhamou, Y., Di Martino, V., Bochet, M., Colombet, G., Thibault, V., Liou, F., Katlama, K., Poynard, T., & and for the Multivir C Group. (2001). Factors Affecting Liver Fibrosis in Human Immunodeficiency Virus and Hepatitis C Virus Co-infected Patients: Impact of Protease Inhibitor Therapy. *Hepatology,* 34(2), August, 283-287.

[15] Martinez-Sierra, C., Arizcorreta, A., Diaz, F., Roldán, R., Martin-Herrera, L., Pérez-Guzmán, E., & Girón-González, J. (2003). Progression of Chronic Hepatitis C to Liver Fibrosis and Cirrhosis in Patients Coinfected with Hepatitis C Virus and Immunodeficiency Virus. *Clinical Infectious Diseases,* 36(2), 491-498.

[16] Poynard, T., Mathurin, P., Ching-Lung, Lai., Quyader, D., Poupon, R., Tainturier, M. H., Myers, R., Muntenau, M., Ratziu, V., Manns, M., Arndt, V., Capron, F., Chedid, A., & Bedossa, P. (2003). for the Panfibrosis Group. (A Comparison of Fibrosis Progression in Chronic Liver Diseases. *Journal of Hepatology,* 38(3), 257-265.

[17] Menghini, G. (1958). One-Second Needle Biopsy of the Liver. Gastroenterology August), 0016-5085 , 35(2), 190-199.

[18] Menghini, G., Lauro, G., & Caraseni, M. (1975). Some Innovations in the Technic of the One- Second Needle Biopsy of the Liver. *American Journal of Gastroenterology*, 64(3), 175-180.

[19] Knodell, R., Ishak, K., Bkack, W., Chen, T., Graig, R., Kaplowitz, N., Kiernan, T., & Wollman, J. (1981). Formulation and Application of a Numerical Scoring System for Assessing Histological Activity in Asymptomatic Chronic Active Hepatitis. *Hepatology*, 1(5), September/October, 431-435, 0270-9139.

[20] French METAVIR Cooperative Study Group. (1994). Intraobserver and Interobserver Variations in Liver Biopsy Interpretation in Patients with Chronic Hepatitis C. *Hepatology*, 20(1), 15-20.

[21] Ishak, K., Baptista, A., Bianchi, L., Callea, F., De Groote, J., Gudat, F., Denk, H., Desmet, V., Korb, J., Mac, Sween. R., Phillips, M., Portmann, B., Poulsen, H., Sheuer, P., Schmid, M., & Thaler, H. (1995). Histological Grading and Staging of Chronic Hepatitis B. *Journal of Hepatology*, 22(6), 696-699.

[22] Inglesby, T., Rai, R., Astemborsky, J., Gruskin, L., Nelson, K., Vlahov, D., & Thomas, D. (1999). A Prospective Community Based Evaluation of Liver Enzymes in Individuals With Hepatitis C after Drug Use. *Hepatology*, 29(2), 590-596.

[23] Green, R., & Flamm, S. (2002). AGA Technical Review on the Evaluation of Liver Chemistry Tests. *Gastroenterology*, 123(4), 1367-1384.

[24] Kim, W., Flamm, S., Di Bisceglie, A., & Bodenheimer, H. (2008). Serum Activity of Alanin Aminotransferase (ALT) as an Indicator of Health and Disease. Hepatology. , 47(4), 1363-1370.

[25] Williams, A., & Hoofnagle, J. (1988). Ratio of Serum Aspartate to Alanin Aminotransferase in Chronic Hepatitis: Relationship to Cirrhosis. Gastroenterology. 0016-5085 , 95, 734-739.

[26] Sheth, S., Flamm, S., Gordon, F., & Chopra, S. AST/ALT Ratio Predict Cirrhosis in Patients with Chronic Hepatitis C Virus Infection. *American Journal of Gastroenterology*, 93, 44-48.

[27] Petrovic, L. (2007). HIV/HCV Co-infection: Histopathological Findings, Natural History, Fibrosis, and Impact of Antiretroviral Treatment: a Review Article. *Liver International*, 598-606.

[28] Mohsen, A. N., Eastbrook, P. J., Taylor, C., Portman, B., Kulasegaram, R., Murad, S., et al. (2003). Impact of Human Immunodeficiency Virus (HIV) Infection on the Progression of Liver Fibrosis in Hepatitis C Virus Infected Patients. *Gut*, 52(7), July, 1035-1040.

[29] Rullier, A., Trimoulet, P., Neau, D., et al. (2004). Fibrosis is Worse in HIV/HCV Patients with Low-level Immunosuppression Referred for HCV Treatment than in HCV-matched Patients. *Human Pathology*, 35, 1088-1094.

[30] Kelleher, T., & Afdhal, N. (2006). Assessment of Liver Fibrosis in Co-infected Patients. *Journal of Hepatology*, 44(1), S126-S131.

[31] Vallet-Pichard, A., & Pol, S. (2006). Natural History and Predictors of Severity of Chronic Hepatitis C Virus (HCV) and Human Immunodeficiency Virus (HIV) Co-infection. *Journal of Hepatology*, 44, 528-534.

[32] Thomas, D. L., Shih, J. W., Alter, H. I., et al. (1996). Effect of Human Immunodeficiency Virus on Hepatitis C Virus Infection among Injecting Drug Users. *Journal Infectious Diseases*, 174, 690-695.

[33] Di Martino, V., Rufat, P., Boyer, N., Renard, P., Degos, F., Martinot-Peignoix, M., Matherov, S., Le Moins, V., Vachin, F., Degott, C., Valla, D., & Marcellin, P. (2001). The Influence of Human Immunodeficiency Virus Coinfection on Chronic Hepatitis C in Injection Drug Users: a Long-term Retrospective Cohort Study. Hepatology December , 34(6), 1193-1199.

[34] Tennant, F. (2001). Hepatitis C, B, D and A: Contrasting Features and Liver Function Abnormalities in Heroin Addicts. *Journal of Addictive Diseases*, 20(1), 9-17.

[35] Ilic, G., Karadzic, R., Kostic-Banovic, L., & Stojanovic, J. (2005). Chronic Intravenous Heroin Abuse: Impact on the Liver. *Facta Universitats Series: Medicine and Biology*, 12(3), 150-153.

[36] Espinal, M., Peréz, E., Baéz, J., Hénriguez, L., Fernández, K., Lopez, M., Olivo, P., & Reingold, A. (2000). Infectiousness of Mycobacterium tuberculosis in HIV-1-infected Patients with Tuberculosis: a Prospective Study. *The Lancet*, 355(9200), January, 275-280.

[37] Sharma, S., Mohan, A., & Kadhitavan, T. (2005). HIV-TB Co-infection: Epidemiology, Diagnosis and Management. Indian Journal of Medical Research. 0971-5916 , 121, 550-567.

[38] Sterlig, T. R., Pham, P. A., & Chaisson, R. E. (2010). HIV Infection-Related Tuberculosis: Clinical Manifestations and Treatment. *Clinical Infectious Diseases*, 50(3), May, S223-S230.

[39] Jones, R., Dunning, J., & Nelson, M. (2005). HIV and Hepatitis C Co-infection. *International Journal Clinical Practice.*, 59, 1082-1092.

[40] Theise, N. D. (2007). Liver Biopsy Assessment in Chronic Viral Hepatitis: a Personal, Practical Approach. *Modern Pathology*, 20(7), July 2006, S3-S14.

[41] Shiha, G., & Zalata, K. (2011). Ishak versus MERAVIR: Terminology, Convertibility and Correlation with Laboratory Changes in Chronic Hepatitis C. *In: Liver Biopsy. Ed by Hirokazu Takahashi, INTECHWEB.ORG*, 155-170.

[42] Tokin, I. B., Hussar, P., Filimonova, G., Hussar, U., Jarveots, T., Suuroju, T., & Tokin, I. I. (2008). Features of the Liver Apoptosis in Patients with Chronic Hepatitis C Viral Infection (HCV). *In: Proceedings of the 7th International Cell Death Society Symposium "Targeting cell death pathway for human diseases", Shanghai Mega City, China,* 127.

[43] Tokin, I. B., Hussar, P., Filimonova, G., Hussar, U., Jarveots, T., Suuroju, T., & Tokin, I. I. (2009). Features of Liver Apoptosis in Chronic Hepatitis C Virus (HCV) Infection. Papers on Anthropology Tartu, Estonia., 1406-0140 , XVIII, 361-371.

Chapter 12

Future Aspects of Liver Biopsy: From Reality to Mathematical Basis of Virtual Microscopy

Ludmila Viksna, Ilze Strumfa, Boriss Strumfs,
Valda Zalcmane, Andrejs Ivanovs and
Valentina Sondore

Additional information is available at the end of the chapter

http://dx.doi.org/10.5772/52753

1. Introduction

Tissue investigation remains one of the most reliable diagnostic ways in both general medical practice and liver pathology. At present, the routine liver biopsy investigation should include obtaining a representative tissue sample, adequate technological processing and application of histochemical stain panel [1-5]. The evaluation must be done in accordance with up-to-date disease classifications and validated diagnostic criteria [6]. Protocol approach is recommended in order to decrease the variability in description. In case of chronic inflammatory liver disease, semiquantitative evaluation of inflammatory activity by Knodell, Ishak, METAVIR or Scheuer score, or analogous system [7-11] must be applied. Additional methods as immunohistochemistry or polymerase chain reaction are applied by necessity. The morphological evaluation of biopsy is a part of medical teamwork. It should be preceded by clinical and laboratory investigations and biopsy findings must be incorporated in the general patient's information. Many of these principles will remain in use in the nearest future. However, both clinical diagnostics and medical research undergo almost unlimited progress. The upcoming innovations in liver biopsy analysis include incorporation of digital image analysis, genetic investigations and immunohistochemistry for functionally important molecules as cytokines, cell cycle markers and viral life cycle markers into everyday practice.

2. Morphological evaluation of liver: Today's reality

Despite the fact that the histological assessment of liver tissues plays an essential role in the diagnosis of liver diseases and the histological conclusion serves quite often as a basis for establishing the diagnosis, there are factors or reasons to be taken into consideration which can negatively influence the results obtained in morphological evaluation of liver biopsy.

We have "assessed" the percentage of each factor's influence on the final result– description and conclusion regarding diagnosis, where "0" is considered a factor that does not affect the evaluation and its outcome, but "100%" – the factor which actually hinders the correct diagnosis of the disease. The factors that may affect the liver tissue morphological assessment and diagnosis of disease are summarized in Table 1.

No.	Factors affecting liver tissue morphologic assessment	Evaluation of impact on final outcome in % *	Comments
1.	Biopsy site selection in liver tissues	100 – 0	It can be completely non-representative site, such as subcapsular
2.	Fixation and transfer of biopsy sample	100 – 0	Chemical environment (composition) and temperature of fixation can affect the biopsy specimen
3.	Selection of certain section out of the whole sample	50 – 0	If the whole sample is used, then the error theoretically is not possible
4.	Selection and quality of staining (panel of visualization methods) of the sample	100 – 0	If the sample is not stained for the reason to label a certain substance, e.g., Fe, the error can reach 100%
5.	Quality of biopsy specimen sections or microtomy	30 – 0	Thick or disrupted tissue sections can hinder the pathology from the observer. The thickness should not exceed 3-4 micrometres.
6.	Number of viewable visual fields	80 – 0	Inaccuracies can occur if only some separate visual fields are examined
7.	Technical condition of the microscope	80 – 0	Incomplete quality of optical system can hinder the pathology from the observer.
8.	Selection of evaluation scale	100 – 0	If the specimen where the basic pathology relates to fatty changes (steatosis) is assessed according to Knodell scale, then the assessment is inadequate if compared to the actual liver tissue damage

* 100% - affecting

0% - not affecting

Table 1. Factors affecting liver tissue morphologic assessment

Further we will have a look at each factor separately. The first reason which may significantly affect the final result is the incidental character of biopsy specimen collection by means of "blind" biopsy. In case of diffuse liver damage, it is important to obtain liver specimen from a representative site (which is not subcapsular) or under ultrasonographic (USG) control. If the liver specimen is obtained during invasive procedure (laparoscopy or open abdominal surgery), it is of high importance to give information about preferable biopsy site to the colleague obtaining liver specimen. The liver specimens obtained during surgery are certainly more targeted. More or less qualitative methodological performance of tissue collection may also cause certain imperfections affecting quality of specimen evaluation.

Presuming that the biopsy specimen is obtained from the site typical for the certain liver pathology, one more important issue is the quality of biopsy specimens' fixation and slicing.

The aspect of „special" tissue staining must also be looked at, because in case of absence of examination request or list of preliminary diagnosis provided by clinician, that emphasizes the need for particular staining, morphologist is unable to give an adequate diagnostic assessment of biopsy specimen. Thus diagnosis like haemochromatosis and other pathologies known as "storage diseases" can be missed.

The next factor, i.e., selection of certain section out of the whole biopsy specimen, is an issue arising only in case if the biopsy specimen is not examined throughout or along its horizontal length. The cross-sectioning gives the chance to analyze tissues on different "depths" or „levels" of the biopsy specimen.

The technical condition or quality of the microscope and number of viewable visual fields are to be considered seriously. Nowadays, the usual practice of the pathologist is a general overview of the material to gain insight into overall picture, noticing the most typical and important peculiarities. Inaccuracies can occur if only some separate visual fields are examined.

The subjective component of the morphological assessment of liver specimens and interpretation of the observed changes and their compliance or adherence to one or the other pathology is essential also. The problem could be the qualification and experience of clinician to put together or combine visual insight in the particular biopsy specimen and clinical diagnosis made up of biochemical, immunological and genetic parameters, and to use the interpretation of morphologist properly for establishing the diagnosis.

Selection of morphological or histological evaluation scale is significant. These scales are very advantageous for standardizing expert's assessment, converting it into measurable characteristics and helping the clinician to make final decision about patient's diagnosis. In case of light microscopy the issue of selection of evaluation scale is a factor with up to 100% error probability. For example, the use of the Knodell scale for patient with steatohepatosis, HAI = 0, leads to incorrect conclusion that the patient is healthy, especially if the biochemical parameters of blood are not altered.

If in addition the electron microscopic investigation of sequential liver biopsy specimens are done, obtained results and conclusions are also affected by the whole process of the above mentioned biopsy specimen collection and processing. The electron microscopy is currently considered as an auxiliary method or technique, yet in the age of high-tech medicine, processes ongoing on the level of organelles are the ones which by characteristic ultrastructural changes frequently refer to or indicate a particular pathology. The following must be strictly observed in electron microscopy: 1) liver tissue sampling and slicing into 1 mm^3 pieces without mechanically squeezing them and immediate immersion in fixing solution; 2) chemical composition of fixing solution, temperature, sample fixation and rinsing time; 3) embedding of liver tissue samples in mixture of epoxy resins in accordance with polymerization time of these resins; 4) quality of sample cutting with ultramicrotome and contrasting with uranyl acetate and lead citrate; 5) all cells and their organelles visible in the ultra-thin slices under the electron microscope have to be examined. It should be noted that resolution of transmission electron microscope (TEM) is within the range of 0.2 to 2 nm and resolution of scanning electron microscope is 4 nm.

3. Virtual microscopy: The general principles

To reduce the potential inaccuracies in the processing and evaluation of biopsy specimens it is important to look for modern solutions in order to maximize the efficiency of use of biopsy specimens. One of the solutions could be application of virtual microscopy having extensive mathematical basis with fractal and entropy considerations as well as technological support by appropriate software and hardware. Implementation of innovations into practice could significantly increase the effectiveness of liver biopsy specimens.

The digital image analysis [12-14] and computed morphometry in general is considered an important tool in pathology. It can decrease the workload of voluminous repeated measurements and increase the accuracy and objectiveness of the results. In several fields, e.g., immunohistochemical and molecular typing of breast cancer, the application of digital image analysis is already highly practical [13].

In virtual microscopy, the demands for mathematical basis are higher than in routine histology. This is illustrated by examples of entropy considerations, Delaunay's triangulation or fractal geometry and general non-Euclidean geometry for irregularly shaped biological objects [14-16]. Sophisticated software must be elaborated as well. Additional technical requirements exist for image resolution and size, fast wide-band data transfer as well as digital data storing [12, 13]. The slide scanners and visualisation software are available and improve continuously [12].

Computed morphometry becomes more practical in association with virtual microscopy and digital image analysis as well. As postulated in reference [16] the natural development of science occurs from the ability to recognize, name and classify the object (corresponding to the diagnosis, e.g., chronic viral hepatitis C) to semiquantitative, ordering measurements (e.g., the activity assessment by Knodell or any analogous scale), finally reaching quantitative characteristics. Descriptive diagnoses and semiquantitative estimates are widely used in the „classic" liver pathology. In order to gain sufficient reliability and fastness, scalar measurements would require digital assessment [16]. Computed morphometry on the basis of virtual microscopy is a way towards scalar measurements.

http://dx.doi.org/10.5772/52753

The virtual microscopy can be performed in two different ways. Interactive virtual microscopy by whole slide imaging leaves the conclusion in the hands of pathologist. It changes significantly the working tools from optical microscopy and subjective decisions to computer screen and objective measurements. The automated virtual microscopy is even more exciting as computer system should evaluate the diagnoses [14].

In liver pathology, the software develops regarding assessment of steatosis [17-19] and fibrosis [20-24]. Necroinflammatory changes can be quantified as well [16].

Regarding liver ultrastructure, morphometric evaluation of hepatocyte volume can have prognostic significance predicting survival as shown in liver cirrhosis associated with portal hypertension [25]. Morphometric analysis of liver parenchyma in different alcohol-related pathologic conditions has been tested with good results [26]. Thus, changes in the volume fraction of parenchymal interstitial space and in the surface density of hepatocyte plasma membrane, rough endoplasmic reticulum and outer mitochondrial membrane can be of importance for distinguishing between cirrhosis and non-cirrhotic states. Hepatocyte nuclear volume fraction measurement can predict the survival in case of cirrhosis. Interestingly, few images are necessary to perform these measurements thus helping to characterise even scarce tissue material [26].

Combination of multiplex quantum dot immunostaining with high resolution whole-slide digital imaging and automated image analysis has been described [27].

At present, the two most frequently studied targets for computer-assisted and/or digital image analysis in liver biopsies include steatosis and fibrosis.

4. Digital assessment of liver steatosis

Among Western population, liver steatosis is a frequent finding [28-29] as it is associated with such common factors as chronic viral hepatitis [19], alcohol drinking, diabetes mellitus or obesity [17]. It has been considered a risk factor for liver fibrosis [18, 19]. Steatosis, including non-alcoholic steatohepatitis [19] has become an important target in diagnostics and scientific research therefore highly reproducible measurements are necessary to evaluate the course of disease, outcome and effect of treatment. The biopsy is still considered a gold standard in the diagnosis and assessment of steatosis as the imaging including ultrasonography, computed tomography and magnetic resonance imaging can be affected by lower sensitivity [17, 30]. The severity of steatosis in liver biopsies can be graded by several semiquantitative systems (Table 2) assessing the eyeballed proportion of affected cells [30-35].

The present semiquantitative estimates are subjective and limit the possibilities of statistic analysis [18]. Numerical value, expressing the exact percentage of affected cells would be more reliable if an adequate biopsy is analysed. Such measurement is possible, especially in computer-assisted way, but it would require architecturally arranged count of nuclei and fat vacuoles per biopsy. Thus, the measurement would be time-consuming and accordingly expensive. On the other hand, steatosis is relatively easy target for digital quantification of the general fat amount due to the regular shape and distinct colour of fat vacuoles [18, 19]. The digital quantification of steatosis shows high reproducibility exceeding the quality of manual estimate [19]. Commercial software for image analysis has been recently employed and novel automated procedures are under development [18]. The estimate is more reliable if both morphological and chromatic operators are used in order to characterise lipid particles [18]. The fat vacuole is optically and geometrically simple object – optically empty after routine processing and deparaffinisation, thus white and rounded. If colour only is used for identification, however, the sinusoids, empty portal vessels and bile ducts [30] as well as glycogen nuclei in hepatocytes might be undertaken as false positives (Figure 1). The rounded shape of fat vacuole helps to exclude longitudinal or tangential sections of sinusoids, blood vessels and portal bile ducts. In haematoxylin-eosin stained sections, the colour contrast can be used to identify glycogen nuclei as in this case the optically empty space is surrounded by basophilic nuclear membrane in contrast to fat vacuole located in eosinophilic cytoplasm. Thus, the conclusion at present is to include both chromatic, size and shape assessment [18, 30]. Manual check can improve the accuracy in case of perpendicular sections of small vessels and fat cysts [30]. However, such control would increase the workload. The benefits of objectiveness and numerical value of continuous variable still remain. More studies would be necessary to determine how accurate the control must be for practical means; theoretically the significant vascular changes in cirrhosis point towards the idea that accurate identification of fat vacuoles is a must to avoid non-random errors.

Grading	Reference
Mild: less than 30% hepatocytes involved Moderate: 30-60% hepatocytes involved Severe: more than 60% hepatocytes involved	[31]
Grade 0 (no or minimal steatosis): less than 5% hepatocytes involved Grade 1: at least 5% but less than 25% hepatocytes involved Grade 2: at least 25% but less than 50% hepatocytes involved Grade 3: at least 50% but less than 75% hepatocytes involved Grade 4: at least 75% hepatocytes involved	[32]
Estimating the percentage of affected hepatocytes in 5% bands	[30]
Grade 0: less than 1% Grade 1: at least 1% but less than 6% hepatocytes involved Grade 2: at least 6% but less than 34% hepatocytes involved Grade 3: at least 34% but less than 67% hepatocytes involved Grade 4: at least 67% hepatocytes involved	[34] [35]
Grade 1: less than 33% Grade 2: at least 33% but less than 66% hepatocytes involved Grade 3: more than 66% hepatocytes involved	[33]

Table 2. The different grading systems of liver steatosis

http://dx.doi.org/10.5772/52753

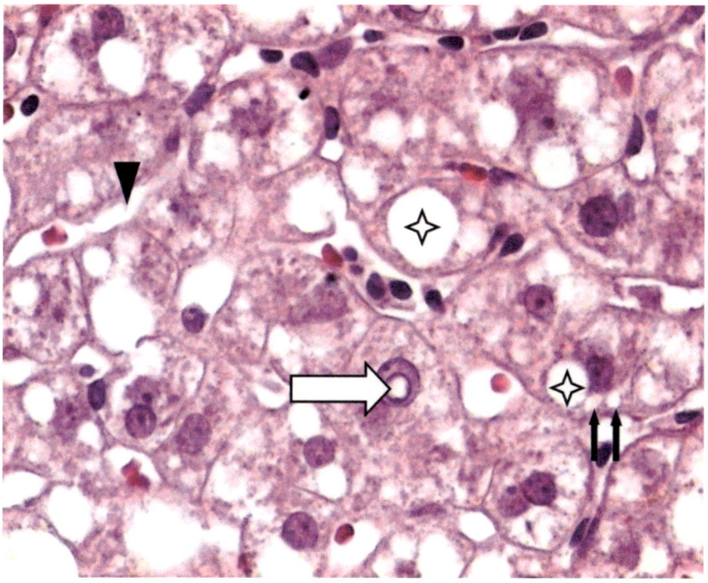

Figure 1. Liver steatosis. Note the macrovesicular steatosis (stars) characterised by size of fat vacuole exceeding the diameter of hepatocyte nucleus, and the microvesicular steatosis (small arrows) caused by fat vacuoles smaller than hepatocyte nucleus. The optically empty fat vacuoles must be promptly distinguished from glycogen nuclei (large arrow) and sinusoids (arrowhead). Haematoxylin-eosin stain, original magnification 400x

The fat stains as Sudan IV are well-known [4]. However, several researchers have reported technical problems. The artifacts can include deformation of lipid vacuoles as well as sinusoidal and background staining [17, 36-38]. The non-lipid positivity would limit the possibilities of colour analysis, and the deformation – of shape analysis. The practicality of osmium tetroxide stain is negatively affected by the necessity to use frozen tissue and by the toxicity of reagents [4].

Several research groups have reported that manual assessment of steatosis leads to significantly higher estimates than computer-obtained data [17, 19] regardless if area measurement or stereological point counting is used [30]. The coefficient can be as high as 3.78 [19]. Practicising physicians should remember that association between degree of steatosis and risk of cirrhosis is proved using manual assessments and thus the scales are adjusted for manual use. Consequently, interpretation of digital data cannot involve the use of unadjusted previous scales as risk classes.

It should be noted that the principal meaning of diagnosing steatosis is not affected by the evaluation method. Increasing steatosis percent is associated with advancing fibrosis stage both manually and digitally [19]. The data obtained by pathologist and automated software show close correlation [17]. After liver transplantation, aspartate aminotransferase, alanine aminotransferase and prothrombin time have shown better correlation with automated measurements in 4 of 5 posttransplant time points but the total bilirubin level correlated better with manual assessment in 3 of 5 time points. The graft survival showed a significant association with macrovesicular steatosis both in automated and manual measurements although the p value was less for automated measurement [17].

When analysing liver steatosis, the observations of higher accuracy in resin-embedded samples [18] request more technological progress in order to create methodology for easy use in routine samples.

Digital stereological point counting has been employed in liver steatosis evaluation as well [33]. The researchers have observed the same fact that manual semiquantitative assessment tends to be significantly higher. The lack of precision in manual evaluation can be related to the physiology of vision and processing of the visual information [19, 39].

Some researchers have also come to the conclusion that automated assessment of liver steatosis is more time-consuming than manual [30]. The time input for digital measurement is found to be threefold greater than for manual evaluation [19]. Although this opinion is based on trustable experience, half of the problem is solved already as the whole slide imaging eliminates the need to choose appropriate number of representative fields submitted for analysis and the necessity for human participation in the obtaining and archiving of digital images. Besides the whole slide imaging, the degree of automatisation must be further increased: optimal software abolishes the manual correction of object inclusion into measurements. However, this deserves morphologically correct mathematical model. Other groups have considered computer-aided morphometry to be fast and objective [16].

5. Digital assessment of inflammation in liver biopsy

The computer-aided assessment of necroinflammatory processes in chronic viral hepatitis has been tested. To perform this, immunohistochemical visualisation is necessary in order to highlight inflammatory cells. The application of immunohistochemistry increases the expenses. This drawback can be counterbalanced by gains of rapid measurement, resulting in rigorous results expressed in scalar numbers as well as by complete characteristics more exactly reflecting the status of the whole organ [16].

The assessment of hepatic fibrosis and the closely related architectural deformities as bridging fibrosis and liver cirrhosis have important role in the diagnostics, treatment and prognostic evaluation of chronic liver diseases [24]. The studies of liver fibrosis are facilitated by standard use of special stains for the routine evaluation of liver biopsies in case of diffuse liver disease. Masson's trichrome is an efficient method to highlight fibrosis [3]. The sharp contrast between blue collagen and red parenchyma allows visualisation of even small excess amounts of collagen [23]. Sirius red stain has also been employed [21, 40]; it has the benefit of selective staining of collagen but not proteoglycans [22]. Not surprisingly, comparatively many authors have applied digital image analysis to quantify fibrosis in liver tissue [24]. Validation studies of computer-assisted morphometry have also been performed [21]. Besides the well-developed methodology including software, the application of computer analysis has resulted in exact numerical data allowing detection of interesting biological relationships. For instance, the correlation of fibrosis burden with end-stage liver disease score, serum total bilirubin and international standard ratio of prothrombin has been shown in hepatitis B-related decompensated cirrhosis. Thus, the correlation between the amount of connective tissue in cirrhotic liver and

http://dx.doi.org/10.5772/52753

hepatic functional reserve was demonstrated [24]. The problem was insufficient accuracy of computer-assisted morphometry [21] manifesting as inter-observer differences. Poor correlation of the fibrosis area with Ishak staging score has been observed as well [21]. Other scientists have also found that analysis of early fibrosis necessities qualitative assessment despite the general correlation between amount of connective tissue and Ishak grade of fibrosis [20]. Tissue geometry differences in subsequent sections also can be more accurately classified by human eye [22]. Full section digital analysis seems to be important [20].

Digital image analysis for the evaluation of fibrosis in chronic viral hepatitis C has been studied also as mentioned in references [41-42]. Automatic quantification of liver fibrosis including the validation of the method has been performed as described in reference [43]. Other investigators have employed computerised image analysis for the evaluation of fibrosis as well [44-47]. In most investigations, correlation between digital and manual semiquantitative score has been shown [20, 44-47]. However, the digital data do not allow to differentiate between low stages of fibrosis [20, 45, 47].

6. Digital biopsy analysis for inflammatory liver lesion: Future begins today

The incorporation of Mandelbrot's fractal geometry [48] into the digital evaluation of liver biopsy for chronic hepatitis has brought revolutionary changes [40].

The short description of fractal is provided in Table 3; detailed characteristics can be found in recent reviews [49].

Definition and essential features of fractal	The fractal is a mathematical object characterised by self-similar patterns. At every scale, fractal shows (infinitely) either the same structure or is at least similar to other scales. The complexity is retained independently of magnification. Thus, although fractal curve is one dimensional similarly to regular line, the fractal dimension is greater than topological dimension. Due to the infinite similarity, fractals cannot be measured in traditional ways. Although fractals have got significant popularity due to their beauty, the importance of fractal theory is in the mathematical basis and the ability to describe, among other processes, the biological phenomena.
Fractals in nature: selected examples	Beds of rivers, irregularity of coastline, profiles of mountain chain, clouds
Fractals in biology: selected examples	Branching of blood vessels or bronchi, the invasive edge of tumour, neurons. See also Figure 2-6
Peculiarities of fractals in biology	Biological fractal-like objects have limited range of self-similarity upon magnification thus behaving as random fractals, in contrast to mathematical/geomaterical constructs with unlimited level of complexity (self-exact fractals)

Table 3. The characteristics of fractals

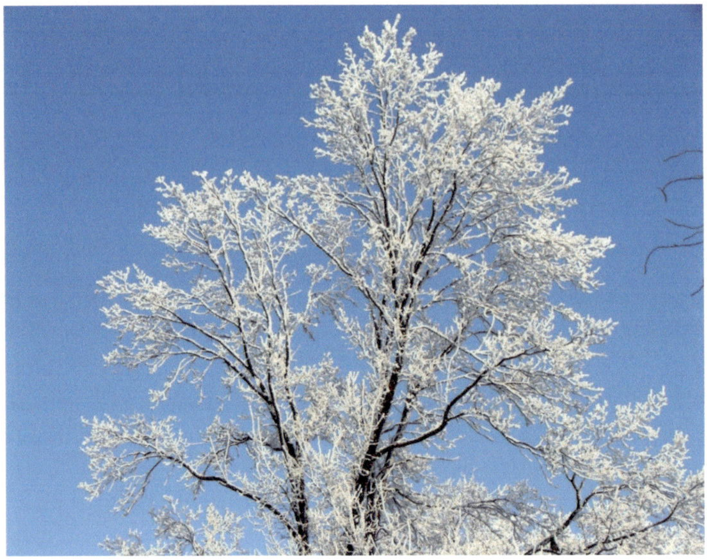

Figure 2. Highly irregular structure of biological object. Use of Mandelbrot's fractal geometry is suggested to describe targets with remarkable degree of complexity and irregularity. Note also the similarity of complex, branching outline with Figures 4 and 5

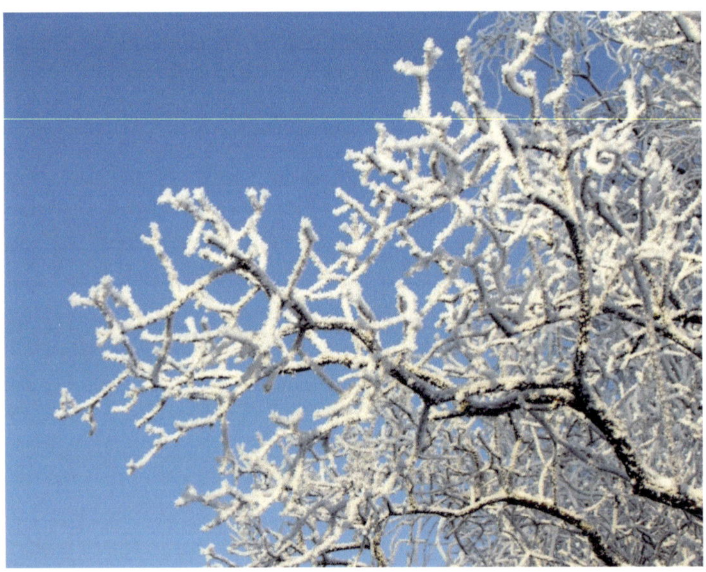

Figure 3. Retained irregularity of the biological structure at higher magnification: note the remarkable similarity with Figure 2. The persisting complexity at different levels of magnification is another feature suggesting the necessity for fractal analysis. The inflammation in liver biopsy (shown in Figures 4 and 5) depicts analogous features

Hurst's exponent is another albeit related mathematical construct with major meaning in the digital analysis of liver biopsy. It was first used to study the variation in water flow in Nile basin during the construction of the Aswan dam [16, 50]. In general, it can be used to detect the irregularity – a key parameter analysing the activity of inflammation in the liver as the active inflammation manifests with periportal piecemeal necrosis causing irregularity in the normally smooth border of portal field. Hurst's exponent also can be detected by fractal mathematics. It can describe quantitatively the deviation from smooth contour in natural fractal objects.

To detect the border of inflammatory cell cluster, Delaunay's triangulation can be used with success. In general, Delaunay's triangulation involves set of points in such way that no point is inside the circle drawn through 3 points. It maximizes the minimum angle avoiding narrow triangles. If circle drawn through 2 input points contain the third point in the outside, these points form Delaunay's triangle. The method can be used to mesh the space. By this triangulation, lines were drawn in the scanned image of liver biopsy through each pair of adjacent inflammatory cells resulting in network of triangles showing common border. The most external triangle short sides formed the border of inflammatory cell infiltrate. The triangle side was defined as appropriately short if it was equal of less than 20 microns based on empiric analysis. After the cluster has been outlined, both the amount (by area) of inflammatory cells and the border irregularity and area of cluster-affected tissue can be evaluated [16].

The mathematical basis of so-called geometry of irregularity (Figure 2-3) has allowed to detect the amount of residual liver parenchyma, inflammation (Figure 4-5) and fibrosis (Figure 6-7) as well as to provide index characterising the appropriateness of liver tissue structure (named tectonic index by the authors).

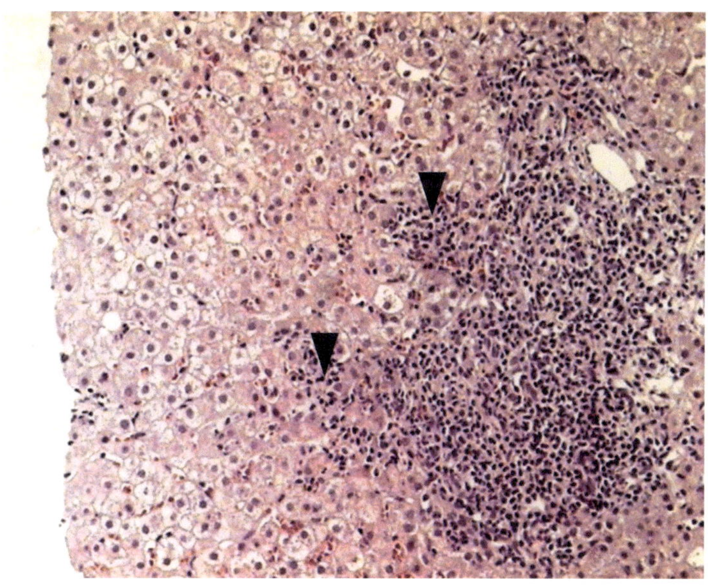

Figure 4. Irregular outline (arrowheads) of portal field in chronic active hepatitis. Haematoxylin-eosin stain, original magnification 100x

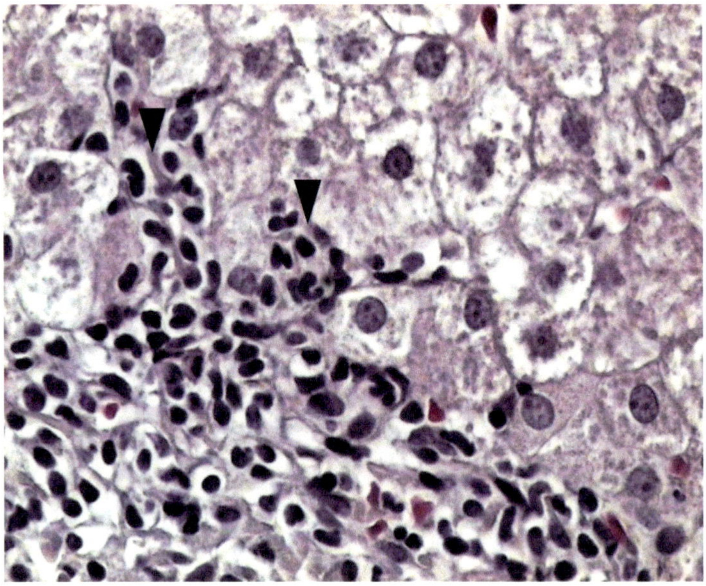

Figure 5. Branching pattern (arrowheads) of periportal inflammatory infiltrate. Note the remarkable similarity with Figure 4 analogous to the relationship between Figures 2-3. The fractal nature of inflammation is thus highlighted. Haematoxylin-eosin stain, original magnification 400x

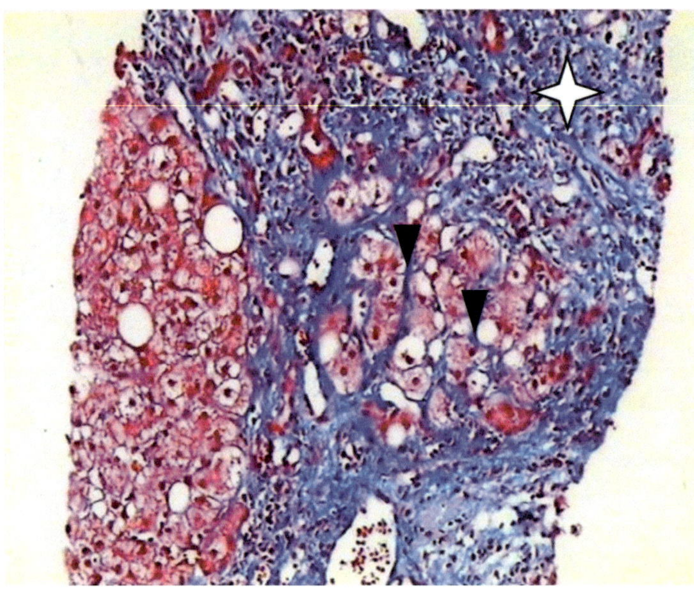

Figure 6. Branching outline of connective tissue fields in liver cirrhosis. Note both the large areas of connective tissue (star) and the thin septa (arrowheads). Masson's trichrome stain, original magnification 100x

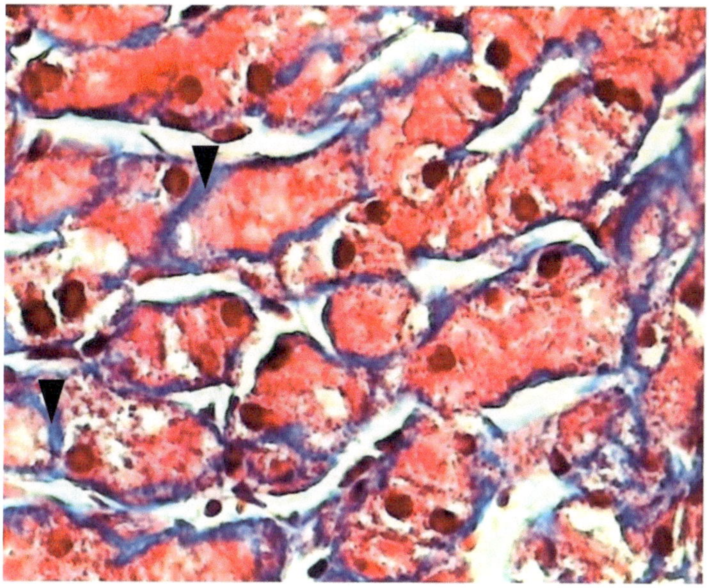

Figure 7. Branching pattern of connective tissue fields in arachnoid liver fibrosis (arrowhead). Masson's trichrome stain, original magnification 400x

The Dioguardi Histological Metriser machine, described in reference [40] is able to produce measurements and even simple diagnoses, working with reasonable speed. The relevant equipment ensures microscope focusing and full slide scanning, and determines the above mentioned parameters excluding any unfilled spaces as vessels, sinusoids, biliary ducts and artifactual holes. The system is able to identify and exclude the Glisson's capsule from the analysis. Colour thresholds are used to select the areas of interest. The inflammatory cells are identified by immunohistochemical visualisation of leukocyte common antigen. For the analysis, the inflammatory cell clusters are outlined by imaginary line connecting the centres of the outermost cells; after that the area of clusters is measured. Thinking in the usual terms, the portal and periportal infiltrates are characterised by this measurement; the portal fibrosis also can influence this measurement providing homing space for inflammatory infiltrate. The area of extra-cluster inflammatory cells is measured separately; these could mostly correspond to intralobular infiltrate. When analysing fibrosis, area of fibrotic tissue is measured. The wrinkledness is detected as the ratio between the perimeter and area of an object. As portal field in healthy liver is smooth, the concept of wrinkledness is an efficient way to detect periportal inflammation and portal fibrosis. The irregularity of collagen islets necessitates the correction by fractal dimension; the fibrotic foci are considered truncated planar fractals. The residual parenchyma is characterised by the tissue area that is not occupied by inflammatory cells and fibrosis. Finally, the loss of order is characterised mathematically. In order to characterise the course of the disease in analogue with the usual staging, the individual fibrosis scalar is compared with the curve of fibrosis development over the course of disease detecting the percentage of the disease course before collagen deposition reaches the maximal tolerated level of 32% [40] or approximately 36% in liver cirrhosis necessitating liver transplantation [24]. Thus, three approaches are combined: the outlines of regular structures as vacuoles are characterised by traditional, non-fractal geometry, the area of fibrosis and parenchyma are detected using the traditional measurements corrected by the fractal dimension, and the tectonic index is based on the relationships between the Euclidean and fractal dimensions of liver tissue. One of the many positive features of this system is the ability to generate continuous scalar variables. When analysing dynamics in repeated liver biopsies by scalar data, naturally, less biopsies are characterised as lacking significant changes.

Although fractal concept is used in medicine, including at least microscopy, neuroscience and ophthalmology as well as automated measurements not limited to pathology [49, 51, 52], the study described in reference [40] is remarkable as it is highly sophisticated and practical; it is understandable that the research group considers their machine as an intelligent collaborator – and this is exactly the way how future biopsy analysis should proceed.

7. Functional liver tissue analysis in biopsy

The diagnostic evaluation of liver biopsy is mostly based on panel of histochemical stains including hematoxylin-eosin [2], Masson's trichrome [3], PAS [5] and Perl's [1] stains as well as others by necessity. These visualisation techniques should be complemented by various "- omics" tools [27] to gain more data on the function of liver cells. The cytokines, inflammatory mediators, viral proteins, cell cycle proteins and apoptosis markers can be detected; metabolic pathways can be investigated as well. At present, most or proteomic and genetic studies are carried out for scientific research in order to outline the pathogenesis of different diseases. However, in future it could be advisable to include such studies with validated value in the routine investigation as technically the amount of tissue in liver biopsy is sufficient.

Cytokine expression can be analysed, e.g., TGF, EGFR and others [25]. When studying interleukin-6 (IL-6) expression in liver biopsies, higher IL-6 expression was found in non-alcoholic steatohepatitis than in steatosis. Correlation between IL-6 expression and degree of inflammation and stage of fibrosis was detected as well [53]. Due to the complex nature of cytokine action, wide spectrum of different molecules and their receptors must be analysed in details in order to avoid insignificant or contradictory results. This leads to a clear-cut necessity for virtual microscopy and digital image analysis. Toll-like receptor-4 (TLR4) expression can be analysed in liver biopsy by immunohistochemistry. The expression of TLR4 has been shown in hepatic progenitor cells and interlobular bile duct epithelium in correlation with stage of liver disease, grade of liver inflammation and activity of portal/septal myofibroblasts [54]. The expression of interferon stimulated gene 15 can be analysed by IHC at protein level; up-regulation in hepatocytes is more pronounced in patients not responding to interferon / ribavirin treatment in contrast to predominant expression in Kuppfer cells in treatment responders [55]. Proteomic studies including immunohistochemistry in liver biopsy have targeted cell structure-associated proteins - actin, tropomyosin, transgelin and human microfibril-associated protein 4 in order to identify biomarkers of liver cirrhosis [56]. COX-2 is over-expressed in chronic hepatitis C and the expression decreases following treatment with interferon alpha regardless of sustained virological response [57]. Increased endoglin and TGF beta 1 expression is significantly associated with progressive hepatic fibrosis in chronic viral hepatitis C [58].

Cell cycle analysis can add valuable information [59]; digital image analysis should be added in the logistics again. Arrested cell cycle status has been demonstrated in chronic hepatitis C infection analysing the expression of mini-chromosome maintenance protein-2 as higher sensitivity proliferation marker, G1 phase marker cyclin D1, S phase marker cyclin A, cell cycle regulators p21 and p53, apoptotic protein caspase 3 and anti-apoptotic protein Bcl-2 [60, 61]. When analysing liver biopsies from patients with chronic viral hepatitis C, higher G1 and lower S phase fractions has been found also by Werling *et al.*, employing image analysis method [59]. Apoptosis-related pathways can be explorated including evaluation of Bax, Bcl-xL and Bcl-2 proteins [62]. Thus, hepatitis C virus infection can deregulate the cellular processes [63] and it can be practical to reveal the way and degree of the regulatory shift.

Viral antigens including hepatitis C antigen can be detected in liver tissue by immunohistochemistry [64]; the finding can be helpful in cases with difficult differential diagnosis or combined liver pathology. The association of expression pattern with fibrosis may suggest pathogenetically important information as well [64].

Metabolic pathways can be evaluated in liver biopsy. For instance, widespread expression of vitamin D receptor has been shown in the hepatocytes and inflammatory cells in case of chronic liver disease including non-alcoholic steatohepatitis and chronic viral hepatitis C. The expression decreases as the liver histology is damaged [65].

Inflammatory cells are as important components in diffuse liver disease as the hepatocytes. Thus, higher numbers of intrahepatic follicular T-helper lymphocytes in conjunction with IL28B polymorphism analysis is found to be strongly predictive of treatment response using pegylated interferon and ribavirin [66]. CD4+ regulatory T cells can be evaluated [67].

Logistic structures have been implemented to develop next generation toolkits for automated image analysis to enable quantification of molecular markers. The group of researchers [27] have collaborated within open source image analysis project [68] to reach effective output by combination of quantitative analysis, multiplex quantum dot (nanoparticle) staining and high resolution whole slide imaging to detect nine different fluorescent signals for multiple antigens [27].

DNA microarray technology has enabled genome-wide analysis of gene transcript levels. This technology has been applied in order to compare gene expression profiles at different stages of chronic hepatitis C and hepatocellular carcinoma in the setting of hepatitis virus C infection [63, 69]. Hundreds of genes involved in carcinogenesis, cell growth, proliferation and death are differently expressed in advanced viral hepatitis C in comparison to early viral hepatitis C or non-viral hepatitis [63]. In chronic hepatitis C, the up-regulation involves genes related to metabolism and immune responses. In hepatocellular carcinoma arising in hepatitis C patients, genes associated with cell cycle, growth, proliferation and apoptosis are up-regulated [69]. Chronic hepatitis B and autoimmune liver disease have been studied by this technology as well [70]. In advanced chronic viral hepatitis B, genes associated with extracellular matrix turnover, cell growth and DNA repair are up-regulated but the expression of genes regulating complement activation and innate immune response is decreased. In early disease stages, the gene expression is different in case of chronic viral hepatitis B, autoimmune hepatitis and primary biliary cirrhosis. Chronic viral hepatitis B is associated with expression of genes considering chemotaxis and cell homeostasis; autoimmune hepatitis – with down-regulation of genes associated with protein binding, but primary biliary cirrhosis in early stages involves the actin and myosin gene expression. As chronic viral hepatitis B progresses, the expression of genes regarding signalling pathway, cell communication, collagen turnover, chemokine ligands and metallothionein changes [70]. The findings are of major interest displaying the pathogenesis of different inflammatory liver diseases and neoplastic transformation. Diagnostic consequences should follow soon as the differential diagnosis of inflammatory liver diseases regarding aetiology can represent a difficult task.

The level of mRNA can be post-transciptionally regulated by micro RNA (miRNA). The regulation of biological processes by miRNA is shown also in case of such canonical diffuse liver disease as chronic viral hepatitis C. Technological studies have been conducted using biopsy material [71]. Transcriptome analysis has shown prognostic value, e.g., in order to predict the severity of fibrosis progression after liver transplantation in recurrent viral hepatitis C patients [72].

8. Conclusions

Liver biopsy investigation could soon shift from routine light microscopy to digital image analysis by virtual microscopy and incorporation of numerical measurements in conjunction with integrated analysis of cell functions at DNA, RNA, protein and signalling level. This shift could lead from static to dynamic tissue evaluation. The technological logistics should include the best standards of tissue fixation, processing, microtomy and visualisation complemented by automated immunostaining, full slide scanning to ensure complete digital analysis and optimal choice of software considering the biological appropriateness of the analysis algorithm.

As the diagnostic electron microscopy is continually developing, we expect that in future it will be used in hepatology as an auxiliary method, based on digital analysis of electronograms. Liver biopsy analysis using transmission and scanning electron microscope could continue to provide important additional information in diagnostic hepatology and scientific research of liver diseases, as well as it could help to study unresolved molecular mechanisms regulating liver cells' functions. In future the ultrastructural studies of liver biopsy in hepatology will probably be associated with assessment of liver tissues in cases of liver transplantation, with studies of new medicinal products – detection or exclusion of their po-

http://dx.doi.org/10.5772/52753

tential hepatotoxic effect, with identification of viruses, as well as with determination of influence of various environmental hazards.

Author details

Ludmila Viksna[1,2], Ilze Strumfa[1], Boriss Strumfs[3], Valda Zalcmane[1], Andrejs Ivanovs[1] and Valentina Sondore[2]

1 Riga Stradins University, Riga, Latvia

2 Riga Eastern Clinical University Hospital, Riga, Latvia

3 Latvian Institute of Organic Synthesis, Riga, Latvia

References

[1] Churukian CJ. Pigments and minerals. In: Theory and practice of histological techniques, 5th ed. Ed. by Bancroft JD, Gamble M. Churchill Livingstone, Edinburgh, 2002. p243-267.

[2] Gamble M, Wilson I. The hematoxylins and eosin. In: Theory and practice of histological techniques, 5th ed. Ed. by Bancroft JD, Gamble M. Churchill Livingstone, Edinburgh, 2002. p125-138.

[3] Jones ML. Connective tissues and stains. In: Theory and practice of histological techniques, 5th ed. Ed. by Bancroft JD, Gamble M. Churchill Livingstone, Edinburgh, 2002. p139-162.

[4] Jones ML. Lipids. In: Theory and practice of histological techniques, 5th ed. Ed. by Bancroft JD, Gamble M. Churchill Livingstone, Edinburgh, 2002. p201-230.

[5] Totty BA. Mucins. In: Theory and practice of histological techniques, 5th ed. Ed. by Bancroft JD, Gamble M. Churchill Livingstone, Edinburgh, 2002. p163-200.

[6] Kanel GC, Korula J. Atlas of liver pathology, 3rd ed. Elsevier Saunders, USA, 2011.

[7] Knodell RG,Ishak KG, Black WC, Chen TS, Craig R, Kaplowitz N, Kiernan TW, Wollman J. Formulation and application of a numerical scoring system for assessing histological activity in asymptomatic chronic active hepatitis. Hepatology, 1981; 1:431-435.

[8] Scheuer PJ. Classification of chronic viral hepatitis: a need for reassessment. J Hepatol, 1991; 13:372-374.

[9] Ishak K, Baptista A, Bianchi L, Callea F, De Groote J, Gudat F, Denk H, Desmet V, Korb G, MacSween RN. Histological grading and staging of chronic hepatitis. J Hepatol, 1995; 22:696-699.

[10] Bedossa P, Poynard T. An algorithm for the grading of activity in chronic hepatitis C. The METAVIR Cooperative Study Group. Hepatology, 1996; 24:289-293.

[11] Shiha G, Zalata K. Ishak versus METAVIR: terminology, convertibility and correlation with laboratory changes in chronic hepatitis C. In: Liver Biopsy, ISBN: 978-953-307-644-7. Ed. by Takahashi H. InTech, 2011.

[12] Giansanti D, Grigioni M, D'Avenio G, Morelli S, Maccioni G, Bondi A, Giovagnoli MR. Virtual microscopy and digital cytology: state of the art. Ann Ist Super Sanita, 2010; 46(2):115-122.

[13] Pantanowitz L, Valenstein PN, Evans AJ, Kaplan KJ, Pfeifer JD, Wilbur DC, Collins LC, Colgan TJ. Review of the current state of whole slide imaging in pathology. J Pathol Inform, 2011: 2:36, doi:10.4103/2153-3589.83746.

[14] Kayser K, Gortler J, Borkenfeld S, Kayser G. How to measure diagnosis-associated information in virtual slides. Diagn Pathol, 2011; 6 (Suppl 1):S9.

[15] Grizzi F, Ceva-Grimaldi G, Dioguardi N. Fractal geometry: a useful tool for quantifying irregular lesions in human liver biopsy specimens. Ital J Anat Embryol, 2001; 106(2 Suppl 1):337-346.

[16] Dioguardi N, Franceschini B, Russo C, Grizzi F. Computer-aided morphometry of liver inflammation in needle biopsies. World J Gastroenterol, 2005; 11(44):6995-7000.

[17] Marsman H, Matsushita T, Dierkhising R, Kremers W, Rosen C, Burgart L, Nyberg SL. Assessment of donor liver steatosis: pathologist or automated software? Hum Pathol, 2004; 35:430-435.

[18] Liquori GE, Calamita G, Cascella D, Mastrodonato M, Portincasa P, Ferri D. An innovative methodology for the automated morphometric and quantitative estimation of liver steatosis. Histol Histopathol, 2009; 24(1):49-60.

[19] Rawlins SR, El-Zammar O, Zinkievich JM, Newman N, Levine RA. Digital quantification is more precise than traditional semiquantitation of hepatic steatosis: correlation with fibrosis in 220 treatment-naive patients with chronic hepatitis C. Dig Dis Sci, 2010; 55(7):2049-2057.

[20] O'Brien MJ, Keating NM, Elderiny S, Cerda S, Keaveny AP, Afdhal NH, Nunes DP. An assessment of digital image analysis to measure fibrosis in liver biopsy specimens of patients with chronic hepatitis C. Am J Clin Pathol, 2000; 114(5):712-718.

[21] Maduli E, Andorno S, Rigamonti C, Capelli F, Morelli S, Colombi S, Nicosia G, Boldorini R, Abate M, Sartori M. Evaluation of liver fibrosis in chronic hepatitis C with a computer-assisted morphometric method. Ann Ital Med Int, 2002; 17(4):242-247.

[22] Wright M, Thursz M, Pullen R, Thomas H, Goldin R. Quantitative versus morphological assessment of liver fibrosis: semi-quantitative scores are more robust than digital image fibrosis area estimation. Liver Int, 2003; 23:28-34.

[23] Dahab GM, Kheriza MM, El-Beltagi HM, Fouda AMM, El-Din OAS. Digital quantification of fibrosis in liver biopsy sections: description of a new method by Photoshop software. J Gastroenterol Hepatol, 2004; 19:78-85.

[24] Xie SB, Ma C, Lin CS, Zhang Y, Zhu JY, Ke WM. Collagen proportionate area of liver tissue determined by digital image analysis in patients with HBV-related decompensated cirrhosis. Hepatobiliary Pancreat Dis Int, 2011; 10(5):497-501.

[25] Khan S, Dodson A, Campbell F, Kawesha A, Grime JS, Critchley M, Sutton R. Prognostic potential of hepatocyte volume and cytokine expression in cirrhotic portal hypertension. J Gastroenterol Hepatol, 2005; 20(10):1519-1526.

[26] Ryoo JW, Buschmann RJ. Morphometry of liver parenchyma in needle biopsy specimens from patients with alcoholic liver disease: preliminary variables for the diagnosis and prognosis of cirrhosis. Mod Pathol, 1989; 2(4):382-389.

[27] Isse K, Grama K, Abbott IM, Lesniak A, Lunz JG, Lee WM, Specht S, Corbitt N, Mizuguchi Y, Roysam B, Demetris AJ. Adding value to liver (and allograft) biopsy evaluation using a combination using a combination of multiplex quantum dot immunostaining, high-resolution whole-slide digital imaging, and automated image analysis. Clin Liver Dis, 2010; 14(4):669-685.

[28] Bellentani S, Tiribelli C, Saccoccio G, Sodde M, Fratti N, De Martin C, Cristianini G. Prevalence of chronic liver disease in the general population of northern Italy: The Dionysos Study. Hepatology, 1994; 20(6):1442-1449.

[29] Hornboll P, Olsen TS. Fatty changes in the liver: the relation to age, overweight and diabetes mellitus. Acta Pathol Microbiol Immunol Scand A, 1982; 90(3):199-205.

[30] Turlin B, Ramm GA, Purdie DM, Laine F, Perrin M, Deugnier Y, Macdonald GA. Assessment of hepatic steatosis: comparison of quantitative and semiquantitative methods in 108 liver biopsies. Liver Int, 2009; 29(4):530-535; doi:10.1111/j.1478-3231.2008.01874.x

[31] Ploeg RJ, D'Alessandro AM, Knechtle SJ, Stegall MD, Pirsch JD, Hoffmann RM, Sasaki T, Sollinger HW, Belzer FO, Kalayoglu M. Risk factors for primary dysfunction after liver transplantation: A multivariate analysis. Transplantation, 1993; 55:807-813.

[32] Turlin B, Mendler MH, Moirand R, Guyader D, Guillygomarc'h A, Deugnier Y. Histologic features of the liver in insulin resistance-associated iron overload. A study of 139 patients. Am J Clin Pathol, 2001; 116:263-270.

[33] Franzen LE, Ekstedt M, Kechagias S, Bodin L. Semiquantitative evaluation overestimates the degree of steatosis in liver biopsies: a comparison to stereological point counting. Mod Pathol, 2005; 18(7):912-916.

[34] Lok AS, Everhart JE, Chung RT, Padmanabhan L, Greenson JK, Shiffman ML, Everson GT, Lindsay KL, Bonkovsky HL, Di Bisceglie AM, Lee WM, Morgan TR, Ghany MG, Morishima C; HALT-C Trial Group. Hepatic steatosis in hepatitis C: Comparison of diabetic and nondiabetic patients in the hepatitis C antiviral long-term treatment against cirrhosis trial. Clin Gastroenterol Hepatol, 2007; 5(2):245-254.

[35] Lok AS, Everhart JE, Chung RT, Kim HY, Everson GT, Hoefs JC, Greenson JK, Sterling RK, Lindsay KL, Lee WM, Di Bisceglie AM, Bonkovsky HL, Ghany MG, Morishima C; HALT-C Trial Group. Evolution of hepatic steatosis in patients with advanced hepatitis C: results from the hepatitis C antiviral long-term treatment against cirrhosis (HALT-C) trial. Hepatology, 2009; 49(6):1828-1837.

[36] Markin RS, Wisecarver JL, Radio SJ, Stratta RJ, Langnas AN, Hirst K, Shaw BW Jr. Frozen section evaluation of donor livers before transplantation. Transplantation, 1993; 56(6):1403-1409.

[37] Trevisani F, Colantoni A, Caraceni P, Van Thiel DH. The use of donor fatty liver for liver transplantation: a challenge or a quagmire? J Hepatol, 1996; 24(1):114-121.

[38] Fukumoto S, Fujimoto T. Deformation of lipid droplets in fixed samples. Histochem Cell Biol, 2002; 118:423-428.

[39] Redden JP, Hoch SJ. The presence of variety reduces perceived quantity. J Consum Res, 2009; 36:406-417.

[40] Dioguardi N, Grizzi F, Fiamengo B, Russo C. Metrically measuring liver biopsy: A chronic hepatitis B and C computer-aided morphological description. World J Gastroenterol, 2008; 14(48):7335-7344.

[41] Standish RA, Cholongitas E, Dhillon A, Burroughs AK, Dhillon AP. An appraisal of the histopathological assessment of liver fibrosis. Gut, 2006; 55:569-578.

[42] Calvaruso V, Burroughs AK, Standish R, Manousou P, Grillo F, Leandro D, Maimone S, Plequezuelo M, Xirouchakis I, Guerrini GP, Patch D, Yu D, O'Beirne J, Dhillon AP. Computer-assisted image analysis of liver collagen: relationship to Ishak scoring and hepatic venous pressure gradient. Hepatology, 2009; 49:1236-1244.

[43] Masseroli M, Caballero T, O'Valle F, Del Moran RM, Perez-Milena A, Del Moral RG. Automatic quantification of liver fibrosis: design and validation of a new image analysis method: comparison with semi-quantitative indexes of fibrosis. J Hepatol, 2000; 32(3):453-464.

[44] Chevallier M, Guerret S, Chossegros P, Gerard F, Grimaud JA. A histological semi-quantitative scoring system for evaluation of hepatic fibrosis in needle liver biopsy specimens: comparison with morphometric studies. Hepatology, 1994; 20(2):349-355.

[45] Kage M, Shimamatu K, Nakashima E, Kojiro M, Inoue O, Yano M. Long-term evolution of fibrosis from chronic hepatitis to cirrhosis in patients with hepatitis C: morphometric analysis of repeated biopsies. Hepatology, 1997; 25(4):1028-1031.

[46] Duchatelle V, Marcellin P, Giostra E, Bregeaud L, Pouteau M, Boyer N, Auperin A, Guerret S, Erlinger S, Henin D, Degott C. Changes in liver fibrosis at the end of alpha interferon therapy and 6 to 18 months later in patients with chronic hepatitis C: quantitative assessment by a morphometric method. J Hepatol, 1998; 29(1):20-28.

[47] Pilette C, Rousselet MC, Bedossa P, Chappard D, Oberti F, Rifflet H, Maiga MY, Gallois Y, Cales P. Histopathological evaluation of liver fibrosis: quantitative image analysis vs. semi-quantitative scores. J Hepatol, 1998; 28(3):439-446.

[48] Mandelbrot BB. The fractal geometry of nature. Freeman, San Francisko, 1982.

[49] Landini G. Fractals in microscopy. J Microsc, 2011; 241(1):1-8.

[50] Hurst HE. Lon-term storage capacity of reservoirs. Trans Amer Soc Civ Eng, 1951; 116:770-808.

[51] Karperien AL, Jelinek HF, Buchan AM. Box-counting analysis of microglia form in schizophrenia, Alzheimer's disease and affective disorder. Fractals, 2008; 16(2):103, doi: 10.1142/S0218348X08003880.

[52] Karperien A, Jelinek HF, Leandro JJ, Soares JV, Cesar RM Jr., Luckie A. Automated detection of proliferative retinopathy in clinical practice. Clin Ophthalmol, 2008; 2(1): 109-122.

[53] Wieckowska A, Papouchado BG, Li Z, Lopez R, Zein NN, Feldstein AE. Increased hepatic and circulating interleukin-6 levels in human nonalcoholic steatohepatitis. Am J Gastroenterol, 2008; 103(6):1372-1379.

[54] Vespasiani-Gentilucci U, Carotti S, Onetti-Muda A, Perrone G, Ginanni-Corradini S, Latasa MU, Avila MA, Carpino G, Picardi A, Morini S. Toll-like receptor-4 expression by hepatic progenitor cells and biliary epithelial cells in HCV-realted chronic liver disease. Mod Pathol, 2012; 25(4):576-589.

[55] Chen L, Borozan I, Sun J, Guindi M, Fischer S, Feld J, Anand N, Heathcote J, Edwards AM, McGilvray ID. Cell-type specific gene expression signature in liver underlies response to interferon therapy in chronic hepatitis C infection. Gastroenterology, 2010; 138(3):1123-1133.

[56] Molleken C, Sitek B, Henkel C, Poschmann G, Sipos B, Wiese S, Warscheid B, Broelsch C, Reiser M, Friedman SL, Tornoe I, Schlosser A, Kloppel G, Schmiegel W, Meyer HE, Holmskov U, Stuhler K. Detection of novel biomarkers of liver cirrhosis by proteomic analysis. Hepatology, 2009; 49(4):1257-1266.

[57] Manning DS, Sheehan KM, Byrne MF, Kay EW, Murray FE. Cyclooxygenase-2 expression in chronic hepatitis C and the effect of interferon alpha treatment. J Gastroenterol Hepatol, 2007; 22(10):1633-1637.

[58] Clemente M, Nunez O, Lorente R, Rincon D, Matilla A, Salcedo M, Catalina MV, Ripoll C, Iacono OL, Banares R, Clemente G, Garcia-Monzon C. Increased intrahepatic and circulating levels of endoglin, a TGF-beta1 c-receptor, in patients with chronic

hepatitis C virus infection: relationship to histological and serum markers of hepatic fibrosis. J Viral Hepat, 2006; 13(9):625-632.

[59] Werling K, Szentirmay Z, Szepesi A, Schaff Z, Szalay F, Szabo Z, Telegdy L, David K, Stotz G, Tulassay Z. Hepatocyte proliferation and cell cycle phase fractions in chronic viral hepatitis C by image analysis method. Eur J Gastroenterol Hepatol, 2010; 13(5): 489-493.

[60] Marshall A, Rushbrook S, Daves SE, Morris LS, Scott IS, Vowler SL, Coleman N, Alexander G. Relation between hepatocyte G1 arrest, impaired hepatic regeneration, and fibrosis in chronic hepatitis C virus infection. Gastroenterology, 2005; 128(1): 33-42.

[61] Sarfraz S, Hamid S, Siddiqui A, Hussain S, Pervez S, Alexander G. Altered expression of cell cycle and apoptotic proteins in chronic hepatitis C virus infection. BMC Microbiology, 2008; 8:133, doi:10.1186/1471-2180-8-133.

[62] Piekarska A, Kubiak R, Omulecka A, Szymczak W, Piekarski J. Expression of Bax, Bcl-xL and Bcl-2 proteins in relation to grade of inflammation and stage of fibrosis in chronic hepatitis C. Histopathology, 2007; 50(7):928-935.

[63] Khalid SS, Hamid S, Siddiqui AA, Qureshi A, Qureshi N. Gene profiling of early and advanced liver disease in chronic hepatitis C patients. Hepatol Int, 2011; 5(3):782-788.

[64] Shiha GE, Zalata KR, Abdalla AF, Mohamed MK. Immunohistochemical identification of HCV target antigen in paraffin-embedded liver tissue: reproducibility and staining patterns. Liver Int, 2005; 25(2):254-260.

[65] Barchetta I, Carotti S, Labbadia G, Vespasiani GU, Onetti MA, Angelico F, Silecchia G, Leonetti F, Fraioli A, Picardi A, Morini S, Cavallo M. Liver VDR, CYP2R1 and CYP27A1 expression: Relationship with liver histology and vitamin D3 levels in patients with NASH or HCV hepatitis. Hepatology, 2012, Epub ahead of print on Jun 30, 2012; doi: 10.1002/hep.25930.

[66] Tripodo C, Petta S, Guarnotta C, Pipitone R, Cabibi D, Colombo MP, Craxi A. Liver follicular helper T-cells predict the achievement of virological response following interferon-based treatment in HCV-infected patients. Antivir Ther, 2012; 17(1):111-118.

[67] Yang G, Liu A, Xie Q, Guo TB, Wan B, Zhou B, Zhang JZ. Association of CD4+CD25+Foxp3+ regulatory T cells with chronic activity and viral clearance in patients with hepatitis B. Int Immunol, 2007; 19(2):133-140.

[68] Farsight; http://farsight-toolkit.org (accessed 31.07.2012.)

[69] Furuta K, Sato S, Yamauchi T, Kakumu S. Changes in intrahepatic gene expression profiles from chronic hepatitis to hepatocellular carcinoma in patients with hepatitis C virus infection. Hepatol Res, 2008; 38(7):673-682.

[70] Furuta K, Sato S, Yamauchi T, Ozawa T, Harada M, Kakumu S. Intrahepatic gene expression profiles in chronic hepatitis B and autoimmune liver disease. J Gastroenterol, 2008; 43(11):866-874.

[71] Peng X, Li Y, Walters KA, Rosenzweig ER, Lederer SL, Aicher LD, Proll S, Katze MG. Computational identification of hepatitis C virus associated microRNA-mRNA regulatory modules in human livers. BMC Genomics, 2009; 10:373.

[72] Mas V, Maluf D, Archer KJ, Potter A, Suh J, Gehray R, Descalzi V, Villamil F. Transcriptome at the time of hepatitis C virus recurrence may predict the severity of fibrosis progression after liver transplantation. Liver Transpl, 2011; 17(7):824-835.

Chapter 13

Real-Time Tissue Elastography and Transient Elastography for Evaluation of Hepatic Fibrosis

Hiroyasu Morikawa

Additional information is available at the end of the chapter

http://dx.doi.org/10.5772/52695

1. Introduction

Liver fibrosis develops as a sequel of chronic liver injury of various etiologies, including viral infection, immunological reaction, and toxic and metabolic insults, and is characterized by the accumulation of extracellular matrix(ECM) components produced by fibroblast-like cells including activated stellate cells and myofibroblasts in the hepatic parenchyma. Hepatic fibrosis progresses towards cirrhosis, an end-stage liver injury, leading to hepatic failure, hepatocellular carcinoma, and finally death. Hepatitis C virus (HCV) infection is the most common cause of liver fibrosis. HCV infects approximately 170 million individuals worldwide according to a report from the

World Health Organization [1]. Liver biopsy has been considered the 'gold standard' method for the evaluation of liver fibrosis in chronic hepatitis C [2]. However, liverbiopsy has some limitations, including its invasiveness, risk of complications, sampling error, variability in histopathological interpretation, and the reluctance of patients to subject to repeated examinations [3-11].Because of these disadvantages, there is a growing shift inclinical practice to utilize or develop 'non-invasive'methodologies to evaluate the stage of liver fibrosis. In particular, liver stiffness measurement by Vibration-Controlled Transient Elastography (Fibroscan) has become establishedas an important modality. Recently we and other investigator reported the usefulness of real-time tissue elastography (RTE) for noninvasive, visual assessment of liver stiffness in patients with chronic hepatitis C [12.13]. RTE is a method integrated in a sonography machine and developed in Japan for the visual assessment of tissue elasticity, based on a Combined Autocorrelation Method that calculates rapidly the relative hardness of tissue from the degree of tissue distortion and which displays this information as a color image [14]. This technology has already been proved to be diagnostically valuable in the breast cancer [15]. We show here the additional value of RTE, in comparsion to Fibroscanin patients with chronic liver disease.

2. Principle of elastography imaging

The two major categories of non-invasive hepatic elasticity imaging are dynamic elastography techniques, such as Fibroscan, and static elastography techniques, such as RTE. At present the dynamic elastography techniques have the advantage of allowing a quantitative imaging and better resolution than the static elastography techniques. These techniques require more complex equipment for the generation mode and imaging modalities. Ultrasound and magnetic resonance imaging are the major imaging modalities. The dynamic elastography techniques may be devided into two groups, based on the method of generating the shear wave: remote generation using radiation force and mechanical vibration. Of the static elastography techniques, real time tissue elastography developed by Hitachi Medical is most advanced ultrasound technique and can reveal tissue distortion using the hart beat and pulsing of the aorta. Several elastography techniques are summarized in Table 1.

	Principle	Mode of generation	Imaging modality
Real-time Tissue Elastography (RTE)	Tissue distortion	Pulsing of the aorta	Ultrasound
Vibration-Controlled Transient Elastography (VCTE, Fibroscan)	Propagating shear wave	Mechanical vibration	Ultrasound
Acoustic Radiation Force Impulse (ARFI)	Propagating shear wave	Radiation force	Ultrasound
Magnetic Resonance Elastography (MRE)	Propagating shear wave	Mechanical vibration	Magnetic resonance imaging
Supersonic Shear Imaging (SSI)	Propagating shear wave	Radiation force	Ultrasound

Table 1. Elastography techniques for measurement of liver stiffness.

3. Real time tissue elastography

The principle underlining RTE is shown in Figure 1A, which illustrates this as a spring model [16]. When a spring is compressed, the displacement in each section of the spring depends on its stiffness: a soft spring compresses more than a hard spring. The strain distribution can be measured by differentiating the spatial displacement at each location. Although the tissue displacement usually is generated by manual compression and relaxation of the probe in practice, we were able to improve the acquisition of RTE images representing the distortion of liver tissue as a result of the beating of the heart or pulsing of the abdominal aorta.

http://dx.doi.org/10.5772/52695

RTE is carried out using a high quality ultrasound system (Hitachi AlokaMedical, Chiba, Japan). The software uses a complex algorithm to process in a very short time all the data coming from the lesion as radiofrequency impulses and to minimize the artifacts due to lateral dislocations, allowing accurate measurement of the degree of tissue distortion. We used the Hitachi EUB-8500 and EUP-L52 Linear probe (3–7 MHz; Hitachi AlokaMedical) for RTE.

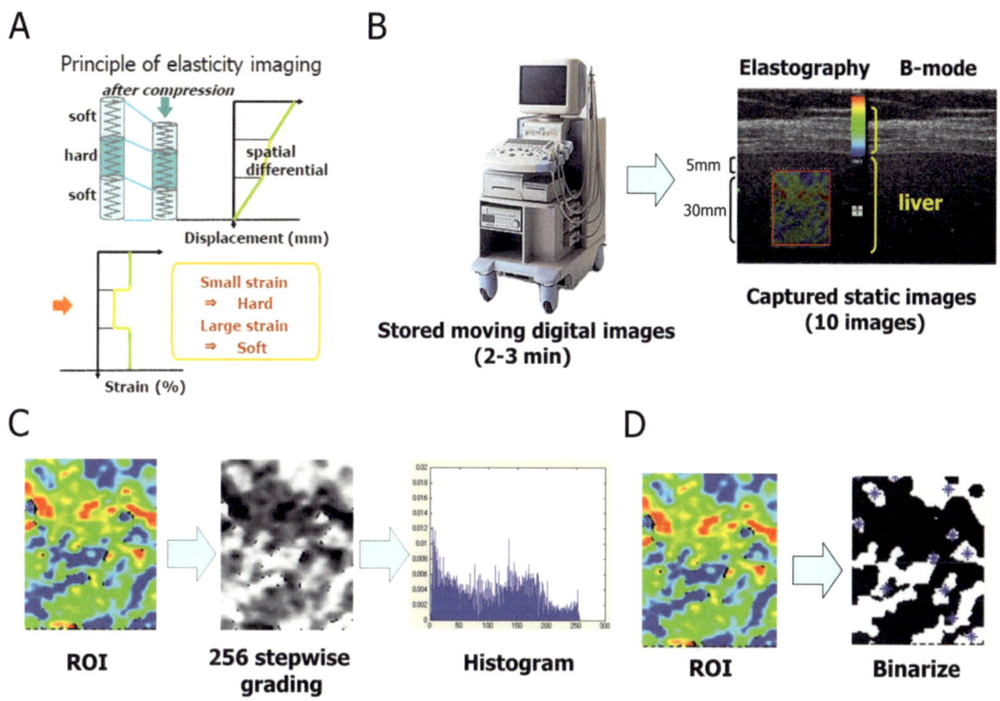

Figure 1. The principle and procedure of image analyses for real-time tissue elastography.(A) When a spring is compressed, displacement in each section of the spring depends on the stiffness of that part of the spring: a soft section compresses more than a hard section. The strain distribution can be measured by differentiating the spatial displacement at each location. (B) The ROI was fixed to a rectangle of approximately 20-30 mm length x 20 mm breadth with a 400–600 mm^2 area located 5-10 mm below the surface of the liver.left; RTE image, right; B-mode image. (C-D) The color-coded images from the ROI of the RTE were analyzed by the software Elasto_ver1.5.1. The colors ranged from blue to red indicating the relative gradients from hardness to softness. The Mean and Standard deviation were calculated by a histogram, which was generated by 256 stepwise grading derived from the color image. The Area and Complexity were calculated from the binary image. Area was derived from the percentage of white regions (asterisks, i.e. hard area). Complexity was calculated asperiphery^2/Area. Median value of the data were recorded as representative of RTE parameters.

This system is currently commercially available for the diagnosis of mammary neoplasm. Patients were examined in a supine position with the right arm elevated above the head, and were instructed to hold their breath. The examination was performed on the right lobe of the liver through the intercostal space, and liver biopsy and Fibroscan also were performed at the same site. The RTE equipment displays two images simultaneously; one shows the regions of interest (ROI) as a colored area and the other indicates the conventional

B-mode image (Fig. 1B). We chose an area where the tissue was free from large vessels and near the biopsy point. The measurement was fixed to a rectangle 30 mm in length and 20 mm in breadth located 5-10 mm below the surface of the liver (Fig. 1B). The color in the ROI was graded from blue (representing hard areas) to red (representing soft areas, Fig. 1B). We stored the RTE images for 2- 3min as moving digital images (Fig. 1B) and ten static images were captured at random from the moving images by the observer using AVI2JPG v6.10 converter software (Novo, Tokyo, Japan) and analyzed on a personal computer using the novel software Elasto_ver 1.5.1,which was developed and donated by Hitachi Medical. Numerical values of pixels were from 0 to 255 (256 stepwise grading) according to color mapping from blue (0) to red (255), and a histogram of the distribution was generated (Fig. 1C). The scale ranged from red for components with the greatest strain (i.e., the softest components) to blue for those with no strain (i.e., the hardest components). Green indicated average strain in the ROI, and therefore intact liver tissue was displayed as a diffuse homogeneous green pattern. An appearance of unevenness in the color pattern was considered to reflect a change in the liver stiffness. For quantification, all pixel data in the colored image were transferred into a histogram and binary image (Fig. 1C, D).

4. Vibration-controlled transient elastography (Fibroscan)

Fibroscan, which has been developed for the measurement of liver stiffness, is currently considered to reflect the degree of liver fibrosis directly and better than other methods. FibroScan502 was developed by ECOSENS (Paris, France) to evaluate liver fibrosis noninvasively in a short examination period by measuring the propagation of low frequency signals of a mechanical shear wave running through the liver tissue. Fibroscan measures liver stiffness in a volume that approximates a cylinder 10-mm wide and 40-mm in length between 25 and 65 mm below the skin surface. This volume is at least 100 times greater than that obtained by liver biopsy and is therefore considered to be far more representative of the condition of the hepatic parenchyma [17-21].The results that were obtained from ten valid measurements with a success rate of at least 60% and an interquartile range under 30% were considered successful. Failure was defined as when fewer than ten valid measurements were obtained. The median of 10 valid measurements was expressed in kilopascals (kPa) and regarded as the liver stiffness of a given subject.

Reports in 2005 from Castera et al. and Ziol et al. were pioneering; the liver stiffness measurements could be useful for assessing the presence of significant fibrosis (F2-4) and for suggesting the presence of cirrhosis in cohorts of patients with chronichepatitis C. The AUROCs ranged from 0.79 to 0.83 for the prediction of F2-4 and were over 0.95 for the identification of cirrhosis [22, 23]. Moreover, reproducibility of Fibroscan has been shown to be excellent for both interobserver and intraobserver agreement with an intraclass correlation coefficient of 0.98 [24, 25]. Friedrich-Rust et al. [26] assessed the overall performance of TE for the diagnosis of liver fibrosis by a meta-analysis that included fifty articles; the mean AUROCs for the diagnosis of significant fibrosis, severe fibrosis, and cirrhosis were 0.84, 0.89, and 0.94, respectively. A recent report from Degos et al. [27] of amulticenter prospective study reported that the

AUROCs for the diagnosis of significant fibrosis and cirrhosis were 0.76 and 0.90, respectively. Table 2 shows concisely the diagnostic accuracy of Fibroscan. The limitations of this method also have been discussed; intraobserver agreement is influenced by variables, such as body mass index (particularly when<28 kg/m2), hepatic steatosis, and flares of transaminases [17.23].

Study	Patients (n)	Prognosis	Cutoff (kPa)	Sen	Spe	PPV	NPV	AUC
Catera et al.	n=183, CHC	≥F2	7.1	67%	89%	95%	48%	0.83
2005		Cirrhosis	12.5	87%	91%	77%	95%	0.95
Zioi et al.	n=251, CHC	≥F2	8.6	56%	91%	88%	56%	0.79
2005		Cirrhosis	14.6	86%	96%	78%	97%	0.97
Friedrich-Rust et al.	50 studies, liver	≥F2						0.84
2008	disease	Cirrhosis						0.94
Degos et al. 2010	n=1307, viral	≥F2	5.2	90%	34%	64%	72%	0.76
	hepatitis	Cirrhosis	12.9	70%	90%	53%	95%	0.79

Sen, Sensitivity; Spe, Specificity; PPV, Positive Predictive Value; NPV, Negative Predictive Value; AUC, Area Under the Receiver-Operator-Characteristic curve; CHC, chronic hepatitis C.

Table 2. Diagnostic accuracies of transient elastography

5. Acoustic Radiation Force Impulse (ARFI) and Magnetic Resonance Elastography (MRE)

The technology applied most recent is acoustic radiation force impulse (ARFI) imaging. ARFI imaging permits evaluation of the elastic properties of a region of interest during real-time B-mode conventional hepatic US examination. Results are expressed in meters per second and the region of interest can be chosen using ultrasound guidance, there by avoiding large blood vessels and the ribs. Previous reports have indicated that the diagnostic power of ARFI imaging for the staging of liver fibrosis is the same as that of Fibroscan [28. 29].

New technological advances have been made in the clinical application of MRI such as diffusion-weighted MRI and MRI elastography. The former measures the apparent diffusion coefficient of water and the parameter is dependent on the tissue structure [30]. The latter measures the propagation characteristic of the shear waves from an acoustic driver within the liver. Although MRI elastography has been shown to be superior to APRI and Fibroscan for determining the stage of fibrosis in patients with various under lying liver diseases [31], it cannot be performed on aniron-overloaded liver because of noise. In addition, MRI takes longer and costs more than the ultrasound-base delastographic examinations.

6. Our results

Patients: Two hundred and one patients with chronic hepatitis received liver biopsy and Fibroscan examination within one week after RTE procedure in the Department of Hepatology, Osaka City University Hospital between 2007 and 2010. Etiologies of chronic liver diseases were hepatitis C virus (CHC; n=129, 64.2 %), hepatitis B virus infection (n=13, 6.5 %), non-alcohol steatohepatitis (n=30, 14.9 %), and others (n=29, 14.4 %). Liver fibrosis was evaluated according to the METAVIR score. Table 3 shows the characteristics of the patients who received these examinations.

Sex: male/ female	**89/112**
Age	55±13 y (21-80)*
BMI (kg/m^2)	22.7±3.5 (14.1-33.2)*
Fibrosis stage(METAVIR Score)	
F0	16
F1	98
F2	33
F3	27
F4	27
Etiology	
HCV	129
NASH	30
HBV	13
Autoimmune hepatitis	9
Primary biliary cirrhosis	6
Others	14

BMI, body mass index.

Table 3. Characteristics of the patients

Results: Histological and laparoscopical examination: 16 (8 %) patients were classified as F0, 98 (49 %) as F1, 33 (16 %) as F2, 27 (13 %) as F3, and 27 (13 %) as F4 (cirrhosis). RTE was performed successfully on all patients but Fibroscan measurements could not be obtained for 14 patients (7.0 %)because of obesity and liver atrophy. The Mean decreased in proportion to the increase of fibrosis score (Jonckheere–Terpstra test, $p<0.0001$). SD, Area, Complexity, and Fibroscan increased in proportion to the increase of fibrosis score (Jonckheere–Terpstra test, $p< 0.0001$).

http://dx.doi.org/10.5772/52695

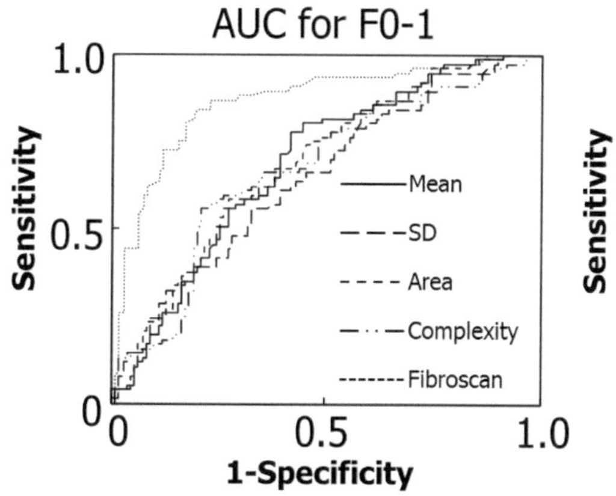

	Cut-off	AUC	Sensitivity [%]	Specificity [%]
Mean	105.6	0.69	62.3	63.1
SD	63.7	0.65	61.0	61.0
Area	31.3	0.69	62.3	65.5
Complexity	25.3	0.67	64.9	65.5
Fibroscan	10.1	0.87	84.4	80.0

Figure 2. Receiver operating characteristic curves of each parameter obtained by RTE and Fibroscan for F0-1.

Table 4 shows linear regression analysis of the values obtained by RTE compared to the liver stiffness values obtained by Fibroscan. Although simple regression analyses indicated that Mean, SD, Area, and Complexity were all significantly correlated with liver stiffness measured by Fibroscan, the *r* value did not indicate a high correlation.

Mean	r=0.458
SD	r=0.377
Area	r=0.487
Complexity	r=0.451
p<0.001)	

Table 4. Correlation between fibroscan and the image features of RTE

The area under the receiver operating characteristic curve (AUC) for stage F0-1 were 0.69, 0.65, 0.69, 0.67, and 0.87 for Mean, SD, Area, Complexity, and Fibroscan, respectively (Fig 2).The AUC for stage F0-2 were 0.79, 0.70, 0.77, 0.73, and 0.87 for Mean, SD, Area, Complexity, and Fibroscan, respectively (Fig 3). The AUC for cirrhosis (F4) were 0.78, 0.68, 0.77, 0.76, and 0.84 for each of respective values (Fig 4).

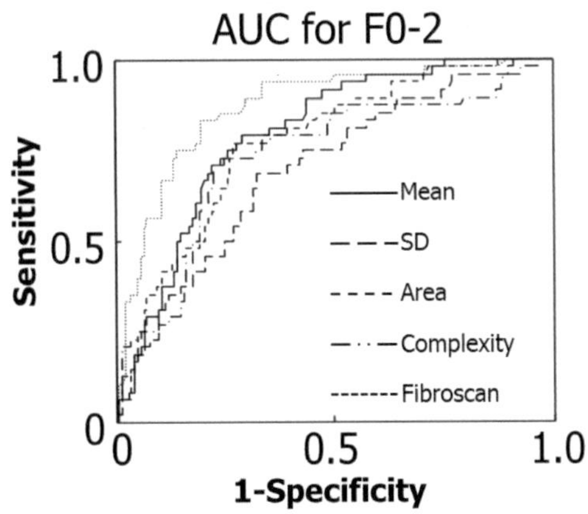

	Cut-off	AUC	Sensitivity [%]	Specificity [%]
Mean	101.5	0.79	75.0	74.1
SD	65.5	0.70	68.8	67.6
Area	33.4	0.77	72.9	73.4
Complexity	26.4	0.73	72.9	75.5
Fibroscan	13.1	0.87	83.3	79.9

Figure 3. Receiver operating characteristic curves of each parameter obtained by RTE and Fibroscan for F0-2.

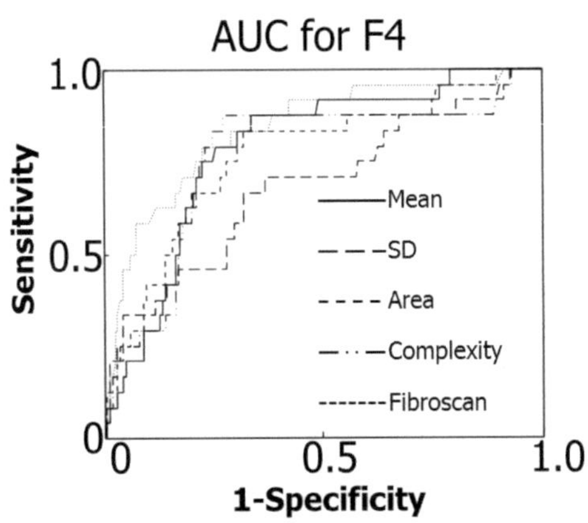

	Cut-off	AUC	Sensitivity [%]	Specificity [%]
Mean	98.1	0.78	75.0	77.3
SD	66.2	0.68	66.7	68.1
Area	35.5	0.77	70.8	73.0
Complexity	28.6	0.76	75.0	77.9
Fibroscan	14.3	0.84	79.2	77.3

Figure 4. Receiver operating characteristic curves of each parameter obtained by RTE and Fibroscan for F4.

7. Further research

Although our results showed that RTE was inferior to Fibroscan in determining the early stage of liver fibrosis(Fig 2 and 3), Figure 4 indicated that the performance of RTE compares favorably with that of Fibroscan for detecting liver cirrhosis in patients with chronic hepatitis. Unfortunately the best method for the analysis and quantification of RTE remains unclear, but this may be determined by future multicenter studies using larger patient cohorts and the combination of these parameters will enable improvement of the accuracy of assessing hepatic fibrosis.

Fibroscan has been reported to have several limitations and disadvantages in evaluating patients with obesity and ascites. In fact, in our study, we evaluated successfully all patients with RTE, while Fibroscan measurements could not be obtained for fourteen patients because of obesity and liver atrophy (data not shown).

In the future, a combination of imaging modalities and serological parameters or of different imaging modalities will improve further the accuracy in differentiating fibrosis stages. Interestingly, Castera et al. reported that the best results were achieved by a combination of Fibroscan and the Fibro Test [22]. Although ARFI, the most recent technology, Fibroscan, and MRE are all based on shear wave propagation, RTE is constructed by an original theory which is based on tissue distortion. The best diagnostic accuracy will be obtained by combining the RTE elasticity score with shear wave propagation.

8. Conclusion

We have described a static elastography technique, RTE, for the "noninvasive" visual assessment of liver stiffness. Although RTE was inferior to Fibroscan in determining the early stage of liver fibrosis, the performance of RTE compares favorably with that of Fibroscan when detecting liver cirrhosis in patients with chronic liver disease. We suggest that RTE could also be used as a routine imaging method to evaluate the degree of liver fibrosis in patients with other liver diseases. Future studies of larger patient cohorts will be necessary for the validation of RTE analysis, and the combination of RTE with other clinical values including dynamic elastography techniques (i.e. Fibroscan, ARFI and MRE) and serum biomarkers will enable improvement of the accuracy of assessing hepatic fibrosis.

Acknowledgments

We thank Ms. Akiko Tonomura and Mr. Junji Warabino, Hitachi AlokaMedical Co., for the technical support for RTE. Hiroyasu Morikawa was supported by a research grant from the Cannon Foundation (2011-12).

Author details

Hiroyasu Morikawa

Department of Hepatology, Graduate School of Medicine, Osaka City University, Osaka, Japan

References

[1] Global surveillance and control of hepatitis C. Report of a WHO Consultation organized in collaboration with the Viral Hepatitis Prevention Board, Antwerp, Belgium. J Viral Hepat. 1999;6:35–47.

[2] Bravo AA, Sheth SG, Chopra S. Liver biopsy. N Engl J Med.2001;344:495–500.

[3] Sporea I, Popescu A, Sirli R. Why, who and how should performliver biopsy in chronic liver diseases. World J Gastroenterol.2008;14:3396–402.

[4] Castera L, Negre I, Samii K, Buffet C. Pain experienced during percutaneous liver biopsy. Hepatology. 1999;30:1529–30.

[5] Castera L, Negre I, Samii K, Buffet C. Patient administer ednitrous oxide/oxygen inhalation provides safe and effective analgesia for percutaneous liver biopsy: a randomized placebo controlled trial. Am J Gastroenterol. 2001;96:1553–7.

[6] Piccinino F, Sagnelli E, Pasquale G, Giusti G. Complications following percutaneous liver biopsy. A multicentre retrospectivestudy on 68, 276 biopsies. J Hepatol. 1986;2:165–73.

[7] Bedossa P, Darge`re D, Paradis V. Sampling variability of liver fibrosis in chronic hepatitis C. Hepatology. 2003;38:1449–57.

[8] Regev A, Berho M, Jeffers LJ, Milikowski C, Molina EG, Pyrsopoulos NT, et al. Sampling error and intraobserver variation in liver biopsy in patients with chronic HCV infection. Am J Gastroenterol.2002;97:2614-8.

[9] Rousselet MC, Michalak S, Dupre F, Croue A, Bedossa P, SaintAndre JP, et al. Sources of variability in histological scoring of chronic viral hepatitis. Hepatology. 2005;41:257–64.

[10] Bedossa P, Carrat F. Liver biopsy: the best, not the gold standard.J Hepatol. 2009;50:1–3.

[11] Cadranel JF, Rufat P, Degos F. Practices of liver biopsy inFrance: results of a prospective nationwide survey. For the Groupof Epidemiology of the French Association for the Study of theLiver (AFEF). Hepatology. 2000;32:477–81.

[12] Morikawa H, Fukuda K, Kobayashi S, Fujii H, Iwai S, Enomoto M, et al. Real-time tissue elastography as a tool for the noninvasive assessment of liver stiffness in patients with chronic hepatitis C. J Gastroenterol. 2011;46:350–8.

[13] Koizumi Y, Hirooka M, Kisaka Y, Konishi I, Abe M, MurakamiH, et al. Liver fibrosis in patients with chronic hepatitis C: noninvasive diagnosis by means of real-time tissue elastographyestablishment of the method for measurement. Radiology. 2011;258:610–7.

[14] Shiina T, Nitta N, Ueno E, Bamber JC. Real time tissue elasticity imaging using the combined autocorrelation method. J MedUltrason. 2002;29:119–28.

[15] Itoh A, Ueno E, Tohno E, Kamma H, Takahashi H, Shiina T,et al. Breast disease: clinical application of US elastography fordiagnosis. Radiology. 2006;239:341–50.

[16] Ophir J, Céspedes I, Ponnekanti H, Yazdi Y, Li X. (1991) Elastography: a quantitative method for imaging the elasticity of biological tissues. Ultrason Imaging. 1991;13:111-34.

[17] Pinzani M, Vizzutti F, Arena U, Marra F. Technology insight:noninvasive assessment of liver fibrosis by biochemical scoresand elastography. Nat ClinPractGastroenterol-Hepatol. 2008;5:95–106.

[18] Sandrin L, Tanter M, Gennisson JL, Catheline S, Fink M. Shearelasticity probe for soft tissues with 1D transient elastography. IEEE Trans UltrasonFerroelectrFreq Control. 2002;49:436–46.

[19] Ganne-Carrie´ N, Ziol M, de Ledinghen V, Douvin C, Marcellin P, Castera L, et al. Accuracy of liver stiffness measurement for the diagnosis of cirrhosis in patients with chronic liver diseases. Hepatology. 2006;44:1511–7.

[20] Yeh WC, Li PC, Jeng YM, Hsu HC, Kuo PL, Li ML, et al. Elastic modulus measurements of human liver and correlation with pathology. Ultrasound Med Biol. 2002;28:467–74.

[21] Sandrin L, Fourquet B, Hasquenoph JM, Yon S, Fournier C, Mal F, et al. Transient elastography: a new noninvasive method for assessment of hepatic fibrosis. Ultrasound Med Biol. 2003;29: 1705–13.

[22] Castera L, Vergniol J, Foucher J, Le Bail B, Chanteloup E, Haaser M, et al. Prospective comparison of transient elastography, Fibrotest, APRI, and liver biopsy for the assessment of fibrosis in chronic hepatitis C. Gastroenterology. 2005;128:343–50.

[23] Ziol M, Handra-Luca A, Kettaneh A, Christidis C, Mal F, Kazemi F, et al. Noninvasive assessment of liver fibrosis by measurement of stiffness in patients with chronic hepatitis C. Hepatology. 2005;41:48–54.

[24] Fraquelli M, Rigamonti C, Casazza G, Conte D, Donato MF, Ronchi G, et al. Reproducibility of transient elastography in the evaluation of liver fibrosis in patients with chronic liver disease. Gut. 2007;56:968–73.

[25] Boursier J, Konate A, Guilluy M, Gorea G, Sawadogo A,Quemener E, et al. Learning curve and interobserver reproducibility evaluation of liver stiffness measurement by transient elastography. Eur J GastroenterolHepatol. 2008;20:693–701.

[26] Friedrich-Rust M, Ong MF, Martens S, Sarrazin C, Bojunga J,Zeuzem S, et al. Performance of transient elastography for the staging of liver fibrosis: a meta-analysis. Gastroenterology.2008;134:960–74.

[27] Degos F, Perez P, Roche B, Mahmoudi A, Asselineau J, Voitot H,et al. Diagnostic accuracy of FibroScan and comparison to liver fibrosis biomarkers in chronic viral hepatitis: a multicenter prospective study (the FIBROSTIC study). J Hepatol. 2010;53:1013–21.

[28] Friedrich-Rust M, Wunder K, Kriener S, Sotoudeh F, Richter S, Bojunga J, et al. Liver fibrosis in viral hepatitis: noninvasive assessment with acoustic radiation force impulse imaging versustransient elastography. Radiology. 2009;252:595–604.

[29] Yoneda M, Suzuki K, Kato S, Fujita K, Nozaki Y, Hosono K,et al. Nonalcoholic fatty liver disease: US-based acoustic radiationforce impulse elastography. Radiology. 2010;256:640–7.

[30] Lewin M, Poujol-Robert A, Boe°lle PY, Wendum D, Lasnier E,Viallon M, et al. Diffusion-weighted magnetic resonance imaging for the assessment of fibrosis in chronic hepatitis C. Hepatology.2007;46:658–65.

[31] Huwart L, Sempoux C, VicautE, Salameh N, Annet L, Danse E, et al. Magnetic resonance elastography for the noninvasive staging of liver fibrosis. Gastroenterology. 2008;135:32–40.